*To my parents who believed in me
from the beginning and to my partner, Nan, who will believe
in me until the end*

Handbook of ICU EEG Monitoring

Edited by

Suzette M. LaRoche, MD
Associate Professor of Neurology
Emory University School of Medicine
Atlanta, Georgia

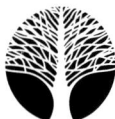

demosMEDICAL
New York

Visit **our website at www.demosmedpub.com**

ISBN: 9781936287390
e-book ISBN: 9781617050787

Acquisitions Editor: Beth Barry
Compositor: Techset

Medicine is an ever-changing science. Research and clinical experience are continually expanding our knowledge, in particular our understanding of proper treatment and drug therapy. The authors, editors, and publisher have made every effort to ensure that all information in this book is in accordance with the state of knowledge at the time of production of the book. Nevertheless, the authors, editors, and publisher are not responsible for errors or omissions or for any consequences from application of the information in this book and make no warranty, express or implied, with respect to the contents of the publication. Every reader should examine carefully the package inserts accompanying each drug and should carefully check whether the dosage schedules mentioned therein or the contraindications stated by the manufacturer differ from the statements made in this book. Such examination is particularly important with drugs that are either rarely used or have been newly released on the market.

Library of Congress Cataloging-in-Publication Data

Handbook of ICU EEG monitoring/[edited by] Suzette LaRoche.
    p. ; cm.
    Includes bibliographical references and index.
    ISBN 978-1-936287-39-0 – ISBN 978-1-61705-078-7 (e-book)
I. LaRoche, Suzette.
    [DNLM: 1. Electroencephalography. 2. Intensive Care Units. 3. Monitoring, Physiologic.
    WL 150]
    616.8′047547–dc23

                                                                    2012029356

Special discounts on bulk quantities of Demos Medical Publishing books are available to corporations, professional associations, pharmaceutical companies, health care organizations, and other qualifying groups. For details, please contact:
Special Sales Department
Demos Medical Publishing, LLC
11 West 42nd Street, 15th Floor
New York, NY 10036
Phone: 800-532-8663 or 212-683-0072
Fax: 212-941-7842
E-mail: rsantana@demosmedpub.com

Printed in the United States of America by IBT-Hamilton
12 13 14 15 / 5 4 3 2 1

Contents

III: EEG INTERPRETATION

Contributors

Nicholas S. Abend, MD, Assistant Professor of Neurology and Pediatrics, Children's Hospital of Philadelphia, Departments of Neurology and Pediatrics, The University of Pennsylvania School of Medicine, Philadelphia, Pennsylvania

Thomas P. Bleck, MD, FCCM, Professor of Neurological Sciences, Neurosurgery, Medicine, and Anesthesiology, Rush Medical College; and Associate Chief Medical Officer (Critical Care), Rush University Medical Center, Chicago, Illinois

Gretchen M. Brophy, PharmD, BCPS, FCCP, FCCM, Professor of Pharmacotherapy & Outcomes Science and Neurosurgery, Virginia Commonwealth University, Medical College of Virginia Campus, Richmond, Virginia

Rhonda Cadena, MD, Assistant Professor, Department of Neurology and Emergency Medicine, University of North Carolina, Chapel Hill, North Carolina

Jan Claassen, MD, PhD, Assistant Professor of Neurology and Neurosurgery, Division of Critical Care Neurology, Columbia University College of Physicians & Surgeons, New York, New York

Frank W. Drislane, MD, Professor of Neurology, Harvard Comprehensive Epilepsy Program, Beth Israel Deaconess Medical Center, Boston, Massachussetts

J. Andrew Ehrenberg, BS, R EEG T, CNIM, Director of Neurophysiology Emory University School of Medicine, Atlanta, Georgia

Nathan B. Fountain, MD, Professor of Neurology, Director, Dreifuss Comprehensive Epilepsy Program, University of Virginia, Charlottesville, Virginia

William David Freeman, MD, Assistant Professor, Departments of Neurology and Critical Care, Mayo Clinic, Jacksonville, Florida

Daniel Friedman, MD, Assistant Professor, Department of Neurology, New York University Medical Center, New York, New York

Nicolas Gaspard, MD, PhD, Post-doctoral Research Fellow, Neurology Department and Comprehensive Epilepsy Center, Yale University School of Medicine, New Haven, Connecticut

Elizabeth Gerard, MD, Assistant Professor of Neurology Northwestern University, Chicago, Illinois

Emily J. Gilmore, MD, Fellow, Neurocritical Care and Continuous EEG Monitoring, Department of Neurology, Columbia University College of Physicians and Surgeons, New York-Presbyterian Hospital/Columbia University Medical Center, New York, New York

Cecil D. Hahn, MD, MPH, Staff Neurologist, The Hospital for Sick Children, Toronto, Assistant Professor, Department of Paediatrics (Neurology), University of Toronto, Toronto, Ontario, Canada

Stephen Hantus, MD, Associate staff, Department of Neurology, Cleveland Clinic Epilepsy Center, Cleveland, Ohio

Susan T. Herman, MD, Assistant Professor of Neurology, Beth Israel Deaconess Medical Center, Harvard University, Boston, Massachusetts

Lawrence J. Hirsch, MD, Professor of Neurology, Yale University, New Haven, Connecticut

Aatif M. Husain, MD, Professor, Department of Medicine (Neurology), Duke University Medical Center, and Neurodiagnostic Center, Veterans Affairs Medical Center, Durham, North Carolina

John Richard Ives, BSc, Adjunct Research Professor, Department of Neuroscience, University of Western Ontario, London, Ontario, Canada

Peter W. Kaplan, MB, FRCP, Professor of Neurology, Johns Hopkins Bayview Medical Center, Baltimore, Maryland

Suzette M. LaRoche, MD, Associate Professor of Neurology, Emory University School of Medicine, Atlanta, Georgia

Ram Mani, MD, Assistant Professor, UMDNJ-Robert Wood Johnson Medical School, Department of Neurology, New Brunswick, New Jersey

Marc R. Nuwer, MD, PhD, Professor, Department of Neurology, David Geffen School of Medicine at UCLA, Reed Neurological Research Center, Department Head, Clinical Neurophysiology, Ronald Reagan UCLA Medical Center, Los Angeles, California

Leisha Osburn, MS, MHA, DABNM, REEG/EPT, CNIM, CLTM, Indiana University Health, Bloomington, Indiana

Sebastian W. Pollandt, MD, Neurocritical Care Fellow, University of Cincinnati Health, Cincinnati, Ohio

James J. Riviello, Jr, MD, Professor of Neurology and Director of Division of Pediatric Neurology, New York University Comprehensive Epilepsy Center, New York University Langone Medical Center, Department of Neurology, New York University School of Medicine, New York

Leslie Rudzinski, MD, Assistant Professor of Neurology, Emory University School of Medicine, Atlanta, Georgia

Sarah Schmitt, MD, Assistant Professor of Neurology, University of Pennsylvania, Philadelphia, Pennsylvania

Lori Shutter, MD, Professor, Departments of Critical Care Medicine, Neurology, and Neurosurgery, Director, Neurocritical Care Fellowship Program, and Co-Director, Neurovascular ICU, University of Pittsburgh School of Medicine, Pittsburgh, Pennsylvania

Saurabh R. Sinha, MD, PhD, Assistant Professor of Medicine (Neurology), Duke University Medical Center, Durham, North Carolina

Michael A. Stein, MD, Assistant Professor of Neurological Sciences, Rush University Medical Center, Murdock, Chicago, Illinois

Christa Swisher, Department of Medicine (Neurology), Duke University Medical Center, Durham, North Carolina

Jerzy P. Szaflarski, MD, PhD, Associate Professor of Neurology, Neuroscience, Psychiatry and Psychology, University of Cincinnati Academic Health Center, Cincinnati, Ohio

William O. Tatum IV, DO, Professor of Neurology, Mayo Clinic, Jacksonville, Florida

Eljim P. Tesoro, PharmD, BCPS, Clinical Assistant Professor, Department of Pharmacy Practice, University of Illinois at Chicago, Chicago, Illinois

Tammy N. Tsuchida, MD, PhD, Assistant Professor of Neurology, Department of Neurology, Children's National Medical Center, George Washington University, Washington, DC

Elizabeth Waterhouse, MD, Professor of Neurology, Virginia Commonwealth University, Richmond, Virginia

Adam Webb, MD, Assistant Professor, Department of Neurology, Emory University, Atlanta, Georgia

Matthew H. Wong, MD, Epilepsy and EEG Fellow, University of Virginia, Charlottesville, Virginia

Wendy L. Wright, MD, Medical Director, Neuroscience Intensive Care Unit, Emory University Hospital Midtown, Assistant Professor of Neurology, Neurosurgery and Pediatrics, Emory University Hospital, Atlanta, Georgia

Courtney J. Wusthoff, MD, Perinatal Neurology Consultant, Hammersmith Hospital, Imperial College NHS Trust

Preface

When I was a clinical neurophysiology fellow learning the science and art of EEG interpretation, one of my favorite tasks was being called bedside to render an "on the spot" decision about whether a particular EEG pattern was of clinical concern. Most of these encounters occurred in the intensive care unit, where I enjoyed working as a resident even though I decided that a lifetime of critical care was not for me. So it seemed natural that I would jump at the chance to venture away from the EEG reading room to review STAT EEGs of critically ill patients when the opportunity arose, something many of my mentors and colleagues did not find as appealing. This was a time in the not too distant past when EEG recording in the ICU meant rolling a behemoth cart stacked with a bulky monitor and full-size CPU to the patient's bedside. And what if we found something concerning on the 20-minute EEG? Order a repeat EEG for the next morning, and we'll take another look.

At the risk of sounding like my grandmother, "Times have changed!" But I have been lucky to grow up in the midst of it, and to be part of the development of ICU EEG monitoring as a specialty in its own right. In just the past decade, advances in technology have given us multiple hardware options for EEG acquisition designed to fit into the ICU environment and electrodes that don't have to be removed for every neuroimaging procedure. EEG reading software comes equipped with alarms, email or pager notifications, and remote networking that will allow you to look at an EEG on your smartphone (although I wouldn't recommend this as routine practice). The most significant technological advance in ICU EEG monitoring has been the development of quantitative EEG software programs that allow hours of raw EEG to be condensed into a few screen shots for rapid identification of seizures or other significant changes. More importantly, however, neurophysiologists and neurointensivists across the country have recognized the significant role of continuous EEG in the detection of secondary causes of injury, such as nonconvulsive seizures and vasospasm and just how prevalent these conditions are. Consequently, the field of ICU EEG monitoring has grown into a significant aspect of neurocritical care.

This book grew out of questions from scores of residents, fellows, EEG technologists, and colleagues looking for advice on texts they could purchase to learn more about ICU EEG monitoring. With the exception of the outstanding *Atlas of EEG in Critical Care* by Drs. Hirsch and Brenner, there have been no practical but comprehensive references devoted to this important topic until now.

The *Handbook of ICU EEG Monitoring* was designed to be a resource for anyone caring for patients in the intensive care unit whose care might involve EEG monitoring, including neurologists, neurointensivists, neurosurgeons, nursing staff, and EEG technologists. The goal of the text is not only to provide a review of common ICU EEG patterns and their clinical significance and treatment implications, but to also discuss many practical facets of EEG monitoring in the critically ill that aren't covered elsewhere. This includes technical issues, aspects of billing and coding, effective communication between clinical and EEG teams, and patient selection for EEG monitoring. I am grateful to have had the collaboration of the nation's top experts in the fields of ICU EEG monitoring and neurocritical care in producing a book that covers all of these important topics and more.

My hope is that the Handbook will serve as a guide for a wide range of professionals working in this field, from those with only an initial interest in ICU EEG monitoring to those who have been utilizing it for years.

Suzette M. LaRoche

Acknowledgments

Special thanks to Dr. Linda Logdberg for her outstanding editorial assistance, to Drs. Lawrence Hirsch, Susan Herman, and the entire Critical Care EEG Monitoring Research Consortium for their contributions to the growth of ICU EEG monitoring and for allowing me to be a part of it, and to Drs. Kimford Meador and Page Pennell for their personal mentorship

Abbreviations List

ACNS	American Clinical Neurophysiology Society
AED	antiepileptic drug
BIPDs	bilateral independent periodic discharges; formerly known as bilateral independent periodic lateralized epileptiform discharges (BiPLEDs)
cEEG	continuous EEG monitoring
CNS	central nervous system
CSE	convulsive status epilepticus
CSF	cerebrospinal fluid
DCI	delayed cerebral ischemia
ECMO	extracorporeal membrane oxygenation
FIRDA	frontally predominant intermittent rhythmic delta activity
GCS	Glasgow coma score
GCSE	generalized convulsive status epilepticus aka
GOS	Glasgow outcome scale
GPDs	generalized periodic discharges; formerly known as generalized periodic epileptiform discharges (GPEDs)
HIE	hypoxic–ischemia encephalopathy
ICH	intracranial hemorrhage
ICP	intracranial pressure
ICU	Intensive Care Unit
MMM	multimodality monitoring
NCS	nonconvulsive seizure(s)
NICU	Neurological Intensive Care Unit
NSCE	nonconvulsive status epilepticus
PDs	periodic discharges
LPDs	lateralized periodic discharges; formerly known as periodic lateralized epileptiform discharges (PLEDs)
QEEG	quantitative EEG
RSE	refractory status epilepticus
SAH	subarachnoid hemorrhage
SE	status epilepticus
SIRPIDs	stimulus-induced rhythmic, periodic or ictal discharges
TBI	traumatic brain injury
TH	therapeutic hypothermia

ONE

Equipment for EEG Acquisition and Review

Susan T. Herman

KEY POINTS

- EEG acquisition equipment for ICU continuous EEG monitoring (cEEG) should meet the technical standards outlined in the American Clinical Neurophysiology Society Guidelines.
- ICU cEEG acquisition equipment can be installed as either a fixed (wall-mounted) unit or portable system.
- Simultaneous audio and video recording is strongly encouraged for correlation of behavioral events with underlying EEG patterns and to aid in proper identification of EEG artifacts that can be easily mistaken for electrographic seizures.
- Specialized hardware and software increases the utility of cEEG for monitoring at the bedside. Options include the ability to enter nursing notes, pushbuttons for seizures and other clinical events, software to integrate physiologic data (eg, intracranial pressure, blood pressure), and quantitative EEG software for graphical display of quantitative EEG trends.

I. BACKGROUND

A. The American Clinical Neurophysiology Society has published guidelines for recording routine EEG and video-EEG monitoring for epilepsy, and will soon publish guidelines for continuous monitoring in the intensive care unit. ICU cEEG equipment should meet the technical standards defined in these guidelines. Relevant guidelines (available at www.acns.org) include:

- Guideline 1: Minimum technical requirements for performing clinical electroencephalography (1).
- Guideline 2: Minimum technical requirements for pediatric electroencephalography (2).
- Guideline 8: Guidelines for recording clinical EEG on digital media (3).

- Guideline 12: Guidelines for long-term monitoring for epilepsy (4).
- Upcoming guideline: Technical standards for continuous EEG monitoring in the ICU.

B. There are multiple components of digital ICU cEEG acquisition machines (Figure 1.1).

II. BASICS

A. There are important similarities and differences between routine EEG acquisition equipment, EEG equipment for long-term epilepsy monitoring, and EEG equipment for cEEG in the ICU (Table 1.1).

B. Physical Configuration
- Fixed installation: Wall-mounted equipment has several advantages.
  - It can be mounted out of the way of bedside caregivers and cameras can be placed in the best recording location.
  - Fixed equipment is less likely to be damaged than portable equipment that is rolled around the hospital.
  - However, if only some ICU rooms have mounted cEEG equipment, critically ill patients may need to be moved into a designated room equipped for monitoring.
  - Despite many advantages, wall-mounted cEEG equipment is expensive and therefore may be underutilized.

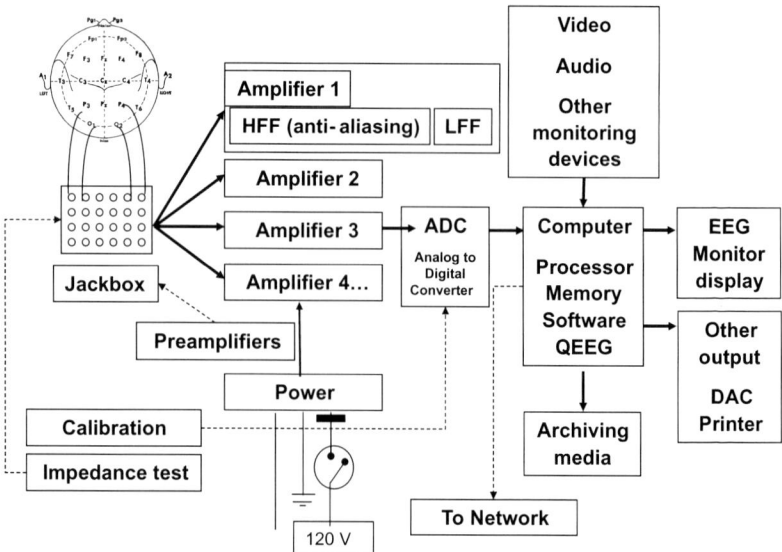

FIGURE 1.1 Components of digital ICU cEEG acquisition machines. See text for details of individual components.

TABLE 1.1   Features of Routine EEG, Epilepsy Monitoring (EMU), and ICU EEG Monitoring Equipment

FEATURE	ROUTINE EEG	EMU	ICU cEEG
Physical configuration	Usually portable	Typically hard-wired	Portable or hard-wired
Number of EEG channels required	16–40	40 to $\geq$ 128	16–32
Sampling rate (per second)	200–512	200 to $\geq$ 2000	200–512
Other physiologic inputs (optional inputs within parentheses)	EOG, EKG, EMG, respiratory effort	EOG, EKG, EMG (oxygen saturation)	EOG, EKG, EMG (BP, ICP, O_2 sat)
Video/audio necessary	Optional	Yes	Yes
Spike and seizure detection	No	Yes	Optional
Quantitative EEG trends	No	Optional	Yes
Network connection for remote monitoring	Optional	Recommended	Yes

Abbreviations: BP: blood pressure; ICP: intracranial pressure; O_2 sat: oxygen saturation.

- Portable equipment: can be configured on a cart or on a small-footprint pole-mount system (approximately 2.5 foot diameter base, height 4–8 feet [taller with camera mount]).
  - Portable cEEG equipment has the advantage of being able to be moved to where it is needed, but it can obstruct patient care and camera views are rarely optimal.
  - Many portable cEEG units now have IP addressable cameras that allow remote camera control over standard network jacks, without the expense of special cabling.
- Some ICU cEEG programs utilize a combination of wall-mounted equipment in high-use areas (eg, neurological intensive care units) and portable equipment for less frequently monitored areas.
- Design of EEG equipment components should take into consideration possible "rough handling" by inexperienced ICU personnel.
  - Delicate cables with fragile connectors, nonwaterproof components (jackboxes and amplifiers), and systems with portable computer components such as laptops and tablets are especially vulnerable to accidental damage.
- Nonproprietary components (cameras, computer components, cables, and connectors) are preferred, as these are generally less expensive.
- A patient event button can be used by family or ICU personnel to mark suspected clinical events.

C. Security and Safety Features
- Failure recovery and protection
  - Some ICU EEG machines have a feature that allows the EEG acquisition to detect an unexpected termination of a study (such as system crash or temporary power outage) and automatically reboot and start recording again when power is restored.
- Uninterruptible power supplies may prevent problems during brief power fluctuations or outages.
- Computers should be securely fastened to the wall or pole mounts to prevent loss of hard drives or other components containing protected health information.
- EEG machines should have security features such as secure log-in, automatic keyboard/screen lock, and firewall and antivirus protection.

D. Jackbox
- In the crowded ICU head-of-the-bed environment, small jackboxes may be beneficial.
- Electrode inputs should be arrayed so that the entire jackbox and electrode pins fit into a waterproof enclosure to prevent accidental damage to the jackbox and inadvertent disconnection of electrodes.
- A long jackbox cable may be necessary if the EEG machine must be placed at a distance from the patient.
- Some jackboxes have wireless connectivity to the amplifier, internal storage, and battery power in the jackbox.
  - Such jackboxes can continue to record EEG while the patient is disconnected from the amplifier (eg, to go to radiology procedures).
  - Disconnected recording time is variable, depending on battery and internal storage size.
  - Before deciding on a wireless solution, ensure that there is no significant overlap in wireless signals from other ICU equipment.

E. Amplifier Specifications (ACNS Guideline #8)
- Inputs:
  - At least 16 referential EEG channels are required.
  - Thirty-two or more EEG channels are preferred for full 10 to 20 electrode placement, as well as additional channels for recording electrocardiogram, electrooculogram (1−2 channels), and electromyogram.
  - Additional channels may be needed if simultaneous intracranial EEG recording is planned.
  - System reference input
  - Ground input
  - DC input channels for connection of other physiologic monitors are preferred (thermistors, oxygen saturation monitors, ICP monitors).
- Full-scale input range greater than ± 2 mV
- Bandpass filters 0.1−0.3 to 70−100 Hz

○ DC or near DC amplifiers required to record infra-slow EEG and cortical spreading depression.
- Noise less than 1 μV rms
- Input impedance at least 10 MΩ
- Common mode rejection at least 100 dB for each input
- Optical isolation for patient safety

F. Analog-to-Digital Converter (ADC) Specifications (ACNS Guideline #8)
- Input range ±1 to 2 mV
- Sampling rate at least 200 samples per second (3 times higher than anti-aliasing filter)
- Resolution at least 12 bit; 16 bit preferred

G. Video and Audio (ACNS Guideline #12)
- Simultaneous video and audio recording is highly recommended to allow correlation of clinical seizures and other behavioral events with EEG patterns as well as to aid in identification of EEG artifacts (eg, patting, chest physiotherapy, suction, ventilator artifact) (5).
- Video is time synchronized with the EEG data.
  ○ Equipment for video recording varies greatly in picture quality, and cost.
  ○ Video may be color or black-and-white.
  ○ Fixed wide-angle cameras may be an option, but may not have adequate resolution for detection of fine motor movements.
  ○ Many modern cEEG units have IP-addressable cameras mounted on a pole. These allow remote pan/tilt and sometimes zoom and focus from remote locations.
- Standard digital video is MPEG 4,320 × 240 or 640 × 480 resolution.
  ○ Higher resolutions are available at the expense of hard disk and server space as well as network bandwidth.
  ○ Video recording size is typically 12 to 20 GB/day.

H. Computer Specifications: Acquisition Machines
- Computers used for EEG acquisition should have sufficient processing capability for simultaneous EEG and video acquisition, spike and seizure detection, quantitative EEG analysis, and network tasks.
- Minimum specifications
  ○ Dual core processor greater than 2 GHz
  ○ 2 GB RAM
  ○ Discrete graphics card
  ○ Network connectivity 100 mbit/sec minimum; Gigabit network interface card preferred
  ○ Hard drive large enough to store at least 1 week of EEG and video data (approximately 2 GB EEG and 12–20 GB video/day = greater than 150 GB)
- Operating system is typically Windows, version is dependent on hospital information technology specifications.
- Some EEG systems run on Macintosh or Linux computers.

I. Computer Specifications: Review Stations

- Computers used for EEG review should have sufficient processing capability for simultaneous EEG and video review, review of automated spike and seizure detection, quantitative EEG analysis, and network tasks.
- Review computers may also have additional functions, such as report generation (office productivity software, voice recognition software), access to hospital clinical information systems, and archiving, which may necessitate additional processing capabilities.
- Recommended specifications
  - Dual or quad core processor greater than 2 GHz
  - 4 GB RAM
  - Discrete graphics card
  - Network connectivity: Gigabit network interface card
  - Hard drive large enough for installation of required software

J. Monitor Display: Acquisition Machines (ACNS Guideline #8)

- Fixed and portable installations should have a monitor in the room for EEG setup and quantitative EEG review by ICU personnel.
- Screen size at least 17″ diagonal (greater than 20″ preferred).
- Monitor resolution at least 1280×1024 pixels

K. Monitor Display: Review Stations (ACNS Guideline #8)

- Review stations require large high-resolution monitors for accurate EEG interpretation.
- Screen size at least 20″ diagonal (greater than 24″ preferred).
- Monitor resolution at least 1600×1200 pixels (widescreen 1920×1200 pixels).
- Dual monitors may be necessary for simultaneous review of EEG and video data, and especially for simultaneous review of raw EEG and quantitative EEG trends.

L. User Interfaces

- Keyboard and mouse remain the standard interface devices for EEG.
- The interface must make it easy for nurses and other ICU personnel to enter annotations, move the camera, and so on without interfering with the ongoing EEG recording.
- Touchscreen monitors with large buttons for common tasks are easier to use but may be difficult to adequately disinfect.
- Security: HiPAA regulations require individual user logons for clinical systems containing protected health information. Bedside systems may include a "transparent screen lock," which locks the computer but allows continued viewing of EEG data, video, and quantitative EEG.

M. Other Hardware and/or Cables

- Inputs for other physiologic monitoring devices are preferred (eg, pulse oximetry, blood pressure, intracranial pressure, temperature, respiratory effort, brain tissue oxygenation).
  - These data streams must be time synchronized with EEG.

- Some ICU EEG machines are true multifunction devices with multimodality monitoring capabilities.
- It is important to ensure that adequate channels are available for EEG recording, and that additional software (seizure detection, QEEG) can be installed on the device.

N. Software
- Patient database
  - A central patient and study database allows management of patient files, archiving, and report generation.
  - Databases can synchronize information across the hospital network, so that all local machines have up-to-date clinical information.
  - Databases may also be linked to the hospital electronic medical record to allow importation of relevant patient demographic data.
- EEG software
  - Should be easy to use by both EEG and ICU personnel.
  - Some systems have separate display modes for EEG and ICU staff, with a simplified interface for ICU personnel.
  - Essential functions include the ability to annotate an ongoing recording as well as move the camera.
  - Software should include a "look-back" feature which is the ability to review already-recorded EEG without the need to interrupt ongoing recording.
  - Many systems now include remote access to the "live" EEG session which allows for instant messaging features as well as system adjustments from remote locations (eg, change montage, move camera).
  - Other useful software features:
    - Ability to automatically stop the EEG recording at a specified interval or time, and automatically beginning a new day's recording.
    - Color-coded displays of 10 to 20 system highlighting electrodes with significant artifact so ICU staff can provide easy maintenance of affected electrodes.
    - Automatic synchronization of common settings (montages, recording protocols) from a central location to local acquisition machines.
  - For research purposes, software should have functions to "de-identify" EEG data and to save in an open-source EEG data format.
- Spike and seizure detection software
  - Current commercially available spike and seizure detection software is not optimal for detection of common seizure patterns seen in the ICU and little data are available on their sensitivity and false-positive rates.
  - May produce many false alerts which prompt inappropriate treatments and are bothersome to ICU personnel.
- Quantitative EEG software
  - Allow graphical display of EEG parameters over long time periods (hours).
  - Can be displayed at the bedside, as well as at a central monitoring station in the ICU or EEG lab.
  - Many types of commercial QEEG software are available and most are proprietary.

○ The main features to consider are ease of use, how well integrated QEEG software is with EEG acquisition software, and accuracy of event detection and artifact rejection algorithms.
○ Some systems can be configured to send alerts and images of corresponding trends and raw EEG via e-mail.

III. FURTHER CONSIDERATIONS/REMAINING QUESTIONS

A. Cost
- The cost of computers and video recording components continues to decrease.
- EEG equipment has become more portable and easier to install, due to development of standard network architecture as opposed to proprietary cabling.
- Software (special features, seizure detection, QEEG) may add a substantial amount to the cost of ICU EEG equipment.
- Information technology and biomedical engineering support is necessary.
  ○ Installing, configuring, maintaining, and updating ICU EEG equipment and software requires significant IT and biomedical resources.
  ○ Large ICU EEG monitoring programs may require dedicated IT and biomedical personnel.

B. Multimodality Monitoring
- Device interoperability is an important issue in ICU EEG.
- Optimally, all physiologic patient data, as well as data from ventilators, cooling devices, and IV pumps would be able to be incorporated into a single time-synchronized data stream.

REFERENCES

1. Guideline one: Minimum technical requirements for performing clinical electroencephalography. *American Clinical Neurophysiology Society [online]*. Available at: https://www.acns.org/
2. Guideline two: Minimum technical requirements for pediatric electroencephalography. *American Clinical Neurophysiology Society [online]*. Available at: https://www.acns.org/
3. Guideline eight: Guidelines for recording clinical EEG on digital media. *American Clinical Neurophysiology Society [online]*. Available at: https://www.acns.org/
4. Guideline twelve: Guidelines for long-term monitoring for epilepsy. *Am J Electroneurodiagnostic Technol.* 2008;48:265–286.
5. Kull LL, Emerson RG. Continuous EEG monitoring in the intensive care unit: Technical and staffing considerations. *J Clin Neurophysiol.* 2005;22:107–118.

ADDITIONAL READING

Guerit JM, Amantini A, Amodio P, et al. Consensus on the use of neurophysiological tests in the intensive care unit (ICU): Electroencephalogram (EEG), evoked potentials (EP), and electroneuromyography (ENMG). *Neurophysiol Clin.* 2009;39:71–83.
Wartenberg KE, Mayer SA. Multimodal brain monitoring in the neurological intensive care unit: Where does continuous EEG fit in? *J Clin Neurophysiol.* 2005;22:124–127.

TWO

Electrodes and Montages

*John Richard Ives**

KEY POINTS

- Patients undergoing EEG monitoring frequently require urgent CT and/or MRI imaging which poses compatibility problems when using traditional electrodes, requiring additional EEG tech time to remove and replace electrodes.
- Reusable electrodes increase cost but can reduce infection and skin breakdown, as well as save EEG technologist time.
- Although most centers use standard 10–20 electrode placement, studies are in progress to determine whether reduced coverage can provide acceptable specificity and sensitivity for detection of seizures and other significant events
- Better designed EEG electrodes are needed to improve signal quality, reduce maintenance time and costs, and allow more efficient software development.

I. BACKGROUND

A. Continuous EEG monitoring (cEEG) in the intensive care unit ICU is a relatively new application of long-term EEG monitoring (LTM) (1).

- Digital EEG recording of patients using computer-based recording hardware and software began in the early 1970s (2).
- Early systems were not capable of continuous recording.
- Early EEG software was only capable of marking push-button events, random time samples, and automatic detection of inter-ictal spikes and seizures but with poor specificity and sensitivity.

Disclosures: J.R. Ives is one of the founders of SleepMed (DigiTrace) and Ives EEG Solutions which manufactures/markets EEG devices. JRI holds various patents associated with EEG technology and is a consultant for Jordan Neuroscience.

B. Now, inexpensive computers with larger memory and expanded storage permit cEEG with or without video.

C. EEG monitoring of critically ill neurological patients has demonstrated the significant contribution of cEEG to patient care by documenting the presence of subclinical epileptic seizures which occur commonly in this population (3,4).

II. BASICS

A. EEG Electrodes and Imaging Compatibility

- Electrodes
    - Early electrodes used for cEEG were the same as those used for routine EEG since the late 1920s.
    - Options included either metal cup or subdermal needle electrodes.
- cEEG patients in the ICU usually require frequent and urgent CT and/or MR imaging which is unique compared to traditional long-term monitoring of patients in the epilepsy monitoring unit.
    - Traditional EEG electrodes are usually not imaging compatible because of their material composition and/or length of lead-wire.
    - Typically, EEG electrodes are removed prior to imaging and replaced afterwards.
    - This significantly increases the work load of the EEG technologist resulting in more on-call and overtime hours.
    - Removing and replacing electrodes also contributes to skin breakdown and infection.
- Electrodes and CT scanners
    - Metal electrodes cause "star-burst" artifact on CT images due to deflection of x-rays.
    - However, the FDA has not identified any patient safety issues associated with EEG electrodes in a CT scanner.
    - The denser the electrode is, the more likely it is that the x-ray can be deflected or blocked, causing significant artifact on the reconstructed images.
    - Figure 2.1 demonstrates the CT artifact (or lack of artifact) associated with three different EEG electrode types.
- Electrodes and MRI scanners
    - Metal electrodes with any ferrous material (or magnetic material), cause susceptibility artifact on MR images.
    - However, pure, noble metals such as silver, gold, copper, and platinum are MRI-compatible (5).
    - Figure 2.2 demonstrates the MRI artifact (or lack of artifact) associated with three different electrode types.
    - Safety concern in MRI: Long leads and ferrous material may lead to heating and burning of the skin and possible physical movement of the electrodes.

(A)

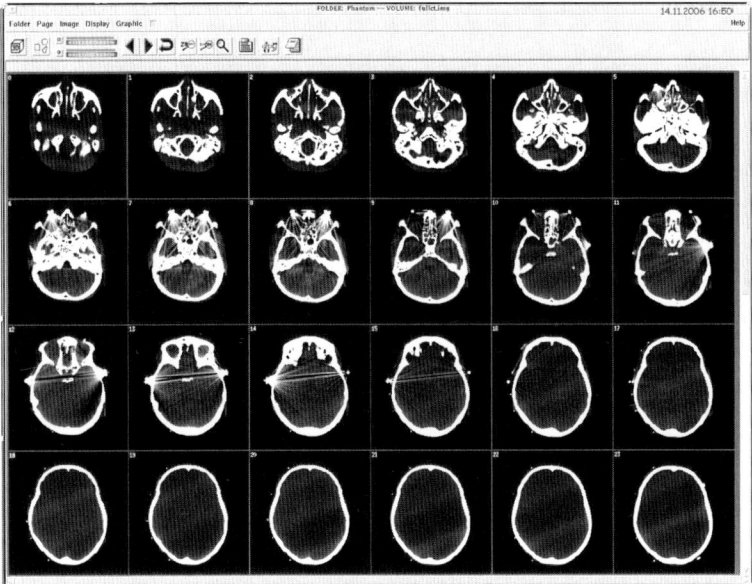

(B)

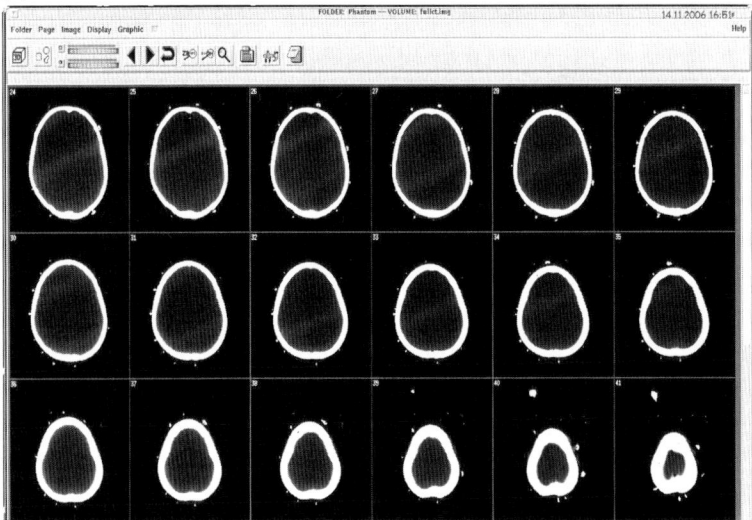

FIGURE 2.1 Comparison of artifact on CT imaging with different three electrode types. (**A**) Gold cup electrodes placed at Fp1/2 and F7/8 show "star-burst" artifact. (**B**) Conductive plastic electrodes over the right hemisphere and subdermal wire electrodes over the left hemisphere demonstrate absence of artifact, only cross-section of lead wire is visible.

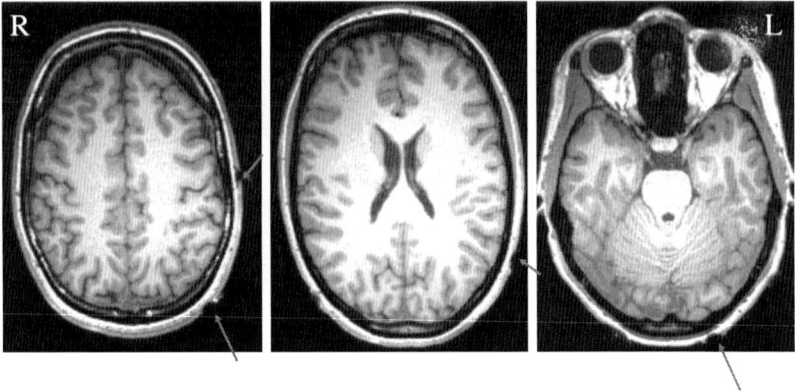

FIGURE 2.2   Comparison of electrode artifact on 3 Tesla MRI from a subject with three different electrode types. Conductive plastic electrodes (CPE) were placed over the left hemisphere (T3, T5, O1, C3, P3). Gold cup electrodes (GCE) were placed over the right hemisphere (T4, T6, O2, C4, P4). Subdermal wire electrodes (SWE) were placed over the left and right frontal area (Fp1, Fp2, F3, F4, F7, F8). Three different slices are shown. Essentially no artifact is seen associated with the SWE over the frontal area. Some obvious artifact (arrows) is associated with the CPE over the left hemisphere, but only involves the scalp and skull, and does not extend into the brain structures. Even less artifact is associated with the GCE over the right hemisphere.

- ○ Coiling of electrode leads (common with longer EEG leads) can also cause artifact on MRI images by acting as an antenna.
- ○ Coiled leads can also permit "eddy-currents" and heating.
- Some electrodes are both CT- and MRI-compatible.
  - ○ Conductive plastic electrodes with a thin silver coat, coupled with very short leads are MRI and CT compatible (6,7).
  - ○ Short-lead, pure silver subdermal wire electrodes (SWE) are also MR and CT compatible (8) and can be used on patients who are comatose and require long duration cEEG (7,9).
  - ○ An advantage of SWE is that once placed, minimal maintenance is required and they can record for months (8,9).
  - ○ Some subdermal needle electrodes are CT compatible, but depending on composition and length of electrode leads, they may or may not also be MRI compatible.
  - ○ There is always some concern for "needle-stick" with subdermal needle electrodes although few complications have been reported.
- Electrode harness system (10)
  - ○ Instead of each electrode connected individually to the head box, an electrode system is available which consists of an electrode array, one set for each hemisphere (Figure 2.3) bundled to a small plastic connector that in turn connects to a single, color-coded harness, again, one per hemisphere (Figure 2.4), which is then attached to the EEG acquisition machine.

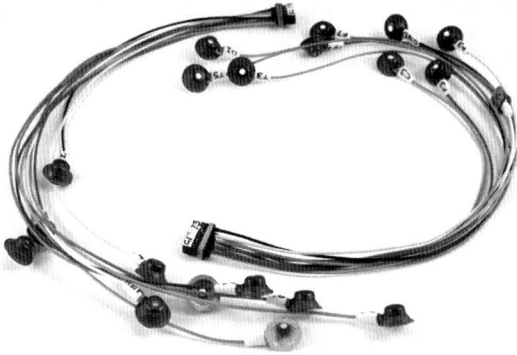

FIGURE 2.3 A 20-electrode array using conductive plastic electrodes with an Ag-Ag/Cl coating. The 10–20 location of each electrode is printed on the label and also identified by lead length and color. The length of the lead to the small mass connector is as short as possible to prevent coiling during MRI imaging.

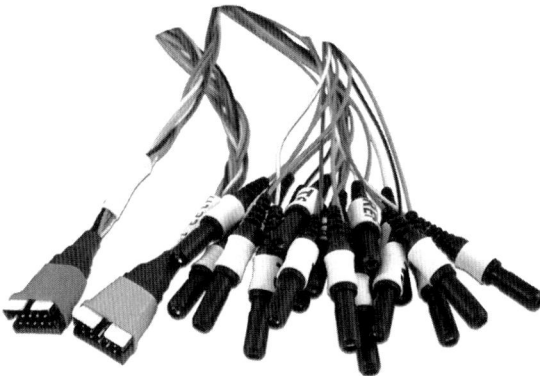

FIGURE 2.4 Matching harness for the electrode set in Figure 2.3, which connects the electrode array to any EEG machine. The small color-coded mass connectors permit nursing staff to disconnect the patient for imaging without requiring the involvement of an EEG technologist.

○ Allows non-EEG technologists (such as ICU nurses) to quickly disconnect and reconnect the harness from the EEG acquisition permitting imaging 24/7, while at the same time reducing lost cEEG monitoring time during imaging procedures.
○ Reduces EEG tech overtime and on-call duties.

B. Reusable Electrodes Versus Disposable Electrodes
- Most EEG labs reuse their EEG electrodes after cleaning and disinfection.
- Patients in the ICU may have head wounds, skin infections, and undergo longer recordings than patients in the epilepsy monitoring unit.

- The EEG electrode may be one of the only pieces of equipment in the ICU that has direct contact with the patient and is commonly reused.
- Disposable EEG electrodes have many advantages.
  - Eliminates concern about cross-infection.
  - Further reduces EEG technologist time by eliminating time needed for cleaning and disinfection.
  - Although disposable EEG electrodes are considerably more expensive than standard electrodes, they can be more cost effective when factoring the cost savings from less EEG tech time spent on cleaning and maintenance.

C. Electrode Caps, Nets, and Templates

- Electrode caps, nets, and templates are designed to allow for quick placement of EEG electrodes, typically by non-EEG trained personnel.
- Electrode caps and nets usually contain the EEG electrodes embedded within the cap while templates provide a colored-coded "map" to ensure accurate placement of disc or needle electrodes without the need for head measurement.
- A single center study evaluated the use of an EEG template system applied by non-EEG personnel (11).
  - Thirty-two critically ill patients underwent up to 8 hours of EEG monitoring with electrodes placed by non-EEG personnel using a template system followed by cEEG with standard electrode placement by EEG technologists.
  - There was no clinically significant differences noted in impedance measures or recording quality for the template applied electrodes versus the technologist applied electrodes.
  - EEG recordings using templates were initiated 3 hours earlier than EEG recordings requiring technologist application.
  - Quality of long-term recordings (greater than 8 hours) using template applied electrodes was not evaluated.
- While these systems may have advantages of permitting non-EEG personnel to obtain EEG data quickly, they are not appropriate for long-term recordings or when scalp access is required for purposes such as management of intraventricular drains, wound care, and so on.

D. Electrode Coverage and Montages

- cEEG, like any long-term monitoring, is recorded with a referential-based montage.
  - The location of the reference electrode is usually specific to the center, usually on the midline.
  - The location of the ground electrode is not critical, but most apply it to the midline on the head.
  - Each active electrode is recorded against a single reference electrode (REF).
- Most EEG systems record each electrode site against a common reference.
  - Exception: It is recommended to refer the EKG electrode to a noncephalic reference such that extraneous activity detected in the EKG electrode can easily be confirmed to be noncerebral.

- Any montage can be generated based on the electrode sites included in the original recording format.
- Review montages are a display of the individual electrodes versus another electrode used for reading.
- Generally, montages are specific to the EEG department and/or the personal preference of the electroencephalographer.
- General guidelines: display left hemisphere over right hemisphere, anterior over posterior, and avoid triangular montages.
- Patterns of EEG electrode use in clinical practice
  - Of 90 centers surveyed that perform cEEG, the majority use the standard 10–20 electrode placement/coverage.
    - This consists of 21 electrodes (Fp1/2, F3/4, C3/4, P3/4, F7/8, T3/4, T5/6, F/C/Pz, A1/2 with a ground/reference pair).
    - Most groups also record single channel EKG.
  - Some centers (45 groups) include extra electrodes (T1/2, M1/2, eye leads, and others) up to a total of 30 electrodes.
  - Advantages of extra electrode coverage
    - Provides redundancy if individual electrodes deteriorate or are displaced.
    - Contributes to improved identification of artifact versus cerebral events.
  - Drawbacks of extra coverage
    - Increases set-up time as well as maintenance time.
    - Increased coverage makes it less feasible for non-EEG personnel to handle the set-up and maintenance.
  - Some centers use significantly less coverage with only 10, 11, or 13 electrodes on selected patients (six of 90 groups).
  - In the ICU, precise seizure localization is lower priority than in the epilepsy monitoring unit, hence, limited electrode arrays may be sufficient.
- Studies have evaluated the sensitivity and specificity of a few select reduced coverage montages.
  - Young et al. evaluated the use of four-channel EEG monitoring system with a "subhairline" montage compared to standard 10 to 20 EEG electrode placement (12).
    - Four-channel recording demonstrated a sensitivity of 68% and specificity of 98% for seizure detection.
  - Kolls et al. used simulated hairline electrode placement by reformatting pre-recorded EEG data (Fp1/2, F7/8, T3/4, T5/6) (13).
    - Data was reformatted in three different six-channel montages.
    - Sensitivity for seizure detection was 72% with seizures frequently misinterpreted as either benign pattern or diffuse slowing.
  - However, in a smaller study utilizing a novel seven-electrode montage (Fp1/2, T3/4, O1/2, and Cz) applied and interpreted by neurology residents, sensitivity for seizure detection was found to be 92.5% with specificity of 93.5% (14).
  - Further studies exploring the reliability of reduced electrode montages are needed before recommending them for widespread use.

III. FURTHER CONSIDERATIONS/REMAINING QUESTIONS

A. Which type of electrodes work best in the ICU?
- Goal: Improved efficiency and simplicity in performing cEEG.
- Properties of an optimally designed EEG electrode for ICU use:
  - Improved signal quality
  - CT and MRI compatible
  - Cost effective
  - Disposable
  - Limited skin breakdown
  - Rapid application
  - Permit software to be more efficient in detecting significant events and rejecting artifact.

B. What is the minimal number of electrodes needed for acceptable sensitivity and specificity and at what locations?
- Montage designs employing reduced electrode coverage are needed.
- New studies should be performed.

C. Can even better electrodes or electrode systems be designed for cEEG that permit faster hookup, better quality signals, and reduced maintenance?
- A recent paper/survey by Schultz covers the pros and cons associated with cEEG and the selection of EEG electrodes.

REFERENCES

1. Jordan KG. Continuous EEG and evoked potential monitoring in the neuroscience intensive care unit. *J Clin Neurophysiol.* 1993;10:445–475.
2. Ives JR, Thompson CJ, Gloor P. Seizure monitoring: A new tool in electroencephalography. *Electroenceph Clin Neurophysiol.* 1976;41:422–427.
3. Vespa PM, Nenov V, Nuwer MR. Continuous EEG monitoring in the intensive care unit: Early findings and clinical efficacy. *Am Clin Neurophysiol Soc.* 1999;16:1–13.
4. Hirsch LJ, Kull LL. Continuous EEG monitoring in the intensive care unit. *Am J Electroneurodiagn Tech.* 2004;44:137–158.
5. Ives JR, Warach S, Schmitt F, et al. Monitoring the patient's EEG during an MRI. *Electroenceph Clin Neurophysiol.* 1993;87:417–420.
6. Das RR, Lucey BP, Chou SH-Y, et al. The utility of conductive plastic electrodes in prolonged ICU EEG monitoring. *Neurocrit Care.* 2009;10:368–372.
7. Vulliemoz S, Perrig S, Pellise D, et al. Imaging compatible electrodes for continuous EEG monitoring in the intensive care unit. *J Clin Neurophysiol.* 2009;26:236–243.
8. Ives JR. New chronic EEG electrode for CCU/ICU monitoring. *J Clin Neurophysiol.* 2005;22:119–123.
9. Martz GU, Hucek C, Quigg M. Sixty day continuous use of subdermal wire electrodes for EEG monitoring during treatment of status epilepticus. *Neurocrit Care.* 2009; 11:223–227.
10. Mirsattari SM, Lee DH, Jones D, et al. MRI compatible EEG electrode system for routine use in the epilepsy monitoring unit and intensive care unit. *Electroenceph Clin Neurophysiol.* 2004;115:2175–2180.

11. Kolls BJ, Olson DWM, Gallentine WB, et al. Electroencephalography leads placed by non-technologists using a template system produce signals equal in quality to technologist-applied, collodion disk leads. *J Clin Neurophysiol.* 2012;29(1):42–49.

12. Young GB, Sharpe MD, Savard M, et al. Seizure detection with a commercially available bedside EEG monitor and the subhairline montage. *Neurocrit Care.* 2009;11:411–416.

13. Kolls BJ, Husain AM. Assessment of hairline EEG as a screening tool for nonconvulsive status epilepticus. *Epilepsia.* 2007;48(5):959–965.

14. Karakis I, Montouris GD, Otis JAD, et al. A quick and reliable EEG montage for the detection of seizures in critical care setting. *J Clin Neurophysiol.* 2010;27(2):100–105.

15. Schultz TL. Technical tips: MRI Compatible EEG Electrodes: Advantages, disadvantages, and financial feasibility in a clinical setting. *The Neurodiagnostic Journal.* 2012;52:1.

ADDITIONAL READING

Hirsch LJ, Brenner RP, eds. *Atlas of EEG in Critical Care.* John Wiley & Sons; 2010.

Varelas P, ed. *Seizures in Critical Care: a Guide to Diagnostic and Therapeutics,* Humana Press; 2010.

Fisch BJ, ed. *Epilepsy and Intensive Care Monitoring: Principles and Practice,* Demos Medical Publishing; 2010.

THREE

Networking, Remote Monitoring, and Data Storage

J. Andrew Ehrenberg

KEY POINTS

- There are various options for network configurations including stand-alone EEG networks, virtual local area networks (VLANs), and facility integrated networks.
- Major considerations when choosing a method of remote access to EEG data include speed and ease of access, security, cost, resources available for maintenance and number of concurrent users. Remote monitoring options include desktop mirroring, terminal services, and virtualized desktops.
- There are various archiving and data storage strategies that can be utilized to store the vast amount of data that is acquired with continuous EEG and video recording. The best method of data storage depends on what resources are available (time and equipment) as well as how much of the data is considered necessary to keep for prolonged periods.

I. BACKGROUND

A. Growth of Networks in Health Care Settings and Clinical Neurophysiology

- Computer networks and remote monitoring have been increasing in use in clinical neurophysiology.
  - Computer networks in the health care setting have become essential. The majority of the growth has been driven by the need to view radiologic images, lab results, and creation of system-wide electronic medical records.
  - Over the past few decades, local networks in Epilepsy Monitoring Units (EMUs) and remote monitoring in Intra-Operative Monitoring (IOM) have become commonplace.
- EMU implementations
  - In the EMU setting, networks are usually physically separate from the hospital or facility network, and have no shared connections. The EMU network usually connects to EEG recording units, data storage servers, and reading stations.

○ This physically separate network configuration allows for collection of large amounts of video and EEG data as well as fast data transmission without impacting the hospital network.

○ The disadvantage to this configuration is the inability to view data remotely, even from physician's offices within the hospital, unless directly connected to the EMU local network.

• Remote monitoring has been utilized in IOM for many years.

○ IOM monitoring is typically arranged in a point-to-point configuration where the reviewer is connected directly to a single data acquisition unit and able to view data in real time.

○ Remote monitoring in IOM was originally accomplished through phone line data connection but is currently through a facility network where viewing takes place from a separate location, either a physician's office or sometimes as distant as other states.

○ This point-to-point configuration is not as effective for prolonged EEG monitoring where there are typically multiple patients, multiple EEG reviewers, and the need to review previously recorded data.

B. Network Configurations

• There are many network configurations and remote monitoring options that can be utilized in ICU cEEG.

○ As with any aspect of clinical neurophysiology, there is no perfect design, any more than there is a perfect montage so applying knowledge of strengths and weaknesses as well as available resources is vital to determining the optimum design.

C. Data Storage

• EEG data storage has undergone many changes over the years.

○ In the past, data storage has ranged from collections of piles of paper in large storage rooms to stacks of video cassette tapes.

○ One of the major benefits of digital EEG is the ease of storing large amounts of data on fairly small media. This began as optical disks, then archiving to CD and later to DVD. More recently, storage to large external USB hard drives and "centralized" network storage has become popular.

• Data file sizes

○ Data file sizes can range from 1 or 2 gigabytes (without video) to 20 or 30 gigabytes (with video) per patient per day.

○ "Clipped" segments are much smaller, with only small time spans of EEG and video data stored, usually for significant events such as seizures or representative samples of background patterns.

○ One of the problems with ICU cEEG data storage is that activity not seen as significant now, might later be decided to be important.

○ However, storing the entire 20 to 30 gigabyte file of patient data each day is cost prohibitive for most institutions.

II. BASICS

A. Network Configurations
- Networks are interconnections between computers and computerized devices, including EEG acquisition units, reading stations, data servers, desktop computers, switches, and routers.
- Network configurations include stand-alone, VLAN, and full integration into a facility network. Each has individual strengths and weaknesses (Table 3.1).
  #### 1. Stand-Alone Networks (Figure 3.1)
  - Stand-alone networks were the most common implementation in EMUs a decade ago. It is a configuration where all of the involved computer devices are connected to each other but not connected to any external network.
  - Early computer EEG systems typically had internal hard drives that could store no more than a few days of continuous data so recording units were connected to large data storage servers that were quite costly and had to be mounted in a large network rack that stood 4 to 5 feet in height.
  - Benefits of a stand-alone network
    - Maximum data speed since bandwidth is not shared with the facility network.
    - Managed within an EEG department without the need for hospital IT resources.
    - Ability to be tailored to the specific needs of the facility.
    - Security of the EEG data from external access.
  - Drawbacks of a stand-alone network
    - No remote monitoring capability.
    - Lack of flexibility since the only recording locations are predefined and separately wired patient rooms.
    - Hospital IT support staff is not usually available to identify and resolve technical issues.
  #### 2. Virtual Local Area Network
  - VLANs are applicable to computers connected within an internal network. This is usually with computers and devices that are physically close to each other, within the same building or on the same campus.
  - Wide area networks (WANs) are applicable to computers that can connect over large distances, such as the Internet, or between different physical campuses of an institution.
  - VLANs would be "in house" networks or hospital intranets, whereas WANs would be access over the Internet using web-based portals for access into the hospital's VLAN.
  - A computer's network cable plugs into the wall and is usually connected on the other end (at some point) into a port on a router. This is somewhat analogous to an old-fashioned telephone switchboard. A router is a fairly simple computer that takes *packets* of information from computers and sends them, or routes them, to where they need to go, either to a system connected to the same router or to a system via a connected router.

TABLE 3.1 Comparison of Different Network Configurations

NETWORK CONFIGURATION	SPEED	TECHNICAL IT STAFF	COST	COMPLEXITY	REMOTE CAPABILITIES	MULTIPLE FACILITIES
Stand alone	High	Low	Moderate	Low	Limited	Limited
VLAN	Moderate	High	High	High	Yes	Yes
Facility network	Fluctuate	Moderate	Low	Moderate	Yes	Yes

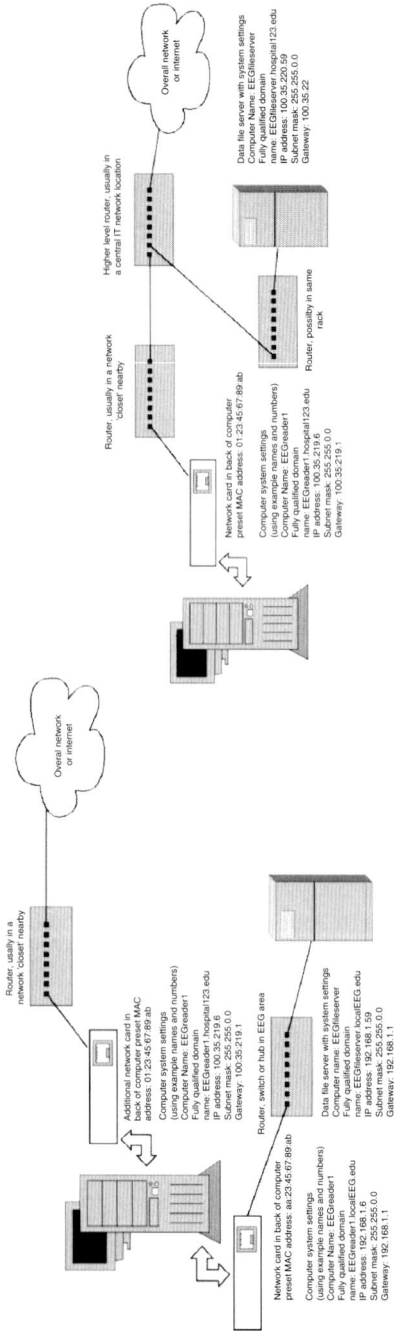

FIGURE 3.1 A graphical representation of stand-alone versus integrated facility EEG networks.

- Advantages
  - Department cost savings by utilizing existing hospital IT support for the network management and troubleshooting.
  - More flexible than a stand-alone network. Recording in additional locations does not require the physical installation of separate network cables.
  - Capable of remote monitoring functions.
- Disadvantages
  - Setting up and managing this type of configuration is relatively complex and requires significant IT resources.

3. Facility Network Integration (Figure 3.1)
  - Most facilities have existing networks connecting to various medical resources, imaging and electronic medical records, as well as e-mail and the Internet. This is referred to being on the facility "backbone."
  - This type of configuration allows for maximum flexibility recording from various locations and remote monitoring, but has some inherent drawbacks, such as fluctuations in speed due to shared bandwidth and increased IT security requirements.
  - Facilities will usually have various rules for systems on their "backbone" to protect the integrity of the network as a whole, including antivirus software, automatic updates for the operating system, and user rights limitations.
  - Other IT regulations include restricted program and system access for users.

B. Network Configuration Summary
- When setting up an ICU EEG monitoring program, it is important to consider network configuration options early in the planning process with consideration of both immediate needs as well as future growth.
- Sometimes a proportionally higher initial cost will ensure that the IT infrastructure is in place to support use in future years.

C. Network Speed
- Modern facility networks speeds range from 100 Mb/sec up to 1 gigabit per second (Gb/sec), with external access at least 4 to 10 Mb/sec, even over wireless connections and the Internet.
- At speeds slower than 10 Mb/sec, only EEG can be seen and not in real time. At speeds of 100 Mb/sec, live EEG can be seen as well as recorded video. At speeds of 1 Gb/sec and faster, true real-time viewing of EEG and digital video is possible (Table 3.2).
- However, in network configurations that are directly on the facility network, these maximum speeds are shared by all the traffic that is concurrently being transmitted, so less than maximum speeds are typically seen.

D. Remote Monitoring
- The definition of remote monitoring in the context of ICU cEEG is the ability to see neurophysiologic data (both real time as well as previously recorded data) from a physically remote location.

TABLE 3.2   Speed Comparisons and the Realistic Expectations for Resulting
Performance and Common Scenarios

NETWORK SPEED	CONNECTION TYPE	REVIEW CAPABILITIES	TYPICAL SCENARIO
28.8 kb/s or 56 kb/s	Modems	Recorded EEG only	Direct connections from review station to acquisition
4–10 Mb/s	Wireless connections across the Internet, CAT3 ethernet	Recorded EEG only	EEG review from home
100 Mb/s	CAT5 ethernet, internal facility networks	Real-time or recorded EEG, recorded video	Facilities with network wiring installed more than 5 years ago
1 Gb/s	CAT5e, CAT6, newer internal facility networks	Real-time EEG and digital video	Modern facility networks

○ There are three major software options for implementation of remote monitoring: desktop mirroring, terminal services, and virtualized native Citrix applications (Figure 3.2).

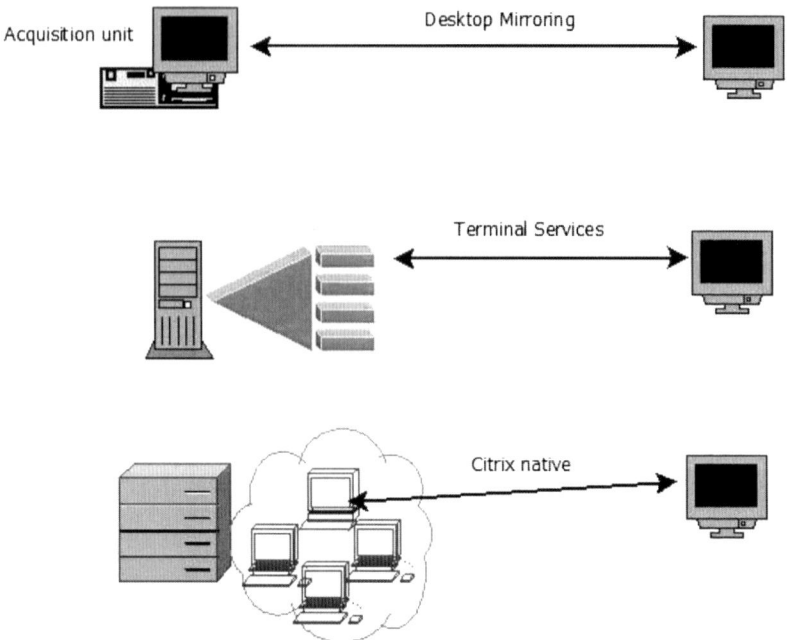

FIGURE 3.2   Remote monitoring options.

- Desktop mirroring refers to the client computer simply viewing and interacting with the desktop running on the host computer.
- Terminal services consist of the client computer logging into a desktop that is running on a remote server. The remote server is also running other desktops.
- Virtualized Citrix native client (or other virtual machine software) is where the client computer connects to a dynamic computer created by the server. Software that is designed specifically to run in this type of environment and security infrastructure is called a *native* application.
- When assessing remote monitoring needs, there are six key aspects to consider: speed of use, ease of use, security, resource requirements, number of users, and functionality (Table 3.3).
- Speed of use
  - Data files are usually physically located on either an acquisition station or a data server. Data files consist of not only the EEG but also of the digital video and other associated files.
  - Remote monitoring requires the ability to run EEG reading software and also access to the EEG data files. If quantitative EEG software is also used, network access to these programs and files is also needed (except in desktop mirroring).
  - Speed of use includes how fast the program opens (or programs in the case of using additional third-party software), how quickly individual EEG page displays can be reviewed and how long it takes for one file to close and the next to open.
  - Example of how speed of use impacts EEG review time
    - Assume that there are 48 hours worth of video EEG data, located in four separate 12 hours files with quantitative EEG (QEEG) data in 2 hours segments, and there are four patients to be reviewed.
    - All QEEG segments are reviewed in addition to three 1-minute samples of raw EEG for each 2 hours QEEG segment.
    - Fastest and slowest times for speed are based on anecdotal but real-world experiences and does not take into account additional time for the EEG reviewer to stop and analyze the EEG recording:
      - Speed for program opening ranged from the fastest scenario at 10 seconds to the slowest scenario of 90 seconds. (The fastest speed of access was with an

TABLE 3.3 Comparison of the Key Aspects of Remote Monitoring Options

	DESKTOP MIRRORING	TERMINAL SERVICES	CITRIX NATIVE
Speed of use	Slow	Fast	Moderate
Ease of use	Poor	Moderate	Good
Security	Poor	Moderate	Good
Resource requirements	Low	Moderate	High
Number of users	1	1–3	Greater than 3
Functionality	Good	Moderate	Low

EEG review program over a terminal services environment with native trending, while the slowest program opening speed was with a Citrix native EEG review program, with third-party trending.)
- Page speed ranged from relatively instant for raw EEG page speed (up to 50×) and QEEG segment speeds of less than 1 second per 2 hours segment to the slowest page speed of 2 pages/second and up to 1 minute per QEEG segment.
- Time to close one file and open the next ranged from 20 seconds in the fastest scenario to over 4 minutes in the slowest.
- Using the above data, the fastest and slowest time to review these patients would be:

FASTEST SCENARIO	SLOWEST SCENARIO
10 s (program opening)	90 s (program opening)
+5 s (to review 1 min of EEG)	+30 s (to review 1 min of EEG)
×3 (1 min epochs reviewed per 2 hr QEEG section)	×3 (1 min epochs reviewed per 2 hr QEEG section)
×24 (2 hr QEEG sections)	×24 (2 hr QEEG sections)
+1 s (to "page" to next QEEG section)	+60 s (to "page" to next QEEG section)
×24 (2 hr sections)	×24 (2 hr sections)
+20 s (to close one file and open the next)	+240 s (to close one file and open the next)
×4 (12 hr files)	×4 (12 hr files)
×4 (patients)	×4 (patients)
Approx 30 min to review (31.27 min)	Approx 5.16 hr to review (310 min)

- Ease of use
  - Ease of use refers to how easy it is to open/access the program and opening data files. This includes the number of times the mouse has to be clicked, and the number of times a user name and password have to be entered, and how many network addresses have to be remembered.
  - The more integrated into the overall facility network, the easier remote monitoring program access will be.
  - In the easiest real-world anecdotal example, a Citrix native application in an integrated networking system allows one entry of a user name and password, opening the application and selecting a patient and double clicking a file to open it.
  - In the most cumbersome example, a VPN is used with remote desktop to a reading station or server, requiring sign-on to the VPN, running remote desktop connection, typing in an IP address, then signing in again through remote desktop connection, running the EEG application and selecting a patient, and double clicking on the file.

- Security
  - Security in remote monitoring encompasses two separate concepts: (1) protecting the privacy of confidential patient data, and (2) controlling the ability of users to modify, or delete data files.
  - Facility networks are usually protected from access by anonymous outside users. Data traffic from outside the facility network that has not been authenticated is blocked.
- Resource requirements
  - Vital resources include hardware, software, and technical staff to both implement and maintain the network.
  - The easiest remote monitoring solution to implement is a desktop mirroring configuration. This usually requires no additional hardware, fairly inexpensive software, and minimal technical staff involvement.
  - Terminal services remote monitoring requires a higher end application server, but software is included in most operating systems. Multiple concurrent users require additional terminal services access licenses. A moderate level of technical staff knowledge is needed but may be shared with hospital IT resources.
  - For Citrix native EEG application implementation, at least one Citrix Presentation server is needed, as well as EEG Citrix native application licenses which are usually more expensive than regular EEG application licenses. In addition, most Citrix native application implementations will require additional servers and software for redundancy in the event of system failure. Configuration and maintenance of Citrix implementations require a high-level IT technical staff.
- Number of users
  - In most large ICU EEG programs, there will likely be many concurrent users (epileptologists, fellows, residents, EEG techs), even more as cEEG services span multiple facilities.
  - To a large degree the number of concurrent users dictates the type of remote monitoring implementation that is warranted.
  - Remote review with desktop mirroring is the slowest option and video review is not realistic. Most software desktop mirroring programs only allow one concurrent user. Therefore, desktop mirroring is only feasible with one remote user, where slow review speed is acceptable, and only one or two patients are reviewed at one time.
  - Terminal services utilizes a review station or application to which the user logs onto. Each user receives a separate desktop presentation, and each desktop presentation sharing the total system resources. The main drawback to a terminal services solution is that with more than three users the shared resources are spread thin and many vendors do not support the configuration. Terminal services applications work best when fiscal and technical resources are available and only one to three concurrent users are expected.
  - Citrix native applications utilize a Citrix presentation server to create "virtual" computers for each user. Programmatic speed is scaled to the speed of the network connection, which can prevent fluctuations in speed when reviewing but also limits maximal review speed. Citrix native remote review

is best for more than three concurrent users, or when viewing EEG across multiple facilities.
- Functionality
  - ○ Functionality refers to what the remote user can accomplish including the ability to see live and recorded video and QEEG as well as perform manipulation of the recording unit or camera.
  - ○ For full functionality, a desktop mirroring scenario is best.
  - ○ Functionality using terminal services is comparable to an in-house EEG reading station.
  - ○ Citrix native implementations have the most limitations, but also have the lowest risk of users disrupting the acquisition unit.

E. Data Storage
- A strategy for data management is essential and involves understanding the size and types of files being acquired.
- It is important to realize that a single EEG recording consists of not just one file, but multiple linked files.
  - ○ There is usually one file for the EEG itself, in a vendor proprietary format, which contains a numeric entry for each electrode for each time sample. This means that for a standard 16-channel montage, with a 500 Hz sample speed, there is an entry every 500th of a second for each electrode.
  - ○ There is also a separate set of digital video files as well as files that include synchronization information, annotations, and QEEG data.
- cEEG files for standard 21 channel montage, at a sample speed of 500 Hz, per 12 hours range from 2 to 6 Gb. The number of electrodes and the sample speed have a significant impact on this size, with a sample speed of 1,000 Hz doubling the file size,
- Digital video in an uncompressed format can run over 100 Gb of data per hour, but with digital compression can reduce file sizes to 5 to 20 Gb per 12 hours.
  - ○ MPEG4 compresses video size by only recording pixels that change from the previous frame. So in a video where a patient is laying completely still and there is no other movement, the file size will be relatively small. A video where there is a lot of constant movement will be much larger.
  - ○ NOTE: Flashing light, either from a monitor or the television, will create constant change in the brightness in the room so an otherwise motionless scene will create a file as large as video with continuous motion.
- Complete video and EEG files should be stored for a period of time, but at some point will need to be archived for long-term storage. Approximately 150 to 200 patient days of data can be kept in entirety on a typical 1 to 2 Tb data server. Most centers keep 30 or 60 days of patient data on local storage before moving to archive, unless the patient is still undergoing monitoring.
- Data storage strategies: How much data to keep?
  - ○ The first data storage strategy is similar to data storage in most typical EMUs. Each patient file is "pruned" to only include certain EEG and video segments of interest; either seizures, other significant events or background samples. All other data are deleted. This leads to the smallest file size for archiving, but is the most limited in terms of later review.

TABLE 3.4 Comparison of Current Data Storage Options and Capabilities

MEDIA TYPE	SIZE	NUMBER OF PATIENT DAYS	COMMENTS
CD	700 Mb	less than 1	Too small to be very useful for cEEG
DVD	4.7 Gb	1–5 depending on how "pruned"	Must include the cost of the tech time involved in pruning (about 1 hr each), no backup of data
External USB hard drive	250 Gb–2 Tb	20–200	No back up of data in the event of drive failure
Network large-scale storage	Relatively unlimited	Relatively unlimited	High cost

○ The second strategy is keeping all EEG and video data. ICU cEEG is a new enough technology that there is no consensus on what aspects of the data might prove important later. However, keeping all EEG and video data on every patient is almost logistically impossible with current storage limitations.

○ The third data strategy is to keep all of the EEG data, but only video for significant events. The EEG is relatively small compared to the size of the digital video, and video data is less likely to be needed for future analysis.

• Data storage media (Table 3.4)

○ There are many options for data storage with a wide range of advantages and disadvantages.

○ External USB hard drives are more expensive than CD/DVD in terms of cost per Mb/Gb. However, when considering EEG tech time for archiving, external USB hard drives are more cost effective.

○ However, with both CD/DVD and external USB hard drives, the risk of file corruption should be considered as well as the possibility of physical loss of the media.

• Data format

○ Most systems record EEG into proprietary formats. To view the data on another system it has to either be bundled with a program to view the data, or if using a different program on another computer, it must be converted into a format that can be imported by the other EEG program.

○ There are three "universal" formats: EDF, ASCII, and TS1.

• EDF stands for European Data Format, and can be imported by most systems. There are related formats, such as BDF and EDF +.

• ASCII is the raw text format of the file which is usually very large since no compression of the data is used.

• Lastly, the American Clinical Neurophysiology Society has published guidance on a universal data format and recommended a standard, referred to as technical standard 1, or TS1. Though not yet in standard use, TS1 is an ideal format that would be extremely beneficial in sharing of EEG data.

III. FURTHER CONSIDERATIONS/REMAINING QUESTIONS

A. Integration With Electronic Medical Records
- HL7 is a standard format for communication between medical systems that can allow orders placed in electronic medical records to populate EEG systems, and then data from the EEG, to populate back to the medical record.
- Though it is relatively simple to implement, the hardware needed and the configuration costs are relatively high. Many hospital IT departments might be accepting of sending data to the EEG systems, but very reluctant to allow data back into the electronic medical record.

B. Rapidly Changing Technology
- Computers, networks, and storage change at a very fast rate.
  - According to Moore's law, computer technology capabilities and speeds double every two years. This theory, developed in 1965 has held true and is expected to continue to hold true through 2015 or 2020 or even later.
  - The current "cutting edge" of wireless networking with gigabit speeds will seem slow by tomorrow's standards. System capabilities will also increase as there is more and more integration of the EEG network and systems into the main networks at facilities.
  - Careful watch must be kept to balance ever increasing costs associated with staying on the "cutting edge" with practical delivery of patient care.

ACKNOWLEDGMENT
My thanks to Sheri Richardson and Dave Huston for their contributions of computer expertise.

FOUR

Staffing an ICU EEG Monitoring Unit

Leisha Osburn

KEY POINTS

- The optimal staffing model for continuous EEG monitoring of ICU patients utilizes neurodiagnostic technologists (CLTM and/or R. EEG T.) who provide real-time EEG review as well as the ability to initiate and maintain quality EEG recordings 24/7.
- Technologists involved in EEG review should have the ability to identify critical EEG patterns that can in turn be viewed and interpreted remotely by the on-call neurologist or neurointensivist.
- However, the current shortage of qualified neurodiagnostic technologists has resulted in "transitional models" in order to provide some level of EEG monitoring for ICU patients.
- Transitional models involve combinations of off-site real-time neurodiagnostic technologist monitoring, on-site nursing involvement, and intermittent neurodiagnostic technologist coverage either in house or on-call from home.
- Continuous EEG monitoring for ICU patients also requires dedicated information services personnel for data management as well as maintenance of the internal cEEG network and remote monitoring applications.
- A neurophysiology director and clinical educator are central to the success of all cEEG programs as well as a coordinator to evaluate outcomes and quality.

I. BACKGROUND

A. Long-term EEG recording for ICU patients has historically been provided for a limited number of patients.

- Data were continuously recorded but often only able to be viewed at the patient's bedside.
- Data review and interpretation occurred intermittently, but often up to 24 hours after the EEG recording.
- Video recording was rarely utilized.

B. Greater use of long-term EEG for ICU patients has revealed its benefits.
- Several studies have provided evidence that subclinical seizures are common in the critically ill population and can only be detected by cEEG.
- EEG monitoring can also provide valuable information for determination of prognosis as well as detection of other clinically significant neurological events such as acute ischemia.
- With these advances, it has become critical to shorten the gap between the occurrence of a significant EEG change and the actual detection of the event by the neurophysiology team and notification of the clinical team caring for the patient.

C. Advances in automated software detection can allow for quicker identification of potentially significant events.
- Health care personnel not specifically trained in EEG review may now be able to provide basic screening of EEG patterns.
- However, automated detection technology is imperfect and false-positive as well as false-negative events are common.
  - High-frequency, rhythmic artifacts are common in the ICU setting which can mimic an electrographic seizure and result in false-positive detections when relying solely on automated detection software.
  - Concurrent review of video often makes the distinction between artifact and cerebral activity obvious, yet automated software programs have no ability to incorporate video data into their detection algorithms.
- Therefore, raw EEG and video review by trained personnel is critical for accurate cEEG interpretation.

II. BASICS

A. Optimal in-house staffing model for continuous video EEG monitoring for ICU patients (Table 4.1)
- On-site neurodiagnostic technologists (CLTM and/or R.EEGT) provide real-time EEG monitoring 24/7 from an on-site central control room.

TABLE 4.1   Optimal Staffing Model for 24/7 Continuous EEG Monitoring (1)

TYPE OF FTE(s)	1–4 PATIENTS	5–8 PATIENTS	9–12 PATIENTS	13–16 PATIENTS	17–20 PATIENTS
EEG real-time monitoring tech	4.2	8.4	12.6	16.8	21
In-house tech	4.2	4.2	8.4	8.4	12.6
IT support	1.0	1.0	1.0	1.0	2.0
Total FTE[a]	9.4	14.6	25	29.2	39.6

[a]Paid time off (PTO) calculation not included.

○ The term "neurotelemetry" (NT) has been used to describe this service in order for care providers across multiple specialties to better understand the role of continuous EEG monitoring.
○ Ideal ratio: One technologist dedicated to monitoring one to four patients simultaneously.
○ Responsible for identifying video and EEG patterns that are considered significant clinical events.
○ The technologist must respond to significant events with a call to the appropriate care provider (on-call neurologist, neurointensivist, or bedside care provider) per established protocols.
○ The technologist keeps a detailed event log for each patient (Figure 4.1).

Running Event Log	Date	Time	Comments
Medication	4/11/2011	23:10	Dr. X confirmed seizures, ordered Ativan
Communicate with RN	4/11/2011	23:00	Informed nurse of second seizure, no clinical signs
Event-Seizure	4/11/2011	22:54	Generalized spike wave, 4min.with no clinical signs
Communicate with RN	4/11/2011	22:37	Nurse informed of seizure, first one in 3 hours
Event-Seizure	4/11/2011	22:36	Face twitching associated with generalized spike wave
When to Call MD	4/11/2011	20:27	Page Dr. X for more than 2 seizures/hour

FIGURE 4.1   Real-time monitoring event log.

- Event log is accessible to the neurologist during on-site and off-site review of the EEG data.
- The most recent entries in each category of the event log populate at the top of the spreadsheet, in addition to a time-stamped running log of events.
- This organization allows the technologist to update physicians and nurses more quickly regarding significant events.
- The event log also provides an accurate summary of events to be shared during patient hand-off between technologists at shift-change.
  - Technologists also assume all data management responsibilities (pruning, archiving, etc.).
- In addition to technologists dedicated to real-time monitoring, other on-site neurodiagnostic technologists initiate and discontinue EEG studies and maintain electrode integrity for existing studies.
  - These technologists may also assist with duties of real-time EEG monitoring as well, provided they hold the appropriate training and experience.
- A dedicated information technology (IT) specialist is required for data management as well as support of the internal EEG network and remote monitoring applications.
- A neurophysiology director and a clinical educator is required if high-volume continuous cEEG monitoring is planned.
  - With an increase in the number of simultaneously monitored beds, other infrastructure support personnel are needed including coordinators to oversee outcomes and quality assessment.
- Neurodiagnostic technologist shift coverage for the optimal in-house staffing model:
  - Similar to nursing models.
  - Two 12.5 hours shifts (12 worked hours and 30 minutes lunch) with 30 minutes overlap of shifts to provide safe patient hand-offs for each 24-hour period.
  - Alternatively, three 8.5 hours shifts per 24-hour period can be employed.
  - Premium pay for night and weekend shifts.
- Currently, no benchmarking models exist for 24/7 real-time neurodiagnostic technologist coverage.

B. Optimal Off-Site Staffing Model
- For EEG monitoring of ICU patients in smaller hospitals and/or without the necessary resources to maintain the optimal on-site staffing model.
  - Off-site technologists provide real-time dedicated monitoring 24/7 from a centralized off-site location.
  - Technologist: Patient ratio, shift coverage, and responsibilities of reporting to the on-call neurologist, maintaining a daily event log and data management are the same as for the "In-house" staffing model.
- On-site technologists provide initiation and discontinuation of studies and maintenance of electrode integrity during regular business hours, and are available on-call from home for the remainder of the 24/7 coverage.
- In this model, nurses providing bedside care for the patients also provide assistance.
  - Perform simple electrode repair and maintenance.
  - Troubleshoot with assistance of the off-site, monitoring technologists.

- A dedicated IT specialist as well as a neurophysiology director and clinical educator would also be required for this model although the off-site service may be able to provide this additional infrastructure support to individual institutions.
- This off-site monitoring service can be provided to the institution as a daily patient charge or monthly charge, based on patient volume.
- With this model, the hospital may desire to provide the in-house and on-call technologists, supplies, and equipment.
  - Usually more cost effective and beneficial for other reasons to have the off-site service provide all other infrastructure and support.
  - In-house IT has to be involved and supportive (though not dedicated) if the off-site service has dedicated IT.

C. Transitional Staffing Models (Table 4.2)

- Can be used while working to transition to 24/7 real-time continuous cEEG monitoring for ICU patients.
- Involves 24/7 recording of continuous cEEG with **delayed** review of the EEG and video data.
- On-site neurodiagnostic technologists
  - Provide initiation and discontinuation of studies.
  - Provide maintenance of electrode integrity on existing studies through in-house coverage during regular business hours and on-call from home for the remainder of the 24/7 coverage.
- Nurses currently providing care for the patients.
  - Monitor trends of quantitative EEG.
  - Page technologists and/or physicians to review patterns that may have clinical significance.
  - May also be trained to perform simple electrode fixes and troubleshooting with the assistance of the on-call technologists over the phone from home.

TABLE 4.2   Transitional Staffing Model for Continuous EEG Recording, No Continuous Monitoring (1)

TYPE OF FTE(s)	1–4 PATIENTS	5–8 PATIENTS	9–12 PATIENTS	13–16 PATIENTS	17–20 PATIENTS
EEG Real-time monitoring tech	0	0	0	0	0
In-house tech	2.6[a]	5.2[a]	7.8[a]	10.4[a]	13.0[a]
IT support	1.0	1.0	1.0	1.0	2.0
Total FTE[b]	3.6	6.2	8.8	11.4	15

[a]Plus call pay and call-in hours.

[b]Paid time off (PTO) calculation not included.

Neither model includes the administrative support roles of technical director, EEG coordinator, or education coordinator.

- EEG and video review is performed by the neurologist or neurointensivist and typically takes place once or twice daily during "rounds" and not in real time.
- This model can result in significant delays between the occurrence of a clinically significant change in the EEG recording and notification of the team caring for the patient.
- A dedicated IT support analyst and neurophysiology director and clinical educator would also be required for this model.
- With an increase in the number of simultaneously monitored beds, other infrastructure support personnel would be needed, specifically coordinators to follow outcomes data and maintain quality measures.

III. FURTHER CONSIDERATIONS/REMAINING QUESTIONS

A. Benefits of Real-Time Neurodiagnostic Technologist Monitoring Model
- Individual cases of identification of seizure and nonseizure events in real time with corresponding treatment decision making suggest that this is the optimal service delivery model for continuous cEEG monitoring in the critical care setting.
- However, data are needed to further establish the benefit of real-time monitoring and corresponding clinical decision making in this patient population.
- This model allows nurses to focus on nursing care for their patients and requires no additional nurse training and no adjustment of nurse-to-patient care ratios.

B. Impact of Transitional Staffing Models
- Data are needed to determine the impact on nurse care providers when they add responsibility for continuous cEEG event identification and electrode maintenance to the services they already provide in the critical care setting.
- Trending and automated event detection utilized to detect some real-time events in this model are imperfect, and false-positive and -negative events are common.
  - False-positive events could lead to excessive calls to on-call neurodiagnostic technologists and/or physicians, or unnecessary use of medications.
  - False-negative events could lead to missed or delayed treatment changes.
- Transitional staffing models allow patients to receive some, but not all, benefits of continuous cEEG monitoring in the ICU.

REFERENCE

1. Modeled after Neurotelemetry Monitoring staffing models at Indiana University Health, Indianapolis, Indiana.

Status Epilepticus

Michael A. Stein and Thomas P. Bleck

KEY POINTS

- Continuous EEG (cEEG) can provide invaluable information and guide appropriate patient management in the setting of status epilepticus (SE).
- cEEG is indicated in the following clinical situations:
  - Following generalized convulsive status epilepticus (GCSE) in patients with persistent encephalopathy to assess for ongoing nonconvulsive status epilepticus (NCSE).
  - For monitoring the response of SE to treatment, especially when using continuous intravenous anesthetic medications.
  - To assess for NCSE in patients with unexplained coma or altered mental status.
  - For determination of whether repetitive, involuntary movements represent SE versus nonepileptic events.

I. BACKGROUND

A. Definitions of SE

- Convulsive Status Epilepticus (CSE)
  - "An acute epileptic condition characterized by continuous generalized convulsive seizures for at least five minutes, or by two seizures without full recovery of consciousness between them" (1,2).
  - Overt CSE is readily diagnosed by clinical presentation and its diagnosis typically does not require cEEG.
  - However, CSE can present with subtle clinical findings which necessitates cEEG monitoring for accurate diagnosis.
- Nonconvulsive Status Epilepticus
  - "Continuous or intermittent ictal discharges without the patient regaining consciousness, and no overt clinical signs of convulsive activity" (3).

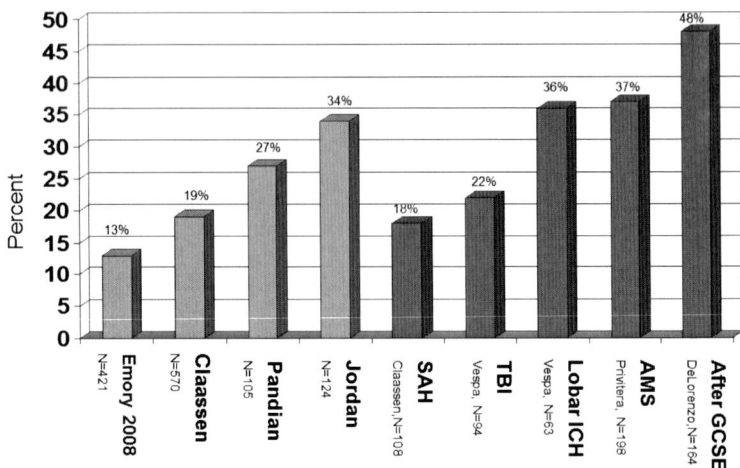

FIGURE 5.1   NCS/NCSE in patients undergoing EEG monitoring in the ICU. Lighter bars on the left represent incidence in series of patients in the ICU regardless of etiology. Darker bars represent incidence separated by underlying etiology. AMS, altered mental status; GCSE, generalized convulsive status epilepticus; ICH, intracranial hemorrhage; SAH, subarachnoid hemorrhage; TBI, traumatic brain injury.

○ In the ICU, NCSE frequently presents as decreased level of consciousness including coma (Figure 5.1).
○ However, other conditions commonly seen in the ICU also present with decreased level of consciousness.
○ Diagnosing NCSE and distinguishing it from these other conditions is a primary indication for cEEG monitoring in the ICU.
○ Because outcomes are strongly related to the duration of SE, prompt identification of SE is critical.

B. Involuntary Movements

• Many types of abnormal involuntary movements are seen in the ICU which may not be epileptic in origin such as tremor, clonus, and dyskinesia.
• If movements are repetitive and/or rhythmic, they can often be assumed to represent epileptic seizures which can lead to addition of unnecessary medications that add potential for adverse effects and drug interactions.
• EEG monitoring is the only method of distinguishing involuntary movements of ictal origin from other physiological or nonphysiological movements.
• Video analysis in addition to EEG is critical to establish that the movements in question have been captured and adequately assessed.
• In addition, video helps aid in the diagnosis of focal motor seizures that may not have an EEG correlate but are highly suggestive of epileptic seizures based on visual analysis of the semiology.

II. BASICS

A. Use of cEEG in the ICU
- It has been suggested that optimal use of cEEG should involve situations in which the underlying condition is treatable, reasonably prevalent, and associated with a high risk for further neurological injury (4).
- SE meets all of these criteria.
- Regarding duration of monitoring, one study of 110 critically ill patients with seizures detected by cEEG showed:
  - The first seizure was detected within the first hour of cEEG in 50% of cases.
  - Amongst comatose patients the first seizure was detected within <24 hours in 80% of cases and within <48 hours in 87% (6).

B. GCSE
- Refractory cases are often treated with anesthetic agents which require cEEG for monitoring treatment response and depth of sedation.
- After cessation of frank clinical seizures, patients frequently have significantly decreased level of awareness, which may be due to:
  - Effects of treatment
  - Effects of underlying cause of SE
  - Post-ictal encephalopathy
  - Conversion to subtle GCSE
  - Evolution to NCSE
- cEEG is necessary to determine whether ongoing alteration in consciousness is due to persistent seizures versus the effects of the treatment, primary neurological condition, or post-ictal state.
- A prospective study evaluated 164 patients with GCSE who underwent cEEG after resolution of overt GCSE (3).
  - 52% had no further electrographic seizures, and EEG was characterized by generalized slowing, focal slowing, attenuation, or lateralized periodic discharges (LPDs).
  - 48% had persistent electrographic seizures, including 14% with NCSE.
  - Controlling for etiology of SE and patient age, those with NCSE following resolution of GCSE had significantly worse outcome.
- Determining adequacy of treatment of GCSE varies but is largely based on:
  - Cessation of clinical seizures
  - Resolution of electrographic seizures
  - Induction of a burst-suppression pattern
  - Suppression of electrographic background activity
- A meta-analysis reviewing refractory SE treatment endpoints showed:
  - A significantly higher rate of breakthrough seizures was seen when cessation of electrographic seizures was used as treatment goal (5).
  - However, a higher rate of treatment-related complications was documented when background suppression was the target.
  - cEEG can therefore be used to optimize treatment by maximizing seizure control and minimizing adverse effects.

C. NCSE

- NCSE is treatable, but may be difficult to detect due to lack of clinical signs.
- Neurological examination in ICU patients often provides very limited information due to decreased level of consciousness from the underlying condition, as well as the effects of sedative and at times, paralytic medications.
- In addition, there are multiple other causes for decreased level of consciousness in ICU patients which are also associated with an increased risk for NCSE.
  - One review (6) stratified the risk of NCSE by clinical condition based on review of several retrospective series:
    - 19% of SAH patients undergoing cEEG monitoring due to decreased mental status were found to have seizures, and of those, 70% had NCSE.
    - In TBI, 8% of patients undergoing cEEG monitoring were found to have NCSE.
    - In one series of patients undergoing cEEG found to have NCSE, 42% had a history of hypoxic–ischemic encephalopathy.
    - In a series of pediatric ICU patients undergoing cEEG, up to one-third were found to be in NCSE.
- Regardless of primary neurological or medical condition, the population most at risk for NCSE are critically ill patients in coma with any of the following (6):
  - A history of epilepsy
  - Fluctuating level of consciousness
  - Acute brain injury
  - Recent CSE

D. Involuntary Movements

- Many patients in the ICU experience abnormal involuntary movements.
- The wide range of these movements further complicate the assessment of SE in ICU patients (6,7).
- One retrospective study analyzed 52 cEEG recordings of adult ICU patients to assess whether involuntary movements represented seizures (7).
  - Seizures were observed in 27%, including 14% with SE with the following distribution:
    - 8% focal motor SE; 4% generalized SE 6% focal clonic seizures; 6% myoclonic seizures; 2% focal tonic seizures; 2% generalized tonic–clonic seizures.
  - Nonepileptic events were seen in 73%.
    - 23% experienced tremor-like movements.
    - 13.5% were documented to have multifocal myoclonus without EEG correlate.
    - 13.5% exhibited slow, semi-purposeful movements, including pedaling, repetitive leg crossing, repetitive adduction/abduction of the lower extremities, repetitive ankle dorsi/plantar flexion; and repetitive flexion and/or extension of the extremities and/or trunk.
    - 20% experienced a variety of other movements including: transient eye movements, repetitive mouth, face, or head movements; psychogenic seizures; repetitive abdominal movements induced by mechanical ventilation; spontaneous clonus; stimulus-induced clonus and shivering.

- Other episodic events that may be seen in the ICU and require cEEG to determine whether epileptic or not include nystagmus as well as autonomic changes (6).

III. FURTHER CONSIDERATIONS/REMAINING QUESTIONS

A. What are the most important questions as the use of cEEG in the ICU increases?
- Large, well-controlled, prospective studies need to assess whether detection and treatment of electrographic seizures and SE in this population is associated with improved outcomes.

B. Seizures: To treat or not to treat?
- Although it has been clearly demonstrated that prolonged seizures, whether convulsive or nonconvulsive, lead to neuronal injury, and that the extent of injury is proportional to the duration of seizure activity, it has not been unequivocally shown that treating electrographic seizures detected by cEEG in comatose ICU patients is associated with improved outcomes.
- Although studies have shown that early detection and treatment of NCSE in comatose ICU patients is associated with decreased mortality, others have shown that treatment of NCSE in elderly critically ill patients leads to increased mortality (6).
- Further work is needed to determine whether some patient subgroups might benefit from treatment more than others.
- The following sequelae of NCS and NCSE support the argument for aggressive treatment:
  - The potential for cerebral edema.
  - Ongoing excitotoxicity leading to increased neuronal injury.
  - Direct neuronal injury and subsequent effects on cognition.
- Conversely, arguments against aggressive treatment include:
  - The potential for serious or life-threatening adverse drug reactions, particularly in at-risk populations with concurrent cardiac, respiratory, and hemodynamic compromise.
  - The potential for drug–drug interactions in patients with multiple medical problems, who typically receive polypharmacy.
  - Prolonged duration of coma from anesthetic medications used to treat SE which is associated with increased length of stay, morbidity, and mortality (7).

C. Obstacles to cEEG
- The ICU setting is prone to unique sources of EEG artifacts many of which appear rhythmic and can be mistaken for SE.
- EEG monitoring requires considerable expense in terms of equipment, personnel, and EEG review time.
- The availability of equipment and human resources for this service is often limited.
- Appropriate indications for the use of cEEG are needed such that it is neither over-utilized nor underutilized.
- Quantitative EEG is an emerging technology that has the potential to reduce the time demands of EEG review.

- ceEG can also provide evidence of other causes of encephalopathy that may coexist with SE such as extension of a vascular process, vasospasm after subarachnoid hemorrhage, or worsening metabolic disturbance.
- In summary, although there appears to be momentum toward continuous monitoring of neurological function with EEG in the ICU setting analogous to the current standard of continuous monitoring of other vital physiologic functions (8), additional studies are needed to determine whether the equipment and personnel costs are warranted for such a change in approach.

REFERENCES

1. Lowenstein DH, Bleck T, Macdonald RL. It's time to revise the definition of status epilepticus. *Epilepsia.* 1999;40(1):120–122.
2. Wasterlain CG, Chen JW. Definition and classification of status epilepticus. In: CG Wasterlain, DM Treiman, eds. *Status Epilepticus: Mechanisms and Management.* Cambridge, MA: The MIT Press; 2006:11–16.
3. DeLorenzo RJ, Waterhouse EJ, Towne AR, et al. Persistent nonconvulsive status epilepticus after the control of convulsive status epilepticus. *Epilepsia.* 1998;39(8):833–840.
4. Young G. Continuous EEG monitoring in the ICU: Challenges and opportunities. *Can J Neurol Sci.* 2009;36(S2):S89–S91.
5. Claassen J, Hirsch LJ, Emerson RG, et al. Treatment of refractory status epilepticus with pentobarbital, propofol, or midazolam: A systematic review. *Epilepsia.* 2002;43(2):146–153.
6. Friedman D, Claassen J, Hirsch LJ. Continuous electroencephalogram monitoring in the intensive care unit. *Anesth Anal.* 2009;109(2):506–523.
7. Benbadis SR, Chen S, Melo M. What's shaking in the ICU? The differential diagnosis of seizures in the intensive care setting. *Epilepsia.* 2010;51(11):2338–2340.
8. Ponten SC, Ronner HE, Strijers RLM, et al. Feasibility of online seizure detection with continuous EEG monitoring in the intensive care unit. *Seizure.* 2010;19(9):580–586.

ADDITIONAL READING

Hirsch LJ, Brenner RP, eds. *Atlas of EEG in Critical Care.* West Sussex: Wiley-Blackwell; 2010.

SIX

Ischemic Stroke

Wendy L. Wright

KEY POINTS

- Acute stroke is a neurologic emergency and a common cause of death and disability.
- Detection and treatment of secondary complications such as seizures is critical to prevent further neurological injury.
- Continuous EEG monitoring is important for identifying subclinical seizures and guiding seizure management but can also be used to monitor for evolving cerebral ischemia.
- Treatment of seizures in ICU patients is recommended to prevent further neurologic damage, although data are insufficient to support use of antiepileptic drugs for primary prevention of seizures after ischemic stroke.

I. BACKGROUND

A. Epidemiology
- Ischemic stroke is a leading cause of death and disability (1).
- The incidence of ischemic stroke is approximately 795,000/yr in the United States with an estimated cost of $73.7 billion in 2010 and lifetime average direct and indirect cost of $140,048 (1).
- Stroke is the most commonly identified etiology of unprovoked seizures and symptomatic epilepsy in older adults (4).
- Rate of seizures after stroke is between 2% and 4%. The incidence varies widely depending upon which patient population is assessed and whether or not cEEG monitoring is used.

B. Diagnosis
- Need to establish time of symptom onset, as reperfusion therapies such as tissue plasminogen activator (tPA) must be administered within a discrete time frame.
- Neurological exam includes NIH stroke scale (NIHSS) score.

- Basic laboratory studies including glucose measurement, since hypoglycemia can mimic focal cerebral ischemia.
- Electrolyte panel, complete blood count, cardiac enzymes, electrocardiogram, PT/PTT/INR.
- CT scan without contrast (2).
- MRI if needed to evaluate for advanced stroke treatment options, but may delay ability to administer IV tPA (2).

C. Treatment
- Reperfusion strategies
  - Intravenous tissue plasminogen activator (tPA, now approved up to 4.5 hours) and intra-arterial tPA (within 6–8 hours, or longer for selected patients) (2).
  - Endovascular options: angioplasty, stenting, mechanical clot disruption, clot extraction, intra-arterial thrombolysis (2).
- Admission to a comprehensive stroke unit has been shown to lessen the rates of morbidity and mortality after stroke. Observe for deterioration in clinical status that may prompt urgent surgical or medical treatment, especially during the high-risk period of 24 to 48 hours after stroke onset (1).
- Provide treatment to reduce bleeding complications, especially after thrombolytic therapy (1).
- Detect and prevent subacute complications, including seizures (1).
- Initiate long-term therapies for secondary prevention of stroke.
  - Includes either antiplatelet or anticoagulant therapy, as well as aggressive risk factor modification (1).
- Temperature control as increased body temperature worsens outcome after stroke (2).
- Cardiac monitoring and treatment of arrhythmias. Atrial fibrillation is the most common arrhythmia after stroke (2).
- Generally allow permissive hypertension to allow blood flow to ischemic penumbra (tissue with decreased blood flow around infarcted stroke core, at risk of stroke), but treat malignant hypertension to avoid hemorrhagic conversion (2).
- Maintain euglycemia (2).

D. Acute Neurological Complications
- Cerebral edema can be treated with hypertonic saline/osmotic diuretics, drainage of cerebrospinal fluid, decompressive surgery, induced coma, therapeutic hypothermia, or paralytic.
  - Induced coma and paralytic therapy often require cEEG monitoring (2).
- Hemorrhagic transformation
- Seizures
  - Detrimental due to increase in brain metabolic demand, possibility of increasing intracranial pressure and possibility of kindling. Can be particularly damaging because seizures can be difficult to detect without cEEG and often go undiagnosed (2).
- The emphasis in neurocritical care units is to detect these secondary complications in time to prevent ongoing neurologic damage (2).

II. BASICS: SEIZURES AND CEEG AFTER STROKE

A. General Considerations

• Seizures after stroke are likely to be partial, with or without secondary generalization.
• Seizures may occur at the onset of stroke.
  ○ From reduced seizure threshold due to cortical excitation and ischemia.
  ○ From an embolic event with transient ischemia and subsequent reperfusion (2).
• Seizure at stroke onset is no longer an absolute exclusion for tPA.
• Seizures that occur within two weeks of stroke are defined as "early" seizures and seizures that occur after that are defined as "late," based on presumably different pathophysiologies.
  ○ Early seizures may result from acute biochemical dysfunction in sensitive neuronal tissue, leading to electrical irritability.
  ○ Metabolic disturbances such as hyperglycemia at the time of infarct may increase the likelihood of seizures (3).
• Late seizures often occur months after ischemic stroke and are likely due to glial scar tissue that acts as an epileptogenic focus.
• Convulsive status epilepticus (SE) is uncommon (less than 1%) (2,3).

B. Risk Factors for Seizures After Ischemic Stroke

• Patients with strokes in a cortical location have the highest risk of seizures (3).
• Seizures can occur after lacunar stroke, which may be a reflection of cortical dysfunction after lacunar infarction (3).
• Stroke severity is an independent risk factor for the development of seizures, but this association may correlate with cortical location (3).
• Younger age, a history of diabetes mellitus, acute infection, and history of TIA have been identified as independent predictors of poststroke seizure (4).
• Cardiogenic embolism is not a clear risk factor for seizure.
• Early postischemic stroke seizures can be an independent risk factor for recurrent and late seizures (3).
• Risk of late seizures is higher in patients with preexisting dementia (2).

C. Impact of Seizures After Stroke

• Stroke severity is the most important determinant in clinical outcome after stroke (3).
• Studies are conflicting, but it is likely that early postischemic seizures are associated with higher mortality, increased length of stay, and greater disability at discharge.
• Early-onset SE is associated with a higher risk of recurrent SE and higher mortality (5).
• Animal data suggest that recurrent seizures may increase infarct size and can impair functional recovery.
• Impact of late-onset seizures is less clear.
• In critically ill patients, seizures can cause secondary neuronal injury by increasing brain metabolic demand in already vulnerable ischemic tissue.

D. Treatment

- There is insufficient evidence to support the use of antiepileptic drugs (AEDs) for primary or secondary prevention of early or late seizures after ischemic stroke.
- However, early seizures after stroke are usually treated due to the unstable neurologic condition of the patients that trigger the ictal event.
- Therefore, most critically ill patients are treated for seizures, even after the first event.
- Late-onset seizures are often treated as well because the glial scar that acts as a seizure focus is likely to cause seizure recurrence.
- Choice of AED should be individualized to the patient.
  - In the ICU, levetiracetam is often considered due to intravenous preparation, favorable side-effect profile, lack of drug interactions, no active metabolites, and minimal effects on cognition.
- Studies are conflicting in that some data suggest that AEDs such as phenytoin, phenobarbital, and benzodiazepines may delay the recovery process after stroke, whereas other studies show that some AEDs have potential as neuroprotectants in hyperacute stroke including phenytoin, benzodiazepines, lamotrigine, topiramate, levetiracetam, and zonisamide (3).
- It is unclear if the use of AEDs impact outcomes in patients with stroke (3).

III. FURTHER CONSIDERATIONS/REMAINING QUESTIONS

A. Early detection and intervention for secondary neuronal damage is a cornerstone of management in neurocritical care units, therefore, using cEEG to detect evolving or worsening cerebral ischemia may be desirable.

- This is particularly important during the highest risk period of 24 to 48 hours within onset of ischemic stroke or transient ischemic attack.
- cEEG could also be used to provide dynamic real-time detection of ongoing ischemic injury.
- Although EEG is a sensitive diagnostic tool for the detection of ischemia, it would be more widely applicable if automated detection systems were available.
- cEEG is not currently used routinely for detection of evolving ischemia in patients with ischemic stroke (5).

B. cEEG Use for Seizure Detection After Ischemic Stroke

- Patients in the ICU with stroke are at risk of subclinical seizures particularly if they are intubated, sedated, or otherwise impaired in a way that limits detection of fluctuating neurologic exam that would alert the health care provider to the presence of seizures.
- Patients with stroke can have lateralized periodic discharges (LPDs) and other EEG findings on the ictal–interictal continuum that put them at risk for developing seizures.
  - Patients with potentially ictal discharges should remain on cEEG monitoring and the clinician should be aware that these patients are at high risk of clinical decline, especially if metabolic and infectious derangements develop.
- It is still unclear whether cEEG monitoring improves outcomes in stroke patients, but awareness of EEG abnormalities is likely beneficial.

- Stroke patients in the ICU who are candidates for cEEG monitoring should include those with:
  - Fluctuating neurologic deficits.
  - Unexplained coma or altered levels of consciousness.
  - Malignant increased intracranial pressure requiring induced coma or paralytics.
  - Treatment modalities that preclude reliable neurologic examination such as paralytics for respiratory indications.
  - Unexplained "spells" such as variations in vital signs or twitching.
  - Seizures or status epilepticus that require active adjustment of therapy.

C. Unanswered Treatment Questions

- There is insufficient evidence to support the use of AEDs for primary or secondary prevention of seizures after stroke.
- It is unclear whether the side effects of some AEDs outweigh the risks of seizures, or whether some AEDs actually worsen outcome after stroke.

REFERENCES

1. Goldstein LB, Bushnell CD, Adams RJ, et al. On behalf of the American Heart Association Stroke Council, Council on Cardiovascular Nursing, Council on Epidemiology and Prevention, Council for High Blood Pressure Research, Council on Peripheral Vascular Disease, and Interdisciplinary Council on Quality Care and Outcomes Research. Guidelines for the primary prevention of stroke: Guideline for healthcare professionals from the American Heart Association/American Stroke Association. *Stroke.* 2011;42:571–584.
2. Adams HP, Zoppo G, Alberts MJ, et al. Guidelines for the early management of ischemic stroke: A guideline from the American Heart Association/American Stroke Association Stroke Council, Clinical Cardiology Council, Cardiovascular Radiology and Interventional Council, and the Atherosclerotic Peripheral Vascular Disease and Quality of Care Outcomes in Research Interdisciplinary Working Groups. *Stroke.* 2007;38:1665–1711.
3. Camilo O, Goldstein LB. Seizures and epilepsy after ischemic stroke. *Stroke* 2004;35:1769–1775.
4. Krakow K, Sitzer M, Rosenow F, et al. Predictors of acute poststroke seizures. *Cerebrovasc Dis.* 2010;30:584–589.
5. Mercarelli O, Pro S, Randi F, Dispenza S, et al. EEG patterns and epileptic seizures in acute phase stroke. *Cerebrovasc Dis.* 2011;31:191–198.

ADDITIONAL READING

Freeman WD, Dawson SB, Flemming KD. The ABCs of stroke complications. *Semin Neurol.* 2010;30:501–510.
Vespa P. Continuous EEG monitoring for the detection of seizures in traumatic brain injury, infarction, and intracerebral hemorrhage: to detect and protect. *J Clin Neurophysiol.* 2005;22:99–106.

SEVEN

Subarachnoid Hemorrhage

Adam Webb

KEY POINTS

- Although subarachnoid hemorrhage (SAH) accounts for only 3% of all strokes, it results in 27% of stroke-related years of potential life lost before age 65.
- Continuous EEG (cEEG) is necessary for detecting nonconvulsive seizures (NCS), which are common in patients with SAH and often associated with nonconvulsive status epilepticus (NCSE).
- cEEG is a potentially valuable tool for detecting cerebral vasospasm and delayed cerebral ischemia (DCI).
- Periodic epileptiform discharges, NCSE, nonreactive background, and the absence of normal sleep architecture are independent predictors of poor outcome in patients with SAH.

I. BACKGROUND

A. Epidemiology

- The incidence of aneurysmal subarachnoid hemorrhage (aSAH) ranges from 2 to 21 per 100,000 persons.
- aSAH accounts for only 3% of all strokes but 27% of stroke-related years of potential life lost before age 65 (1).
- Risk factors include hypertension, smoking, family history, and cocaine use.

B. Intracranial Aneurysms

- Rupture of intracranial aneurysms accounts for approximately 80% of nontraumatic SAH.
- Intracranial aneurysms are acquired lesions that develop predominantly at branching points of the anterior cerebral circulation (Circle of Willis).
- Ruptured and unruptured aneurysms may be treated either by endovascular coiling or by craniotomy with surgical clipping.

C. Clinical Features
- The classic presentation of aSAH is the acute onset of severe headache which may be accompanied by seizure, loss of consciousness, or vomiting.
- Focal neurological deficits, especially cranial nerve palsies, may be associated with certain aneurysm locations, elevation of intracranial pressure (ICP), focal parenchymal hemorrhage, or ischemic infarction.

D. Diagnosis
- Noncontrast head CT is rapid, widely available and has a reported sensitivity of 90% to 100% for detection of SAH.
- MRI or lumbar puncture may be useful in patients with a high clinical suspicion for SAH and equivocal findings on head CT.
- After diagnosis of SAH, CT angiography and catheter angiography are used to evaluate for intracranial aneurysms.

E. Grading Scales
- The Hunt & Hess (Table 7.1) and World Federation of Neurological Surgeons (Table 7.2) grading scales are based upon features of clinical presentation and are predictors of prognosis.
- The modified Fisher grading score (Table 7.3) (2) is a radiographic scoring system based upon the amount and distribution of subarachnoid as well as intraventricular hemorrhage and helps stratify the risk of cerebral vasospasm and delayed cerebral infarction.

TABLE 7.1   Hunt & Hess Grading Scale

GRADE	DESCRIPTION
I	Asymptomatic or mild headache
II	Moderate-to-severe headache, nuchal rigidity, no focal deficit other than cranial nerve palsy
III	Confusion, lethargy, or mild focal deficits other than cranial nerve palsy
IV	Stupor or moderate-to-severe hemiparesis
V	Coma, extensor posturing, moribund appearance

TABLE 7.2   World Federation of Neurosurgeons Scale

GRADE	DESCRIPTION
I	GCS sum score 15 without hemiparesis
II	GCS sum score 13–14 without hemiparesis
III	GCS sum score 13–14 with hemiparesis
IV	GCS sum score 7–12 with or without hemiparesis
V	GCS sum score 3–6 with or without hemiparesis

GCS = Glasgow Coma Score.

TABLE 7.3   Modified Fisher Scale (2)

GRADE	DESCRIPTION	% DCI
0	No SAH or IVH	0
1	Minimal/thin SAH, no IVH in both lateral ventricles	12
2	Minimal/thin SAH, with IVH in both lateral ventricles	21
3	Thick SAH, no IVH in both lateral ventricles	19
4	Thick SAH, with IVH in both lateral ventricles	40

IVH = Intraventricular hemorrhage.
DCI = Delayed cerebral ischemia.

F. Cerebral Vasospasm and DCI

- Approximately 60% of aSAH patients have radiographic vasospasm identified by transcranial Doppler or angiography, although only about 30% develop symptoms of cerebral ischemia.
- Of those patients who survive to definitive treatment of a ruptured aneurysm, cerebral vasospasm and DCI are the major contributors to morbidity and mortality.
- The risk of cerebral vasospasm increases between day 3 and day 7 post-hemorrhage while the peak risk of DCI is between days 5 and 14.
- Risk factors for development of vasospasm and DCI include younger age, poor neurological grade, thick subarachnoid clot, intraventricular hemorrhage, and history of smoking.
- Initial detection of vasospasm and DCI relies primarily on the clinical neurological examination and periodic serial transcranial Doppler measurements of mean cerebral blood flow velocity. CT angiography/CT perfusion and MRI/MRA may aid in the confirmation of vasospasm, but the gold standard is catheter angiography.
- Standard detection techniques are performed on an intermittent basis, at most, occurring once per day. Therefore, real-time detection and intervention is not possible using standard vasospasm detection methods.
- Prophylactic use of nimodipine 60 mg every 4 hours has been shown to reduce the risk of poor neurological outcome from DCI.
- First-line treatments for symptomatic vasospasm are noninvasive and includes volume repletion/expansion and induced hypertension.
- Endovascular management of cerebral vasospasm includes balloon angioplasty and intra-arterial vasodilator (verapamil, nicardipine) administration.

G. Seizures

- The incidence of clinical seizures at any point after SAH ranges from 4% to 21% (3,4,5).
- An estimated 7% to 8% of patients have clinical seizures at the onset of bleeding, although precise measurements are hard to obtain because other abnormal movements such as posturing from elevated ICP can mimic a seizure (5).
- 5% to 11% of patients experience clinical seizures at some time during their hospital course and 7% of patients develop chronic epilepsy (6). Isolated seizures

during the hospital course and the development of epilepsy are associated with poor neurological outcomes.
- The utility of prophylactic antiepileptic drugs (AEDs) for patients with aSAH have not been well established (4). Phenytoin exposure has been shown to be associated with worse neurological and cognitive outcomes (7). However, newer AEDs may have fewer side effects.
- Routine AEDs can be considered in the immediate post-hemorrhage period, but long-term use is not recommended unless patients have experienced seizures (8).

II. BASICS

A. cEEG for the Detection of DCI
- cEEG has great potential as a monitoring modality for detecting DCI secondary to cerebral vasospasm as it is both continuous and noninvasive.
- Because cerebral ischemia often results in very subtle changes in EEG background, quantitative EEG analysis (QEEG) can increase the sensitivity of EEG for detection of ischemia.
- Total power and relative alpha variability are two quantitative parameters that have been associated with the detection of cerebral vasospasm and DCI in awake patients with low Hunt & Hess-grade SAH (9,10).
- A reduction in post-stimulation alpha/delta power ratio has been associated with the development of DCI in Hunt & Hess-grade IV and V patients (stuporous or comatose) (11).
- More recently, another study looking at QEEG parameters of relative alpha power and variability predicted clinical deterioration in patients with SAH one day before the clinical changes occurred. Predictions based on QEEG plus clinical data were more accurate than those based on clinical data alone (12).
- In addition, QEEG of intracortical EEG looking at changes in alpha/delta ratio has shown promise in detecting vasospasm in poor-grade SAH patients and was superior to QEEG of surface recordings (13).

B. cEEG for the Detection of Seizures Following aSAH
- The true frequency of nonconvulsive seizures (NCS) after aSAH is unknown as cEEG is required to detect NCS.
- A majority of aSAH patients with NCS also experience nonconvulsive status epilepticus (NCSE) (14).
- NCSE may contribute to encephalopathy and coma in aSAH patients and is associated with high morbidity and mortality.
- NCSE may be present in 8% to 31% of patients with persistent coma or unexplained neurological deterioration following aSAH (15).

C. cEEG and Prognosis Following aSAH
- The presence of periodic discharges or NCSE, as well as the absence of normal sleep architecture and reactivity, have been independently associated with poor neurological outcomes defined as Modified Rankin Scale greater than 4 (16).

III. FURTHER CONSIDERATIONS/REMAINING QUESTIONS

A. Detection of DCI
- Comparative studies are needed to identify QEEG parameters that are the most sensitive to the initial onset of cerebral ischemia.
- The ability to differentiate QEEG changes that represent ischemia from other common clinical changes such as elevations in intracranial pressure, increases in sedative medications and other metabolic abnormalities is equally important although may not be feasible.
- Ideally, QEEG for the detection of cerebral ischemia would have high enough sensitivity and specificity to enable an "alarm" that would prompt additional diagnostic studies (CTA, MRI/MRA, angiography) to confirm cerebral vasospasm and allow for more timely initiation or escalation of treatment.

B. Current limitations to widespread application of cEEG include technician availability to maintain monitoring over long periods of time and the need for 24/7 real-time EEG review from physicians with experience in cEEG interpretation.

C. Proposed Recommendations for Use of cEEG After aSAH
- Patients with persistent coma or unexplained neurological deterioration following aSAH should have cEEG in order to detect nonconvulsive seizures and NCSE.
- Patients with history of a prior witnessed clinical seizure are at high risk for subsequent subclinical seizures and should undergo cEEG as well.
- The use of cEEG for the detection of DCI may be applied in centers with significant ICU EEG experience and a high volume of aSAH patients as a compliment to the clinical neurological exam, TCD, and radiographic evaluations.
- The duration of cEEG monitoring after aSAH is dependent upon the indication for monitoring. A minimum of 24 to 48 hours of monitoring is required in order to detect nonconvulsive seizures while more prolonged monitoring over several days or weeks is needed to monitor for DCI.

REFERENCES

1. Johnston SC, Selvin S, Gress DR. The burden, trends, demographics of mortality from subarachnoid hemorrhage. *Neurology.* 1998;50:1413–1418.
2. Claassen J, Bernardini GL, Kreiter K, et al. Effect of cisternal and ventricular blood on risk of delayed cerebral ischemia after subarachnoid hemorrhage: The Fisher scale revisited. *Stroke.* 2001;32:2012–2020.
3. Butzkueven H, Evans AH, Pitman A, et al. Onset seizures independently predict poor outcome after subarachnoid hemorrhage. *Neurology.* 2000;55:1315–1320.
4. Rhoney DH, Tipps LB, Murry KR, et al. Anticonvulsant prophylaxis and timing of seizures after aneurysmal subarachnoid hemorrhage. *Neurology.* 2000;55:258–265.
5. Lin CL, Dumont AS, Lieu AS, et al. Characterization of perioperative seizures and epilepsy following aneurysmal subarachnoid hemorrhage. *J Neurosurg.* 2003;99:978–985.
6. Claassen J, Peery S, Kreiter KT, et al. Predictors and clinical impact of epilepsy after subarachnoid hemorrhage. *Neurology.* 2003;60:208–214.
7. Naidech AM, Kreiter KT, Janjua N, et al. Phenytoin exposure is associated with functional and cognitive disability after subarachnoid hemorrhage. *Stroke.* 2005;36:583–587.

8. Bederson JB, Connolly ES, Batjer HH, et al. Guidelines for the management of aneurysmal subarachnoid hemorrhage. A statement for healthcare professionals from a special writing group of the Stroke Council, American Heart Association. *Stroke.* 2009;40:994–1025.

9. Labar DR, Fisch BJ, Pedley TA, et al. Quantitative EEG monitoring for patients with subarachnoid hemorrhage. *Electroencephalogr Clin Neurophysiol.* 1991;78:325–332.

10. Vespa PM, Nuwer MR, Juhász C, et al. Early detection of vasospasm after acute subarachnoid hemorrhage using continuous EEG ICU monitoring. *Electroencephalogr Clin Neurophysiol.* 1997;103:607–615.

11. Claassen J, Hirsch LJ, Kreiter KT, et al. Quantitative continuous EEG for detecting delayed cerebral ischemia in patients with poor-grade subarachnoid hemorrhage. *Clin Neurophysiol.* 2004;115:2699–2710.

12. Rathakrishnan R, Gotman J, Dubeau F, Angle M. Using continuous electroencephalography in the management of delayed cerebral ischemia following subarachnoid hemorrhage. *Neurocrit Care.* 2011;14:152–161.

13. Stuart RM, Waziri A, Weintraub D, et al. Intracortical EEG for the detection of vasospasm in patients with poor-grade subarachnoid hemorrhage. *Neurocrit Care.* 2010;13:355–358.

14. Claassen J, Mayer SA, Kowalski RG, et al. Detection of electrographic seizures with continuous EEG monitoring in critically ill patients. *Neurology.* 2004;62:1743–1748.

15. Dennis LJ, Claassen J, Hirsch LJ, et al. Nonconvulsive status epilepticus after subarachnoid hemorrhage. *Neurosurgery.* 2002;51:1136–1144.

16. Claassen J, Hirsch LJ, Frontera JA, et al. Prognostic significance of continuous EEG monitoring in patients with poor-grade subarachnoid hemorrhage. *Neurocrit Care.* 2006;4:103–112.

ADDITIONAL READING

Claassen J, Mayer SA, Hirsch LJ. Continuous EEG monitoring in patients with subarachnoid hemorrhage. *J Clin Neurophysiol.* 2005;22:92–98.

Bederson JB, Connolly ES, Batjer HH, et al. Guidelines for the management of aneurysmal subarachnoid hemorrhage. A statement for healthcare professionals from a special writing group of the Stroke Council, American Heart Association. *Stroke.* 2009;40:994–1025.

EIGHT

Intracranial Hemorrhage

Rhonda Cadena and Lori Shutter

KEY POINTS

- In patients with intracranial hemorrhage (ICH) early neurological deterioration is associated with poor outcome.
- Seizures have been reported in up to 28% of patients undergoing continuous EEG monitoring (cEEG) following ICH.
- Periodic discharges (PDs) on cEEG have been associated with worse outcome following ICH.
- Any patient with ICH and suspected seizures or abnormal or fluctuating mental status should undergo cEEG.

I. BACKGROUND

A. Epidemiology

- Only 10% of all strokes are due to ICH, but ICH carries a high mortality (almost 40%).
- Risk factors for mortality include advanced age, size, and location of ICH, poor Glasgow coma score at presentation, and presence of accompanying intraventricular hemorrhage (1) (Tables 8.1 and 8.2).
- Several primary and secondary causes of ICH have been identified (Table 8.3).
- Early neurological deterioration after ICH is associated with poor outcome due to hematoma expansion, intraventricular bleeding, elevated blood pressure, and/or local inflammatory changes. Systemic processes (eg, hypotension, fever, hypoxia) also contribute to clinical worsening.

B. ICH Management (2)

- Prevention of hematoma expansion and secondary brain injury.
  - Hematoma expansion is seen in up to 38% of patients, usually within the first hour (3), and is predictive of clinical deterioration as well as increased morbidity and mortality (4).

TABLE 8.1   ICH Score

FACTOR		POINTS
Presenting GCS	3–4	2
	5–12	1
	13–15	0
ICH Volume	≥30 mL	1
	≤30 mL	0
IVH	Yes	1
	No	0
Infratentorial	Yes	1
	No	0
Age	≥80 y	1
	<80 y	0

GCS, Glasgow coma scale; IVH, intraventricular hemorrhage.

TABLE 8.2   Probability of 30-day Mortality Based on
ICH Score

ICH SCORE	30-DAY MORTALITY
0	0
1	13%
2	26%
3	72%
4	97%
5–6	100%

Hemphill CJ, Bonovich DC, Besmertis L, Manley GT, Johnston SC.
The ICH score: A simple, reliable grading scale for intracerebral
hemorrhage. *Stroke*. 2001;32:891–897.

TABLE 8.3   Causes of ICH

PRIMARY	SECONDARY
Hypertension	AVM
Cerebral amyloid angiopathy	Vasculitis
Hemorrhagic diatheses	Drug use (cocaine, alcohol)
	Intracranial neoplasm
	Cerebral venous thrombosis

- Rapid reversal of coagulopathy
  - The current recommendation for patients on oral anticoagulants is the administration of vitamin K and fresh frozen plasma (FFP).
  - Prothrombin complex concentrates (PCCs) are also emerging as a potential treatment, although their impact on outcome is unclear.
  - Recombinant factor VIIa (rfVIIa) increases the risk of thrombotic complications and has not shown a clear benefit in patients with ICH, so current guidelines do not support its use in ICH.
- Blood pressure (BP) management
  - The exact BP target that improves outcomes is not known, but studies have shown that acute lowering of the systolic blood pressure (SBP) to 140 mmHg is probably safe (5).
  - Current guidelines suggest lowering SBP greater than 180 mmHg to a target MAP of 110 mmHg or a SBP of 160 mmHg.
- Maintain euglycemia
  - High blood glucose on admission predicts an increased risk of mortality and poor outcome in patients with ICH (6); however, hypoglycemia can be harmful as well.
  - Until specific serum glucose targets are better characterized, hyperglycemia should be treated and hypoglycemia should be avoided.
- Use of antiepileptic medications (AEDs) in patients with clinical seizures
  - Seizures have been seen in a high percentage of patients with ICH (7–9) despite the use of prophylactic AEDs at therapeutic levels (7,9).
  - A recent study demonstrated worse outcomes in ICH patients without evidence of seizures who received prophylactic phenytoin (10).
  - Prophylactic AEDs are not routinely recommended in the absence of documented seizures. The use of newer AEDs has not been assessed in controlled trials.

II. BASICS

A. Incidence of Seizures in ICH
- Early seizures are up to 4 times as common in ICH as in ischemic strokes. Earlier studies showed clinical seizures in 15.4% of patients with ICH compared to only 6.5% of patients presenting with ischemic stroke (11).
- More recent studies of patients with ICH undergoing cEEG have reported a much higher incidence of seizures: nearly 28% of patients with ICH, versus 6% of patients with ischemic stroke (7). Other studies of patients with ICH undergoing cEEG have shown seizure incidences as high as 31% (9).
- The site of the ICH appears to influence the risk of seizures. The highest incidence of seizures has been seen in hemorrhages with cortical involvement, but seizures have also been reported in up to 31% of patients with subcortical hemorrhages (7–9).
- Most seizures are detected on cEEG within the first few days of monitoring. One study captured up to 89% of seizures within the first 72 hours (7). However, a

recent study monitored all patients presenting with ICH for an average of 3 days and detected 94% of seizures in the first 48 hours of EEG monitoring (9).

- Determining which patients require monitoring is difficult because nonconvulsive seizures (NCS) can present with a wide array of clinical symptoms. In one series of patients with NCS and no history of obvious motor convulsions, the majority was unresponsive to commands (7) or had unexplained or fluctuating mental status without any known cause (9).

B. EEG Abnormalities Associated With ICH (Table 8.4) (9)

- In addition to NCS and nonconvulsive status epilepticus (NCSE), periodic discharges (PDs), frontal intermittent rhythmic delta activity (FIRDA), and burst suppression have been documented.
- PDs are seen more frequently in hemorrhages greater than 60 mL and near the cortex but, after controlling for demographics and clinical factors, only hemorrhages located within 1 mm of the cortex were independently associated with PDs.

C. Impact of Seizures on Outcome in Patients With ICH

- The impact of seizures on outcome in patients with ICH is unclear.
- Patients with NCS after ICH have been shown to incur further neurological deterioration as measured by worsening NIH Stroke Scale (NIHSS). However, the trend toward poorer outcome for ICH patients with NCS was not significantly greater than for patients without NCS (7).
- Changes on neuroimaging have been seen in ICH patients with NCS, including increased cerebral edema and increased midline shift (7). The relevance of this to patient outcome is still unclear, and it is unknown whether these changes are caused by seizures or whether the neuroimaging changes themself lead to seizure development.
- The impact of seizures on hematoma expansion also is unclear. An increase in hematoma volume has been seen in some patients who experience early seizures after ICH; however, no independent association between seizures and hematoma expansion was shown when other clinical variables were controlled (9). Other

TABLE 8.4   Specific EEG Abnormalities in Patients With ICH

EEG ABNORMALITY	% OF PTS WITH ICH
Periodic discharges (PDs) • Lateralized periodic discharges (LPDs) • Generalized periodic discharges (GPDS) • Bilateral independent periodic discharges (BIPDs)	17% 13% 6% 1%
Focal epileptiform discharges	15%
Frontal intermittent rhythmic delta activity (FIRDA)	9%
Burst suppression	9%
Nonconvulsive status epilepticus (NCSE)	7%

Data based on results from Claassen et al. *Neuro.* 2007;69:1356–1365.

observations have shown only a weak tendency toward increased hemorrhage volume following seizures (7).

* Although a trend toward increased mortality has been reported in patients who experience seizures after ICH, no statistical difference has been shown (7,8). However, certain EEG abnormalities do appear linked to poor outcomes.
  ○ A recent study demonstrated that although poor outcome was not different between patients with and without seizures, patients with any periodic discharges (PDs), lateralized periodic discharges (LPDS), or stimulus-induced rhythmic, periodic, or ictal discharges (SIRPIDs), did experience a worse outcome (9). These EEG findings remained independently associated with poor outcome (defined as a Glasgow Outcome Scale of 1–2) after controlling for several clinical variables.

D. Recommendations for cEEG in Patients With ICH
* Any patient with suspected seizure
* Abnormal or fluctuating mental status
* Duration of up to 72 hours

III. FURTHER CONSIDERATIONS/REMAINING QUESTIONS

A. Do prophylactic AEDs modify the risk of early seizures?
* Because the use of AEDs may be harmful (10), it is important to asses benefit versus risk to allow for appropriate patient selection.
* In one study in which all patients with ICH received prophylactic AEDs, the incidence of seizures was 28% (9). A second study documented NCS in 19% of patients on AEDs versus 14% of patients not taking AEDs (9).
* Prophylactic AEDs have demonstrated a decrease in seizures in patients with lobar ICH, but not in patients with ICH in any other location (8).

B. Does the presence of seizures affect outcome?
* A cause and effect relationship between seizures and ICH has not been demonstrated. It is currently not known whether seizures lead to worsening of ICH and thereby worsen outcome, or if worsening of ICH leads to development of seizures.
* Previous studies have shown that seizures can be associated with acute worsening of neurological status and poor outcomes, but the impact of seizures on long-term outcome still needs to be determined.

REFERENCES

1. Hemphill CJ, Bonovich DC, Besmertis L, Manley GT, et al. The ICH score: A simple, reliable grading scale for intracerebral hemorrhage. *Stroke*. 2001;32:891–897.
2. Morgenstern LB, Hemphill JC, Anderson C, et al. Guidelines for the management of spontaneous intracerebral hemorrhage. A guideline for healthcare professionals from the American Heart Association/American Stroke Association. *Stroke*. 2010;41:1–22.
3. Brott T, Broderick J, Rashmi K, et al. Early hemorrhage growth in patients with intracerebral hemorrhage. *Stroke*. 1997;28(1):1–5.

4. Davis SM, Borderick J, Hennerici M, et al. Hematoma growth is a determinant of mortality and poor outcome after intracerebral hemorrhage. *Neurology.* 2006;66:1175–1181.
5. Anderson CS, Huang Y, Wang JG, et al. INTERACT investigators. Intensive blood pressure reduction in acute cerebral haemorrhage trial (INTERACT): A randomised pilot trial. *Lancet Neurol.* 2008;7(5):391–399.
6. Passero S, Ciacci G, Ulivelli M. The influence of diabetes and hyperglycemia on clinical course after intracerebral hemorrhage. *Neuro.* 2003;61:1351–1356.
7. Vespa PM, O'Phelan K, Shah M, et al. Acute seizures after intracerebral hemorrhage. A factor in progressive midline shift and outcome. *Neurology.* 2003;60:1441–1446.
8. Passero S, Rocchi R, Rossi S, et al. Seizures after spontaneous supratentorial intracerebral hemorrhage. *Epilepsia.* 2002;43(10):1175–1180.
9. Claassen J, Jette N, Chum F, et al. Electrographic seizures and periodic discharges after intracerebral hemorrhage. *Neurology.* 2007;69:1356–1365.
10. Messe SR, Sansing LH, Cucchiara BL, et al. Prophylactic antiepileptic drug use is associated with poor outcome following ICH. *Neurocrit Care.* 2009;11:38–44.
11. Kilpatrick CJ, Davis SM, Tress BM, et al. Epileptic seizures in acute stroke. *Arch Neurol.* 1990;47:157–160.

ADDITIONAL READING

Varelas PN, ed. *Current Clinical Neurology: Seizures in Critical Care: A Guide to Diagnosis and Therapeutics.* New Jersey: Humana Press Inc, 2005.

NINE

Encephalitis and Other CNS Infections

Sebastian W. Pollandt and Jerzy P. Szaflarski

KEY POINTS

- Encephalitis is associated with both focal and global neurological dysfunction (eg, focal neurological deficits, seizures, and altered mental status).
- The incidence of nonoutbreak cases of encephalitis is estimated to be 0.07 to 12.6 cases per 100,000. Of the identified causes, 2/3 are infectious and the rest are caused by an immune-mediated process (1).
- The diagnosis of encephalitis is rarely based solely on clinical presentation. However, in some cases, the discrete clinical profile may help focus the diagnostic evaluation (2).
- Symptoms of encephalitis vary depending on the severity of the disease. Most mild cases present with fever, headache, and malaise, whereas severe cases usually present with altered mental status or coma, focal neurological signs and seizures including status epilepticus.
- The majority of seizures in patients with encephalitis have no clinical correlate and can only be detected using continuous EEG monitoring (cEEG).

I. BACKGROUND

- Encephalitis is a common cause of seizures in the intensive care unit (ICU). Patients with CNS infections and seizures have worse outcome compared to patients with CNS infections without seizures (3–5).
- Increased brain metabolism, increased intracranial pressure (ICP), and prolonged ICU stays are all complications seen in association with seizures in patients with CNS infections. Therefore, it is prudent to have a high index of suspicion for seizures in ICU patients presenting with symptoms suggestive of meningitis or encephalitis.

- However, it remains unclear if seizures by themselves contribute to morbidity and mortality in patients with encephalitis, or if they are simply a marker of severity of the underlying disease and neuronal injury especially given that patients with encephalitis and seizures are more likely to experience focal neurological deficits compared to patients without seizures (6).

II. BASICS

A. Infectious Causes of Encephalitis

- Types of CNS infections include meningitis, encephalitis, ventriculitis, and abscess.
- The most commonly encountered CNS infections are due to viral or bacterial organisms and less often fungal or parasitic etiologies.
- CNS infections after neurosurgical procedures are common and usually related to staphylococci, Gram-negative bacilli, and *Streptococcus pneumoniae*.
- One study in California of 334 cases of encephalitis between 1998 and 2000 identified the following etiologies: 9% viral, 3% bacterial, 1% parasitic, and 10% noninfectious. In an additional 12%, an infectious cause was suspected but not confirmed. Despite extensive testing, the etiology of encephalitis in 62% of cases remained unexplained (7).
- In a more recent prospective study using advanced testing methods, 42% (86/203) of encephalitis cases were caused by infectious agents, 21% (42/203) by acute immune-mediated process, and in 37% (75/203) the etiology was not identified (8).
- Enteroviruses are responsible for the majority of viral CNS infections. Less common causes are mumps, arboviruses, herpesviruses, HIV, and lymphocytic choriomeningitis virus. Outside the United States, Japanese encephalitis is the most common CNS infection.
- Recently, other etiologies of infectious encephalitis have been reported including West Nile virus, avian influenza, H1N1, rotavirus, Lyssavirus, and Niaph virus (8–10).
- Availability of more specific tests including DNA assays, has led to the development of improved laboratory evaluation of patients with suspected encephalitis (2,8,11). This has increased the diagnostic yield of serum and cerebrospinal fluid (CSF) analysis from 38% up to 63% (7,8).

B. Noninfectious Causes of Encephalitis

- Noninfectious etiologies include post-infectious as well as autoimmune-mediated or paraneoplastic causes. These etiologies have been reported to be responsible for 21% of encephalitis cases in an English cohort (8).
- Of the noninfectious causes of encephalitis, autoimmune disease, and/or vasculitis is identified in 43% of cases, 27% cases are neoplastic, 6% metabolic, and 25% are related to other disorders (2).
- The predominance of inflammation and/or demyelination along with the absence of a causative organism are the most salient features distinguishing cases of noninfectious encephalitis.

- Post-infectious encephalitis such as acute disseminated encephalomyelitis (ADEM) and acute hemorrhagic leukoencephalitis (AHLE) or autoimmune encephalitis frequently present with seizures or status epilepticus (4,12,13).
  - ADEM has been described following a variety of relatively minor microbial infections or vaccinations. It is primarily a pediatric disease with a reported incidence in children of 0.4/100,000/year (13). There is little data regarding the worldwide distribution of pediatric ADEM as well as the incidence in adult populations, even though numerous case series have been reported (4,14).
  - AHLE is a rare hemorrhagic variant of ADEM with a fulminant clinical course and a high mortality.
- Autoimmune/paraneoplastic encephalitis represents a heterogeneous group of clinical entities that include Hashimoto's and Rasmussen's encephalitis and lupus.
- More recently, anti-*N*-methyl-D-aspartic acid (NMDA) receptor antibody-mediated (12) and anti-voltage-gated potassium channel (VGKC) receptor antibody-mediated (15) encephalitis have been described. The incidence of anti-NMDA and anti-VGKC antibody-mediated encephalitis is felt to be increasing, which may be due in part to increased recognition of these clinical syndromes.

C. Clinical Features

- Infection may enter the brain directly or indirectly via:
  - Contiguous spread from para-nasal sinuses, mastoid processes, teeth, skull (osteomyelitis), or through retrograde venous infection.
  - Open skull trauma or surgical intervention.
  - Hematogenous spread from a distant focus such as infectious endocarditis, lung infections, empyema, or intravenous drug use.
- Symptoms of encephalitis usually include:
  - Fever
  - Headache with or without nuchal rigidity and with or without papilledema
  - Nausea/vomiting
  - Irritability, moodiness, impaired judgment, hallucinations, and other psychiatric symptoms
  - Mental status changes including confusion, lethargy, or coma
  - Focal neurological signs including focal dyskinesias
  - Seizures/status epilepticus

D. EEG and Seizures in Patients With Encephalitis

- The literature on cEEG in ICU populations has demonstrated conclusively that EEG monitoring increases the detection rate of seizures dramatically. One of the first large studies of cEEG in the ICU setting detected seizures or status epilepticus in approximately 35% to 40% of all ICU patients (16).
- In critically ill patients, 88% of seizures are detected within the first 24 hours of cEEG monitoring and an additional 5% in the next 24 hours of monitoring. Seizures are more frequently detected in the first 24 hours of monitoring in patients who are non-comatose compared to patients who are comatose (17).
- A retrospective review study of 42 patients with confirmed CNS infection reported that seizures occurred in 33% of patients. The majority of seizures were seen on EEG only, without any clinical correlate (3).

- In a Dutch Meningitis Cohort Study, seizures occurred in 17% of patients with community-acquired bacterial meningitis confirmed by CSF analysis (18). In that study, death rates were significantly higher in patients with seizures compared to patients without seizures (41% versus 16%; $P < .001$). Further analyses revealed that CSF white count below 1,000 cells/mm^3, higher protein level, higher erythrocyte sedimentation rate, infection with *S. pneumoniae*, focal cerebral abnormalities, and low Glasgow Coma Scale (GCS) were all associated with seizures (18).
- Another study examined acute symptomatic seizures in patients with encephalitis, or bacterial, fungal, or tuberculous meningitis (viral meningitis was excluded) (6). The majority of seizures were secondarily generalized tonic–clonic seizures. Twenty-three percent of patients presented with a seizure during the acute phase of the infection. Of note, acute symptomatic seizures were found in 73% of encephalitis cases, but only 17% of meningitis cases.
- In a 12-year retrospective study of 117 patients with community-acquired bacterial meningitis, 27% of patients were found to have seizures during the course of their illness with 80% of seizures occurring within 24 hours of presentation (5). Approximately, one-third of patients with seizures progressed to status epilepticus. None of the patients without seizures during hospitalization developed epilepsy during follow-up (5).
- Whitley et al. showed that in patients with laboratory-confirmed herpes simplex virus (HSV) encephalitis, seizures occurred in 67% of patients (73/109) (19). Even higher rates of seizures were reported in cases of anti-NMDA-R encephalitis (76%) (12).
- Finally, Claassen et al., found that continuous EEG monitoring detected seizures in 29% of patients with CNS infections; the majority of which were nonconvulsive (17).

E. EEG Characteristics
- Studies evaluating EEG findings in CNS infections are scarce with the majority of them reporting only the incidence of seizures (clinical and/or electrographic).
- A variety of EEG patterns are frequently observed in patients with CNS infections. These include generalized slowing (ranging from mild to severe), focal slowing, focal epileptiform discharges, lateralized periodic discharges (LPDs), generalized periodic discharges (GPDs), bilateral independent periodic discharges (BIPDs), and frontal intermittent rhythmic delta activity (FIRDA) (17).
- The most commonly encountered EEG patterns include generalized background slowing and LPDs, especially in HSV encephalitis where LPDs are observed in up to 65% of patients (19) (Figures 9.1 and 9.2).
- In the Dutch meningitis cohort, EEG was performed in 31% of patients with meningitis and history of clinical seizures. The majority of recordings indicated varying degrees of background slowing, while focal or multifocal abnormalities were noted in 38% of cases. Epileptiform discharges or status epilepticus were recorded in 30% (18).
- In another study, all patients with community-acquired bacterial meningitis and seizures had EEGs performed (31/117). The majority of these EEGs (29/31, 94%) showed diffuse abnormalities, and only 2/31 (6%) demonstrated unilateral

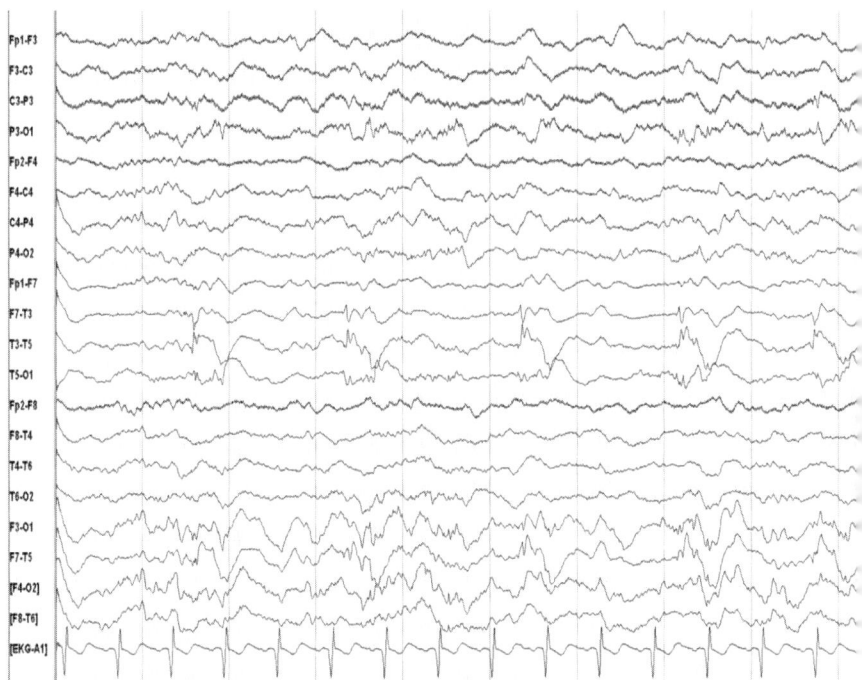

FIGURE 9.1 LPDs in a 31-year-old patient with preexisting multiple sclerosis treated with immunosuppression with superimposed HSV encephalitis. The patient presented with mental status changes and seizures clinically consisting of unresponsiveness, left-gaze deviation, and rhythmic left-leg twitching.

EEG findings, which were attributed to the development of an empyema or abscess (5).

- In a study by Kim et al., 32/34 patients with seizures received EEG with 38% of them showing epileptiform discharges and background slowing. In this study, 41% of patients with acute symptomatic seizures progressed to refractory epilepsy. Status epilepticus during active CNS infection was identified as a significant clinical predictor of subsequent refractory epilepsy (6).

F. Outcome
- The outcome of patients with encephalitis is dependent on the severity of CNS involvement, presence or absence of seizures, and the etiology of the disease (5,6,8).
- The mortality associated with encephalitis ranges from 5% to 30% and is not significantly different between various etiologies whether infectious or noninfectious (2,8,11,20,21). Of the survivors, 26% are reported to be severely disabled, 25% have moderate disability, and 49% have good outcome (8).

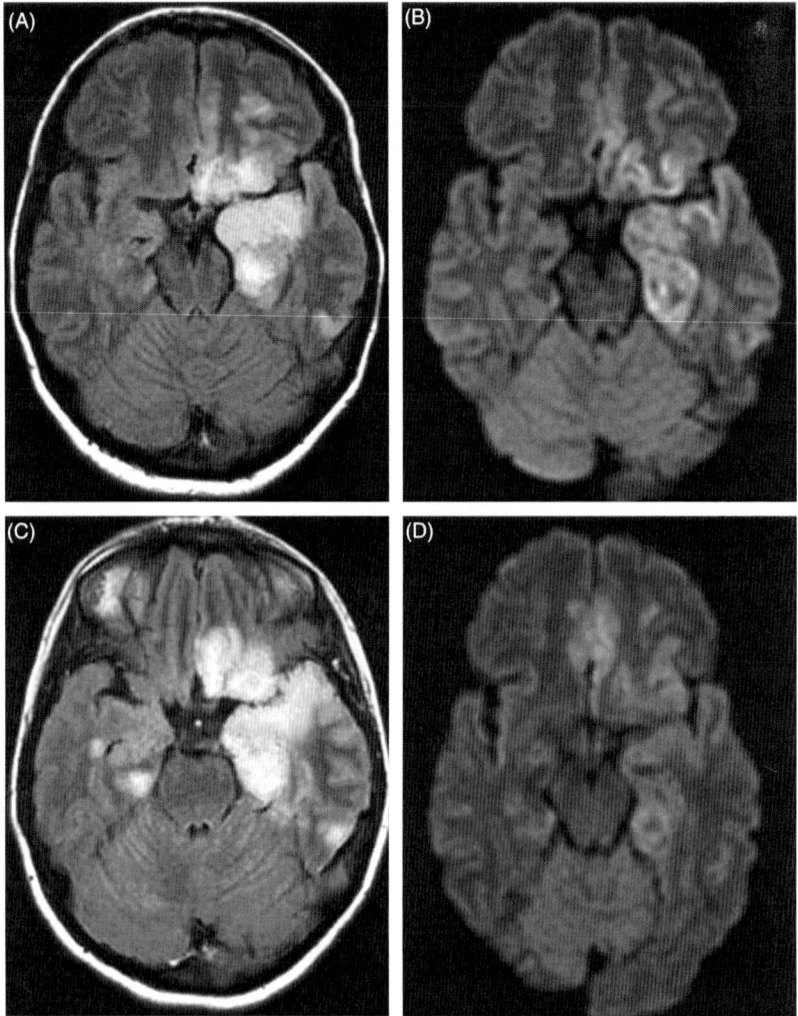

FIGURE 9.2   MRI FLAIR (left) and diffuse weighted imaging (DWI) (right) from the patient whose EEG is shown in Figure 9.1. Images were obtained at presentation (A, B) and 7 days later (C, D).

- Seizures in patients with encephalitis are more likely to be accompanied by focal neurological deficits (6).
- The risk of developing epilepsy after encephalitis is approximately 7 times higher than the risk in the general population. Within the first 20 years, 22% of patients with viral encephalitis and early seizures develop epilepsy while the incidence

of epilepsy in encephalitis patients without early seizures is only 13%. This compares to 2.1% to 2.4% incidence of epilepsy in patients with aseptic or bacterial meningitis (20).

- Approximately 50% of adult patients with acute symptomatic seizures progress to develop chronic epilepsy (6). The course and outcome of encephalitis in children may be somewhat more benign than in adults with seizure incidence only 6% in adults (6,21).

- In a recent retrospective study, multiple seizures or status epilepticus, focal slow waves or continuous generalized delta waves were identified as predictors of an adverse outcome. Children with focal spikes or continuous generalized delta waves on EEG were also more likely to have abnormal brain imaging (21).

- Finally, in most patients, post-encephalitis epilepsy is difficult to control with antiepileptic drugs and these patients may be candidates for epilepsy surgery (22). One study specifically evaluated the outcomes of epilepsy surgery in patients who had developed focal seizures as a result of a CNS infection. Of the 20 patients with history of meningitis and 36 with encephalitis, 64.3% developed mesial–temporal-lobe sclerosis which was unilateral in 27/36; and 20 patients developed neocortical epilepsy. Seizure-freedom rates after surgical intervention were similar in patients with meningitis versus encephalitis (66.7% versus 69.2%) (22).

III. FURTHER CONSIDERATIONS/REMAINING QUESTIONS

- Studies examining the short- and long-term outcomes of patients with encephalitis and seizures are needed to determine whether seizures are a marker of severity of the underlying disease or whether seizures by themselves contribute to morbidity and mortality.

- Current retrospective cEEG studies are limited by considerable selection bias since most patients who present with clinical seizures are likely to receive an EEG study, whereas patients without reported clinical seizures may not. Prospective cEEG studies of all patients admitted to the ICU with CNS infections are needed to truly determine seizure risks, response to medications, and differences in outcomes.

- It is likely that the increased use of cEEG in the ICU setting will result in increased recognition of subclinical seizures in patients with CNS infections including encephalitis.

- Finally, because of the high-incidence of seizures and/or status epilepticus in patients with encephalitis, these patients present an opportunity to study the effects of antiepileptic drugs for seizure prevention as well as their antiepileptogenic potential in this clinical setting.

REFERENCES

1. Granerod J, Tam CC, Crowcroft NS, et al. Challenge of the unknown. A systematic review of acute encephalitis in non-outbreak situations. *Neurology.* 2010;75:924–932.
2. Glaser CA, Honarmand S, Anderson LJ, et al. Beyond viruses: Clinical profiles and etiologies associated with encephalitis. *Clin Infect Dis.* 2006;43:1565–1577.

3. Carrera E, Claassen J, Oddo M, et al. Continuous electroencephalographic monitoring in critically ill patients with central nervous system infections. *Arch Neurol.* 2008;65:1612–1618.
4. Sonneville R, Demeret S, Klein I, et al. Acute disseminated encephalomyelitis in the intensive care unit: Clinical features and outcome of 20 adults. *Intensive Care Med.* 2008;34:528–532.
5. Wang KW, Chang WN, Chang HW, et al. The significance of seizures and other predictive factors during the acute illness for the long-term outcome after bacterial meningitis. *Seizure* 2005;14:586–592.
6. Kim MA, Park KM, Kim SE, et al. Acute symptomatic seizures in CNS infection. *Eur J Neurol.* 2008;15:38–41.
7. Glaser CA, Gilliam S, Schnurr D, et al. In search of encephalitis etiologies: Diagnostic challenges in the California Encephalitis Project, 1998–2000. *Clin Infect Dis.* 2003;36:731–742.
8. Granerod J, Ambrose HE, Davies NW, et al. Causes of encephalitis and differences in their clinical presentations in England: A multicentre, population-based prospective study. *Lancet Infect Dis.* 2010;10:835–844.
9. Glaser C, Bloch KC. Encephalitis: Why we need to keep pushing the envelope. *Clin Infect Dis.* 2009;49:1848–1850.
10. Granerod J, Cunningham R, Zuckerman M, et al. Causality in acute encephalitis: Defining aetiologies. *Epidemiol Infect.* 2010;138:783–800.
11. Mailles A, Stahl JP. Infectious encephalitis in France in 2007: A national prospective study. *Clin Infect Dis.* 2009;49:1838–1847.
12. Dalmau J, Gleichman AJ, Hughes EG, et al. Anti-NMDA-receptor encephalitis: Case series and analysis of the effects of antibodies. *Lancet Neurol.* 2008;7:1091–1098.
13. Leake JA, Albani S, Kao AS, et al. Acute disseminated encephalomyelitis in childhood: Epidemiologic, clinical and laboratory features. *Pediatr Infect Dis J.* 2004;23:756–764.
14. Schwarz S, Mohr A, Knauth M, et al. Acute disseminated encephalomyelitis: A follow-up study of 40 adult patients. *Neurology.* 2001;56:1313–1318.
15. Buckley C, Oger J, Clover L, et al. Potassium channel antibodies in two patients with reversible limbic encephalitis. *Ann Neurol.* 2001;50:73–78.
16. Privitera M, Hoffman M, Moore JL, et al. EEG detection of nontonic–clonic status epilepticus in patients with altered consciousness. *Epilepsy Res.* 1994;18:155–166.
17. Claassen J, Mayer SA, Kowalski RG, et al. Detection of electrographic seizures with continuous EEG monitoring in critically ill patients. *Neurology.* 2004;62:1743–1748.
18. Zoons E, Weisfelt M, de Gans J, et al. Seizures in adults with bacterial meningitis. *Neurology.* 2008;70:2109–2115.
19. Whitley RJ, Soong SJ, Linneman C, Jr, et al. Herpes simplex encephalitis. *Clin Assess JAMA.* 1982;247:317–320.
20. Annegers JF, Hauser WA, Beghi E, et al. The risk of unprovoked seizures after encephalitis and meningitis. *Neurology.* 1988;38:1407–1410.
21. Wang IJ, Lee PI, Huang LM, et al. The correlation between neurological evaluations and neurological outcome in acute encephalitis: A hospital-based study. *Eur J Paediatr Neurol.* 2007;11:63–69.
22. Lancman ME, Morris HH, 3rd. Epilepsy after central nervous system infection: Clinical characteristics and outcome after epilepsy surgery. *Epilepsy Res.* 1996;25:285–290.

TEN

Traumatic Brain Injury

William David Freeman

KEY POINTS

- As many as 22% of patients with traumatic brain injury (TBI) have early post-traumatic seizures (within 7 days of injury), half of which are nonconvulsive seizures (NCS).
- Anticonvulsant prophylaxis is recommended for severe TBI patients (Glasgow Coma Scale 8 or less) within the first 7 days, but not recommended for routine seizure prophylaxis beyond 7 days unless seizures occur.
- Prophylactic barbiturate-induced burst suppression is not recommended in patients with TBI. Although barbiturates may be used to control intracranial pressure (ICP), there is no evidence to suggest that their use improves outcomes.
- Since at least half of all seizures in patients with severe TBI are subclinical, EEG monitoring is a critical tool in the management of these patients.
- Although the association between seizures and clinical outcome is not clear in all TBI patients, early seizures increase with TBI severity and may predict worse outcomes in these patients.

I. BACKGROUND

A. Epidemiology
- Traumatic brain injury (TBI) is a common form of brain injury that can be neurologically devastating, and seen in predominantly younger, male patients.
- TBI typically occurs after blunt head injury such as falls, assault, or motor-vehicle collisions.
- The health care cost of acute care and rehabilitation for TBI patients in the United States is $9 to 10 billion per year, with average lifetime cost per patient ranging from $600,000 to $1,875,000 for severe TBI (1).

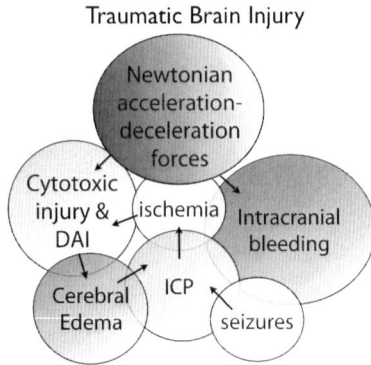

FIGURE 10.1   Pathophysiologic mechanisms of TBI.

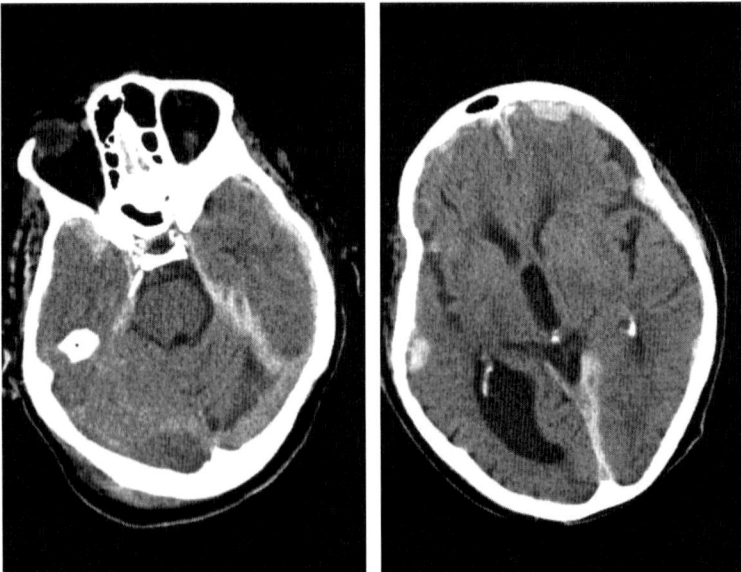

FIGURE 10.2   Traumatic intracranial hemorrhage (ICH) in an 80-year-old female patient after a fall at home. The patient arrived in the emergency department with a GCS of E1M2V1T consistent with severe TBI. Left image demonstrates bitemporal hemorrhagic contusions with subarachnoid hemorrhage, right occipital cephalohematoma with underlying right occipital lobe cerebral edema, left temporal lobe convexity subdural hematoma, and left tentorial subdural hematoma. Right image shows bifrontal hemorrhagic contusions and subarachnoid hemorrhage (right Sylvian fissure), as well as subdural hemorrhage (bihemispheric convexities).

B. Pathology

- TBI consists of vascular, cellular, and parenchymal pathophysiological mechanisms (Figure 10.1).
- Newtonian acceleration–deceleration forces on brain and skull contents cause shearing of axons (diffuse axonal injury, DAI) and tearing of intracranial vessels. These effects result in hemorrhage which can be subdural, epidural, subarachnoid, intraparenchymal, or intraventricular (Figure 10.2).
- Posttraumatic seizures (PTS) may occur early (within 7 days of injury) or late (after 7 days) (1).
- The prevalence of clinical seizures varies with the severity of TBI and ranges from 4% to 22% (2–8).
- In addition, seizures can lead to high brain tissue oxygen demand, poor oxygen and glucose supply, disturbed autoregulation, and raised ICP all of which contribute to metabolic supply:demand mismatch which can induce secondary brain injury (9).

II. BASICS

A. TBI severity is classified by Glasgow Coma Scale (GCS) within 48 hours of injury. Classification is independent of structural CT imaging findings.

- Mild TBI is defined as GCS 13 to 15.
- Moderate TBI is defined as GCS 9 to 12.
- Severe TBI is defined as GCS 3 to 8.

B. Risk Factors for Seizures After TBI (1)

- GCS score less than 10
- Cortical contusion
- Depressed skull fracture
- Subdural hematoma
- Epidural hematoma
- Intracerebral hematoma
- Penetrating head wound
- Seizure within 24 hours of injury

C. Brain Trauma Foundation Evidence-Based Guidelines, 2007 (1)

- An early study by Temkin showed that treatment with phenytoin in the first 7 days following injury decreased the prevalence of clinically evident PTS in patients with TBI from 14.2% to 3.6% (5). Based upon this data, it is recommended that patients with severe TBI should receive anticonvulsant, ie, antiepileptic drug (AED), prophylaxis for the first 7 days following injury.
- Routine AED prophylaxis beyond 7 days post-injury is not recommended unless seizure(s) have occurred.
- Barbiturate therapy has not shown a clear benefit in improving outcome. Prophylactic administration to induce burst suppression on EEG is not recommended for TBI patients.

- High-dose barbiturates can be used to control ICP refractory to maximum standard medical and surgical treatment, but should not be given if hemodynamic stability is compromised.
- Propofol can be used for sedation and control of ICP, but does not reduce mortality or improve 6-month outcomes.

D. cEEG and TBI

- Few studies have assessed the prevalence of seizures in TBI patients undergoing cEEG.
- In a retrospective study of TBI patients undergoing cEEG ($n = 51$), Claassen et al. found that 18% of patients experienced seizures during cEEG, all of which were subclinical and 8% were in nonconvulsive status epilepticus (3).
- In an earlier study, Vespa et al evaluated 91 patients with moderate-to-severe TBI who underwent cEEG and found that 22% of these patients experienced seizures, 57% of which were purely subclinical (2).
- Since at least half of all seizures in patients with severe TBI are subclinical, EEG monitoring is a critical tool in the management of these patients (Figure 10.3).

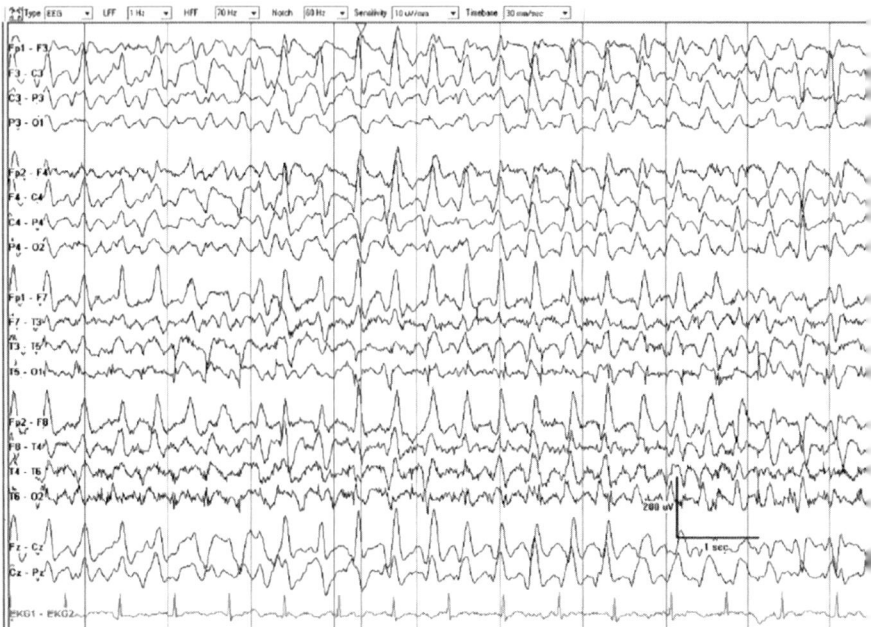

FIGURE 10.3 Same patient as Figure 10.2. EEG recording several days later demonstrated NCSE with unresponsiveness.

E. Effect of Seizures on Outcome in TBI Patients

- NCS and nonconvulsive status epilepticus (NCSE) in TBI patients are increasingly recognized as harmful.
- Vespa et al studied patients with moderate-to-severe TBI using cEEG and cerebral microdialysis 7 days after injury (8). Ten patients with PTS (seven of which were in NCSE) were compared with 10 patients without seizures.
  - Patients with PTS had increased ICP (22.4 ± 7 mmHg versus 12.8 ± 4.3 mmHg, $P < .001$), and increased lactate/pyruvate ratios (LPR) (49.4 ± 16 versus 23.8 ± 7.6; $P < .001$).
  - Elevated ICP and LPR remained persistently elevated up to 100 hours post-injury in the PTS group but not in the control group ($P < .02$).
- In addition, both NCS and NCSE have been associated with subsequent hippocampal atrophy in TBI patients (9).
- Thus, detecting and treating PTS in patients with TBI may represent a therapeutic opportunity to prevent secondary brain injury from seizures.

III. FURTHER CONSIDERATIONS/REMAINING QUESTIONS

A. Seizures and Clinical Outcomes

- The correlation between seizures and clinical outcome in patients with TBI is not entirely clear.
- Seizures are more common with more severe TBI but questions remain regarding what contribution seizures have toward outcome independent of the degree of brain injury.
- However, early posttraumatic seizures are independently associated with poor outcome in both adults and children (10,11).
- Newer AEDs such as levetiracetam and lacosamide have fewer systemic side effects and drug–drug interactions than conventional anticonvulsants and their role in the treatment and prevention of PTS should be studied more extensively.
- One prospective, randomized trial of intravenous levetiracetam versus phenytoin for seizure prophylaxis found that levetiracetam had fewer cognitive effects compared to phenytoin in TBI survivors (12).
- Preliminary studies of quantitative EEG (QEEG) measures such as percent alpha variability after TBI have been shown to predict clinical outcomes (13). Thus, further research is needed into the possible prognostic value of QEEG in this patient population.
- The significance of periodic and rhythmic patterns in TBI patients (eg, LPDS) and whether they should be treated with AEDs requires further study. Risks and benefits of treatment including clinical outcomes versus medication-related side effects (cognitive impairment, prolonged mechanical ventilation, or hypotension from drug-induced burst suppression) should be evaluated.
- Finally, to better characterize NCS in patients with TBI, future studies should assess the impact of NCS on biomarkers such as LPR and brain atrophy, in addition to functional outcomes.

REFERENCES

1. Bratton SL, Chestnut RM, Ghajar J, et al. Guidelines for the management of severe traumatic brain injury. XIII. Antiseizure Prophylaxis. *J Neurotrauma.* May 2007, 24(Suppl 1): S-83–S-86.
2. Vespa PM, Nuwer MR, Nenov V, et al. Increased incidence and impact of nonconvulsive and convulsive seizures after traumatic brain injury as detected by continuous electroencephalographic monitoring. *J Neurosurg.* 1999;91:750.
3. Claassen J, Mayer SA, Kowaski RG, et al. Detection of electrographic seizures with continuous EEG monitoring in critically ill patients. *Neurology.* 2004;62:1743–1748.
4. Annegers JF, Grabow JD, Groover RV, et al. Seizures after head trauma: A population study. *Neurology.* 1980;30:683–689.
5. Temkin NR, Dikmen SS, Wilensky AJ, et al. A randomized, double-blind study of phenytoin for the prevention of post-traumatic seizures. *N Engl J Med.* 1990;323:497–502.
6. Lee S, Lui T, Wong C, et al. Early seizures after moderate closed head injury. *Acta Neurochir.* 1995;137:151–154.
7. Vespa P. Continuous EEG monitoring for the detection of seizures in traumatic brain injury infarction, intracerebral hemorrhage: "To detect and protect." *J Clin Neurophysiol.* 2005;22:99–106.
8. Vespa PM, Miller C, McArthur D, et al. Nonconvulsive electrographic seizures after traumatic brain injury result in a delayed, prolonged increase in intracranial pressure and metabolic crisis. *Critic Care Med.* Dec 2007;35(12):2830–2836.
9. Vespa PM, McArthur DL, Xu Y, et al. Nonconvulsive seizures after traumatic brain injury are associated with hippocampal atrophy. *Neurology.* Aug 31, 2010;75(9):792–798.
10. Wang HC, Chang WN, Chang HW, et al. Factors predictive of outcome in posttraumatic seizures. *J Trauma.* 2008;64:883–888.
11. Chiaretti A, Piastra M, Pulitano S, et al. Prognostic factors and outcome of children with severe head injury: An 8-year experience. *Childs Nerv Syst.* 2002;18:129–136.
12. Szaflarski JP, Sangha KS, Lindsell CJ, et al. Prospective, randomized, single-blinded comparative trial of intravenous levetiracetam versus phenytoin for seizure prophylaxis. *Neurocrit Care.* Apr 2010;12(2):165–172.
13. Vespa PM, Boscardin WJ, Hovda DA, McArthur DL, et al. Early and persistent impaired percent alpha variability on continuous electroencephalography monitoring as predictive of poor outcome after traumatic brain injury. *J Neurosurg.* Jul 2002;97(1):84–92.

ADDITIONAL READING

Wallace BE, Wagner AK, Wagner EP, McDeavitt JT. A history and review of quantitative electroencephalography in traumatic brain injury. *J Head Trauma Rehabil.* Apr 2001;16(2):165–190.

NIH Consensus Development Conference on Rehabilitation of Persons with Traumatic Brain Injury http://www.nichd.nih.gov/publications/pubs/TBI_1999/NIH_Consensus_ Statement.cfm

ELEVEN

Therapeutic Hypothermia in Adults

Ram Mani

KEY POINTS

- Therapeutic hypothermia (TH) is associated with improved survival in comatose adults after cardiac arrest (high level of evidence). TH is occasionally used in other conditions (ie, severe traumatic brain injury (TBI), ischemic stroke, and fulminant hepatic failure) but there is a lack of clinical trial evidence of its utility in these situations.
- EEG offers useful prognostic information in comatose survivors of cardiac arrest in the first 1 to 3 days following arrest and treatment with TH.
- Electrographic seizures are common following cardiac arrest; seen in approximately 20% to 40% of patients. Seizures are difficult to detect as well as treat since they may be nonconvulsive and often present as status epilepticus (SE).
- Myoclonic status epilepticus (MSE) is a common form of SE in post-cardiac arrest comatose patients and is associated with poor outcome.

I. BACKGROUND

A. **Target diseases for which TH in adults has been evaluated are those associated with severe brain injury (often with intracranial hypertension and sometimes with large regions of cerebral ischemia). However, cardiac arrest is the only disease in which TH has been associated with consistent improvement in outcomes based on randomized clinical trials.**

B. **Cardiac Arrest**
- After successful resuscitation, most patients are comatose. Approximately 70% of these patients die (1) and more than 1/3 are left with neurologic deficits (2).
- Four randomized clinical trials found that mild TH instituted in comatose patients within 6 hours of ventricular fibrillation or pulseless ventricular tachycardia reduced mortality by 20% and decreased poor neurologic outcome by 27% (3). Based on these findings, TH is now the standard of care for these patients.

C. Severe TBI (Glasgow Coma Scale less than 9)

- Patients with severe TBI often have intracranial hypertension and high risk of death.
- Most clinical trials involving patients with severe TBI (total of greater than 1,000 patients) show reduction in elevated intracranial pressure (ICP) following TH, but with variable impact on clinical outcome (4).
- A recent meta-analysis of six clinical trials (694 patients) found TH was associated with a nonsignificant reduction in mortality but a significant improvement in functional outcome in patients with severe TBI (5).
- EEG monitoring (cEEG) should be considered in these patients given the relatively high prevalence of nonconvulsive seizures (6,7) (Table 11.1).

D. Ischemic Stroke

- It is difficult to determine the effectiveness of TH in patients with ischemic stroke due to a variety of confounding factors such as presence of rebound intracranial hypertension and the use of hemicraniectomy which often accompanies TH.
- Clinical protocols must be optimized, and further randomized clinical trials conducted, before widespread clinical use of TH can be recommended for these patients.

E. Acute Hepatic Failure

- Acute hepatic failure is defined as the abrupt onset of hepatic injury with coagulopathy and hepatic encephalopathy in patients without preexisting liver disease.
- Increase ICP is the most severe complication from which many patients die while awaiting transplantation (4,9).
- TH led to marked decrease in ICP in one case series, allowing 13/14 patients to receive a liver transplant with neurologic recovery (10).
- It is unclear whether all patients with acute hepatic failure should undergo cEEG but seizure prevalence can be high (11) (Table 11.1). In addition, EEG patterns of uncertain clinical significance (triphasic waves and other periodic discharges that can be difficult to distinguish from ictal activity) are common in these patients making EEG interpretation complex.

TABLE 11.1   Indications for Therapeutic Hypothermia and Seizure Prevalence

ACUTE CONDITION	THERAPEUTIC HYPOTHERMIA DATA	SEIZURE PREVALENCE
Post-cardiac arrest	Good evidence that TH improves mortality and neurologic outcome after ventricular fibrillation and ventricular tachycardia arrest (3).	15%–40%
Severe TBI	Good evidence that TH decreases ICP. Mixed evidence that functional outcome is improved (4,5). TH being used on a case-by-case basis.	20%
Malignant ischemic stroke	Research is ongoing (8).	Unknown (8)
Acute hepatic failure	Small sample sizes. TH used as bridge to maintain survival until liver transplantation (9,10).	2%–33%

II. BASICS

A. Hypothermia Protocols and EEG Basics

- Hypothermia protocols
  - Adult patients are most often cooled with surface cooling devices, as opposed to neonates, who are often cooled with head caps. Other cooling options in adults are endovascular cooling catheters, cold IV solutions, ice packs, and alcohol baths.
  - Patients should be cooled within a few hours of brain injury and maintained at a target temperature. The target temperature varies per study, but 32°C to 34°C is most often used.
  - The duration of TH varies according to the clinical condition and case specifics. Post-cardiac arrest patients are often cooled for 24 hours, while TBI patients may be cooled for 2 to 5 days (4).
  - Rewarming is often done in a controlled manner; often a rate of 0.25°C/hr to prevent rebound intracranial hypertension (4).
  - Shivering is common during the cooling induction phase. It is metabolically counterproductive and often causes a characteristic EEG artifact resembling diffuse low- to high-amplitude repetitive spikes. It may be combated with paralytics, or sedatives.
  - When interpreting the EEG, attention should be paid to the CNS-active drugs that the patient is presently receiving or recently received while being cooled since hypothermia decreases the metabolism of many sedative drugs commonly used in the ICU (12).
- EEG basics
  - cEEG has excellent potential for impact in disease states where seizures are relatively common yet clinically undetected. Post-cardiac arrest and TBI are examples of such disease states. Sedatives and paralytics used to prevent shivering make the neurologic exam less reliable and thus EEG for detection of NCS is vital during this time period.
  - Timing: EEG hookup is ideal when the patient is hemodynamically stable and the head is accessible. If early detection of electrographic seizure activity is a priority, cEEG-monitoring within 12 hours (or earlier) after arrest is desirable. If only routine EEG is available, it may be necessary to repeat the EEG serially as seizures may be missed, especially as high-dose anesthetics are weaned off.
  - EEG is not significantly affected at body temperatures of 32°C to 34°C (13,14). However, other sedative drugs commonly administered during TH can markedly affect the EEG background.
  - Electrode placement and equipment setup is the same with or without TH.
  - Hypothermia presents a theoretically increased risk of coagulopathy. However, scalp breakdown with bleeding or infection has not been observed among more than 150 post-arrest patients treated with TH who underwent up to several days of cEEG with either disposable or reusable versions of the Ives EEG Electrode System (Ives EEG Solutions, Newburyport, MA). Steps to avoid scalp injury include regular electrode maintenance, scalp inspections, keeping the scalp dry, and reducing pressure on scalp from the electrodes.

B. Seizures After Cardiac Arrest

- Clinical seizures occur in 10% to 40% of patients following cardiac arrest, mostly in the first 3 to 5 days after arrest (15,16).
- Seizures most commonly present as diffuse or multifocal myoclonus, but focal and generalized tonic–clonic seizures have also been reported.
- MSE is a clinical diagnosis consisting of unrelenting diffuse myoclonus involving the face, limbs, and torso. It often occurs with stimulation but can also occur spontaneously.
  - MSE is strongly associated with poor outcome if onset is during the first 24 hours post-arrest (17). This strong association remains true even when patients are treated with TH, although the onset of MSE may be delayed 3 to 5 days after cardiac arrest (18).
  - There have been reports of rare survivors (less than 5%) of MSE with good cognitive outcome (19). Most of these patients were treated with at least three to four antiepileptic drugs (including high-dose anesthetics), had preserved brainstem reflexes, intact cortical somatosensory evoked potentials responses and reactive EEG background.
  - The EEG correlate of MSE is often generalized periodic discharges (GPDs) and/or burst suppression pattern. However, MSE has also been observed with nonepileptiform patterns such as diffuse alpha activity (20).
- Electrographic seizures and SE
  - Electrographic seizures are prevalent and often present as SE. SE after cardiac arrest is very difficult to treat, and it is not clear if treatment alters neurologic outcome and mortality.
  - In four studies of post-arrest patients treated with TH and receiving routine EEG or cEEG monitoring, pooled data showed prevalence of SE to be 29% (82/284 patients; 95% CI 23%–35% (21–24).
  - Seizures typically begin within the first 2 days following cardiac arrest but it is not uncommon to see electrographic seizures upon initial EEG hookup.
  - Several studies have shown that initial electrographic seizures are typically not associated with any clinical correlate, although many patients eventually demonstrate a clinical correlate of myoclonus or other motor seizure types by day 2 to 3.
  - In patients with post-arrest SE, special attention should be given to the following:
    - Caution should be used when prescribing intravenous phenytoin loads due to the risk of cardiac dysrhythmia or hypotension in this very susceptible population.
    - Valproate, benzodiazepines, and levetiracetam have shown some efficacy in reducing post-anoxic myoclonus.
    - When using moderate or high-dose barbiturates, it is reasonable to delay prognostication because of their prolonged sedative effect. A randomized trial of refractory SE found a median duration of intubation of 14 days in survivors in the thiopental or pentobarbital infusion arm (median administration, 2 days), versus 4 days for survivors in the propofol arm ($P = .03$) (25). A total of 39% of patients were alive at the study end with no significant difference between the barbiturate and propofol arms.

- Epileptiform activity post-arrest: Many studies assessing EEG features in survivors of cardiac arrest do not differentiate well between electrographic seizures, SE, and interictal epileptiform activity. However, such differences may be important for outcome.
  - In our experience at the Hospital of the University of Pennsylvania, we have seen a trend toward better outcome for those with less epileptiform activity (eg, 0.5 Hz LPDs evolving to brief seizures for a total of a few minutes) compared to those with more frequent epileptiform activity or periodic discharges (2–4 Hz evolving GPDs for a total of days).
  - Varying definitions and terms for sharp, periodic, rhythmic, and evolving patterns has contributed to some of the lack of descriptive EEG analysis in the literature.
  - Standardized terminology for EEG features in comatose patients will aid in future studies of the impact of seizures and epileptiform activity on outcomes following cardiac arrest (26).
- There are specific EEG patterns and findings that have implications for prognostic and other management decisions after cardiac arrest (Table 11.2). The EEG can be particularly helpful in determination of prognosis but only in the absence of confounding effects due to high-dose sedative medications.

TABLE 11.2 Important EEG Features in Patients Undergoing TH

EEG FEATURES	SIGNIFICANCE
Background frequency and voltage	Burst-suppression, discontinuity, and persistent slowing and voltage attenuation (less than 10 μV) are highly associated with poor outcome following cardiac arrest (17,27). High doses of midazolam, propofol, and other anesthetics can induce burst-suppression pattern and severe voltage attenuation interfering with ability to prognosticate (28).
Reactivity and variability	Lack of reactivity is strongly associated with poor outcome when tested in the optimal conditions. Presence of variability excludes diagnosis of alpha coma (22,28).
Discontinuity	Discontinuity is associated with poor outcome (29).
Sleep architecture	May help judge level of coma. Increased prevalence of normal sleep patterns was associated with shorter coma duration and less depressed consciousness in TBI patients (30,31).
Epileptiform activity	GPDs on a severe voltage attenuated background are highly associated with poor outcome. Burst suppression with epileptiform activity is associated with later electrographic seizures (17,27).
EEG artifact (eg, rhythmic theta; repetitive EMG artifact)	Shiver artifact is common. Use of video and ICU team/nurse event reports can avoid misinterpretation and unnecessary treatment (32).

III. FURTHER CONSIDERATIONS/REMAINING QUESTIONS

A. Treatment

- The most clinically relevant questions regarding brain-injured patients treated with TH include: (1) Which epileptiform patterns are responsive to AED therapy? and (2) Does treatment of these patterns improve outcome?
- A well-designed randomized controlled trial is necessary for further evaluation of the significance of various EEG patterns, clinical correlates such as myoclonus, response to treatment, and association with outcome.

B. Prognosis

- Identifying EEG patterns and sequences of patterns with prognostic value at particular times after specific brain injuries is necessary. Controlling for confounding factors (especially sedative medication exposure) will be necessary.

C. Quantitative EEG Analysis

- Studies have shown that some features of EEG measured quantitatively (eg, burst-suppression ratio and various frequency ratios) are associated with outcome (24). Quantitative EEG needs further research before widespread clinical use.

REFERENCES

1. Nolan JP, Laver SR, Welch CA, et al. Outcome following admission to UK intensive care units after cardiac arrest: A secondary analysis of the ICNARC Case Mix Programme Database. *Anaesthesia.* Dec 2007;62(12):1207–1216.
2. Neumar RW, Nolan JP, Adrie C, et al. Post-cardiac arrest syndrome: Epidemiology, pathophysiology, treatment, and prognostication. A consensus statement from the International Liaison Committee on Resuscitation (American Heart Association, Australian and New Zealand Council on Resuscitation, European Resuscitation Council, Heart and Stroke Foundation of Canada, InterAmerican Heart Foundation, Resuscitation Council of Asia, and the Resuscitation Council of Southern Africa); the American Heart Association Emergency Cardiovascular Care Committee; the Council on Cardiovascular Surgery and Anesthesia; the Council on Cardiopulmonary, Perioperative, and Critical Care; the Council on Clinical Cardiology; and the Stroke Council. *Circulation.* Dec 2 2008;118(23):2452–2483.
3. Cheung KW, Green RS, Magee KD. Systematic review of randomized controlled trials of therapeutic hypothermia as a neuroprotectant in post cardiac arrest patients. *Can J Emergency Med.* Sep 2006;8(5):329–337.
4. Marion D, Bullock MR. Current and future role of therapeutic hypothermia. *J Neurotrauma.* Mar 2009;26(3):455–467.
5. Bratton SL, Chestnut RM, Ghajar J, et al. Guidelines for the management of severe traumatic brain injury. III. Prophylactic hypothermia. *J Neurotrauma.* 2007;24(Suppl 1):S21–S25.
6. Claassen J, Mayer SA, Kowalski RG, et al. Detection of electrographic seizures with continuous EEG monitoring in critically ill patients. *Neurology.* May 25 2004;62(10):1743–1748.
7. Vespa P. Continuous EEG monitoring for the detection of seizures in traumatic brain injury, infarction, and intracerebral hemorrhage: "to detect and protect." *J Clin Neurophysiol.* Apr 2005;22(2):99–106.
8. Mecarelli O, Pro S, Randi F, et al. EEG patterns and epileptic seizures in acute phase stroke. *Cerebrovasc Dis.* 2011;31(2):191–198.

9. Trey C, Davidson CS. The management of fulminant hepatic failure. *Prog Liver Dis.* 1970;3:282–298.

10. Jalan R, Olde Damink SW, Deutz NE, et al. Moderate hypothermia in patients with acute liver failure and uncontrolled intracranial hypertension. *Gastroenterology.* Nov 2004;127(5):1338–1346.

11. Friedman D, Claassen J, Hirsch LJ. Continuous electroencephalogram monitoring in the intensive care unit. *Anesth Analg.* Aug 2009;109(2):506–523.

12. Tortorici MA, Kochanek PM, Poloyac SM. Effects of hypothermia on drug disposition, metabolism, and response: A focus of hypothermia-mediated alterations on the cytochrome P450 enzyme system. *Crit Care Med.* Sep 2007;35(9):2196–2204.

13. Stecker MM, Cheung AT, Pochettino A, et al. Deep hypothermic circulatory arrest: I. Effects of cooling on electroencephalogram and evoked potentials. *Ann Thorac Surg.* Jan 2001;71(1):14–21.

14. Michenfelder JD, Milde JH. The relationship among canine brain temperature, metabolism, and function during hypothermia. *Anesthesiology.* Jul 1991;75(1):130–136.

15. Krumholz A, Stern BJ, Weiss HD. Outcome from coma after cardiopulmonary resuscitation: Relation to seizures and myoclonus. *Neurology.* Mar 1988;38(3):401–405.

16. Snyder BD, Hauser WA, Loewenson RB, et al. Neurologic prognosis after cardiopulmonary arrest: III. Seizure activity. *Neurology.* Dec 1980;30(12):1292–1297.

17. Wijdicks EF, Hijdra A, Young GB, et al. Practice parameter: Prediction of outcome in comatose survivors after cardiopulmonary resuscitation (an evidence-based review): Report of the Quality Standards Subcommittee of the American Academy of Neurology. *Neurology.* Jul 25, 2006;67(2):203–210.

18. Fugate JE, Wijdicks EF, Mandrekar J, et al. Predictors of neurologic outcome in hypothermia after cardiac arrest. *Ann Neurol.* Dec 2010;68(6):907–914.

19. Rossetti AO, Oddo M, Liaudet L, Kaplan PW. Predictors of awakening from postanoxic status epilepticus after therapeutic hypothermia. *Neurology.* 2009;72(8):744–749.

20. Thomke F, Marx JJ, Sauer O, et al. Observations on comatose survivors of cardiopulmonary resuscitation with generalized myoclonus. *BMC Neurol.* 2005;5:14.

21. Legriel S, Bruneel F, Sediri H, et al. Early EEG monitoring for detecting postanoxic status epilepticus during therapeutic hypothermia: A pilot study. *Neurocrit Care.* 2009;11(3):338–344.

22. Rossetti AO, Oddo M, Logroscino G, et al. Prognostication after cardiac arrest and hypothermia: A prospective study. *Ann Neurol.* Mar 2010;67(3):301–307.

23. Rundgren M, Westhall E, Cronberg T, et al. Continuous amplitude-integrated electroencephalogram predicts outcome in hypothermia-treated cardiac arrest patients. *Crit Care Med.* 2010;28(9):1838–1844.

24. Wennervirta JE, Ermes MJ, Tiainen SM, et al. Hypothermia-treated cardiac arrest patients with good neurological outcome differ early in quantitative variables of EEG suppression and epileptiform activity. *Crit Care Med.* Aug 2009;37(8):2427–2435.

25. Rossetti AO, Milligan TA, Vulliemoz S, et al. A randomized trial for the treatment of refractory status epilepticus. *Neurocrit Care.* Feb 2011;14(1):4–10.

26. Hirsch LJ, Brenner RP, Drislane FW, et al. The ACNS subcommittee on research terminology for continuous EEG monitoring: Proposed standardized terminology for rhythmic and periodic EEG patterns encountered in critically ill patients. *J Clin Neurophysiol.* Apr 2005;22(2):128–135.

27. Koenig MA, Kaplan PW, Thakor NV. Clinical neurophysiologic monitoring and brain injury from cardiac arrest. *Neurol Clin.* Feb 2006;24(1):89–106.

28. Mahla ME. Anesthetic effects on the electroencephalogram. *Neuro Sci Monitor* 1992;3:2–7.

29. Rundgren M, Westhall E, Cronberg T, et al. Continuous amplitude integrated EEG predicts outcome in hypothermia treated cardiac arrest patients. *Crit Care Med* 2010;38:1838–1844.

30. Kaplan PW, Genoud D, Ho TW. Clinical correlates and prognosis in early spindle coma. *Clin Neurophysiol.* Apr 2000;111(4):584–590.

31. Rumpl E, Prugger M, Bauer G, et al. Incidence and prognostic value of spindles in post-traumatic coma. *Electroencephalogr Clin Neurophysiol.* Nov 1983;56(5):420–429.

32. Young GB. Continuous EEG monitoring in the ICU: Challenges and opportunities. *Can J Neurol Sci.* Aug 2009;36(Suppl 2):S89–S91.

TWELVE

Therapeutic Hypothermia in the Neonatal and Pediatric Population

Nicholas S. Abend and Courtney J. Wusthoff

KEY POINTS

- Therapeutic hypothermia (TH) has been demonstrated to improve outcome in term neonates with hypoxic–ischemic encephalopathy and is being utilized widely as a neuroprotective strategy.
- Nonconvulsive seizures are common in neonates following hypoxic–ischemic brain injury and may worsen outcome.
- TH is feasible in children after cardiac arrest and is sometimes utilized based on adult cardiac arrest data but has not been shown to improve neurodevelopmental outcome.
- Nonconvulsive seizures are common in children following cardiac arrest, but their impact on outcome is unknown.
- TH after traumatic brain injury (TBI) has not been demonstrated to be neuroprotective, but is undergoing further study and is used in some situations.

I. BACKGROUND

A. Neonates With Hypoxic–Ischemic Encephalopathy (HIE)

- HIE is a major cause of morbidity and mortality among term newborns, with acute and chronic consequences.
- Neonates with moderate or severe HIE are at risk for acute symptomatic seizures, which occur in up to one-half of patients.
- EEG monitoring studies show that more than half of electrographic seizures in neonates have no clinical correlate, and thus cannot be detected by clinical observation alone (1,2).
- Administration of phenobarbital or phenytoin may terminate clinically evident convulsions, but nonconvulsive seizures may persist (electroclinical uncoupling) (3).

- Among neonates with HIE, seizures have been correlated with biomarkers of brain injury such as more severe injury on MRI as well as worse clinical outcomes. However, it remains unknown whether this association is causal.
- TH has been demonstrated to improve neurodevelopmental outcome in neonates with HIE.
  - Several large multicenter randomized studies have compared normothermia to TH (34–36°C) in term neonates (4–6).
  - Hypothermia was administered by selective head cooling (head cap) or whole body cooling (cooling blanket) for 72 hours.
  - Neonates treated with TH demonstrated significantly lower death and severe disability at 18 to 22 months of age.
  - On the basis of these data, many neonatal intensive care units now utilize TH treatment pathways for term neonates with HIE.

B. Children Resuscitated From Cardiac Arrest

- Although less common than in adults, cardiac arrest is a major cause of morbidity and mortality in children.
- Causes of cardiac arrest are different in children compared to adults. A substantial number occur in the context of respiratory arrest or in children with preexisting chronic neurodevelopmental and medical conditions.
- On the basis of data that TH improves outcome in adults resuscitated from cardiac arrest, it is sometimes utilized in children, although efficacy data are lacking. Studies in children have demonstrated the feasibility of TH and noted few associated adverse effects.
- In contrast to the 72-hour hypothermia period used in neonates with HIE, children resuscitated from cardiac arrest generally undergo TH for 24 to 48 hours.

C. Children With Traumatic Brain Injury (TBI)

- TBI is a major cause of morbidity and mortality in children.
- The role for TH in children with TBI is unknown.
- A recent prospective multicenter randomized study compared children managed with and without TH and demonstrated no benefit (7).
- Thus, TH is not currently in wide use for pediatric TBI, although studies are ongoing.

II. BASICS

A. Neonates With HIE

- Electrographic seizures are common in neonates with HIE undergoing TH, and most are not accompanied by clinical symptoms.
  - One study evaluated 41 newborns with HIE managed with TH and cEEG. Electrographic seizures occurred in 34% and status epilepticus occurred in 10%. Seizures were subclinical in 43% (8).
  - Another study of 26 newborns with HIE managed with TH and cEEG, demonstrated electrographic seizures in 65% and status epilepticus in 23%. Seizures were subclinical in 47% (9) (Figure 12.1).

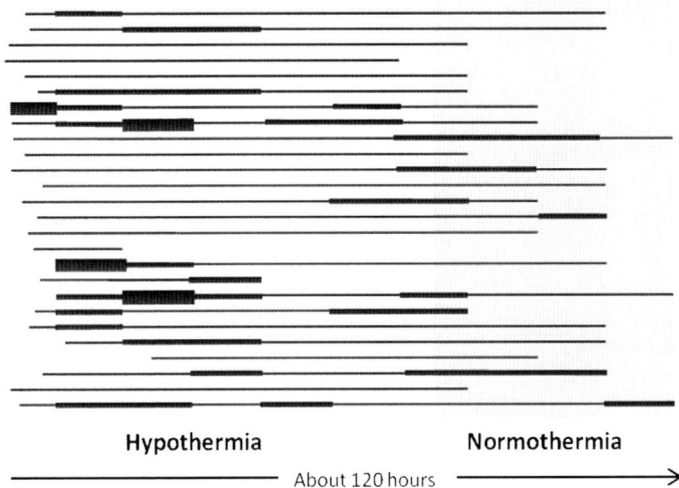

FIGURE 12.1 Seizures during and following therapeutic hypothermia in neonates with hypoxic–ischemic encephalopathy. Each horizontal gray line represents a single patient's continuous EEG recording. Thin black bars represent periods with electrographic seizures and thick black bars represent status epilepticus. Image based on Wusthoff, CW. *J. Child Neuro*, 2011.

- In 107 neonates with HIE, those who underwent hypothermia had fewer electrographic seizures than those who did not receive hypothermia (median of 60 versus 203 min); this reduction in electrographic seizures occurred in those neonates with moderate HIE (10).
- The impact of clinical and subclinical seizures on neurodevelopmental outcome is unclear, although some data suggest that seizures may worsen outcome.
  - In 41 newborns with HIE managed with TH who underwent MRI, seizures were more frequent in neonates with moderate-to-severe injury on MRI compared to those with no or mild MRI-documented injury. Status epilepticus occurred only in newborns with moderate-to-severe injury on MRI (8).
  - In term newborns, clinical seizures have been associated with worse neurodevelopmental outcome, even after controlling for the degree of injury on MRI (11).
- Aside from identifying seizures, serial EEGs or EEG monitoring may provide prognostic information in neonates with HIE.
  - A normal EEG background, especially early during hypothermia, is predictive of a normal MRI and normal neurodevelopmental outcome.
  - A severely abnormal background (severe attenuation, burst suppression), especially when it persists for several days after birth, is predictive of severe MRI injury and abnormal neurodevelopmental outcome.
- Amplitude-integrated EEG (aEEG) monitoring using two or four channels can be applied by bedside caregivers and provides a bedside display of compressed EEG.
  - aEEG has fair-to-moderate agreement with conventional EEG in terms of background description (12).

○ Background categorization has been used to select which neonates might benefit from TH in some studies (Figure 12.2) (4).

○ Conventional full-array EEG monitoring is superior to limited-channel aEEG for seizure detection. However, when interpreted by a skilled user, limited-channel aEEG can identify seizures in many neonates (Figure 12.3) Thus, limited-channel aEEG may play an important role in seizure detection, but only when conventional EEG is not available or feasible.

○ Studies of limited-channel aEEG for seizure identification report that only about half of seizures identified on conventional EEG are identified by aEEG, with the best identification when aEEG electrodes are placed at C3 to C4 (13).

○ One study randomized newborns with HIE to undergo treatment for both clinical and electrographic seizures identified on aEEG versus treatment of clinical seizures only.

• There was a trend toward a reduction in total seizure duration when both clinical and subclinical seizures were treated, compared to when management was directed only at clinical seizures.

• Longer-duration seizures were associated with more severe brain injury on MRI (14).

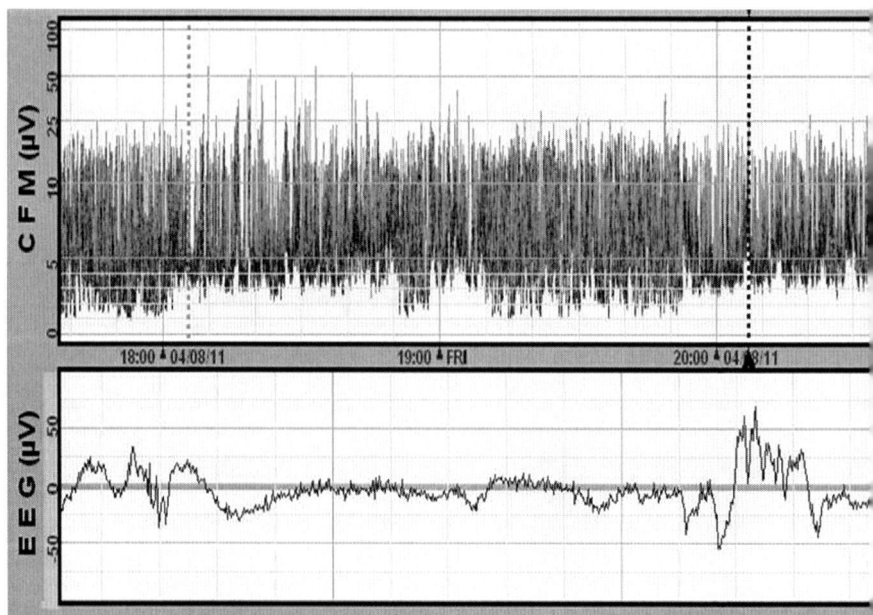

FIGURE 12.2   aEEG tracing from a newborn receiving hypothermia for HIE. The top box shows compressed EEG signal over 3 hours. The lower box gives a snapshot of 15 seconds of source EEG. In this case, the record starts with the lower border of the aEEG band below 5 μV, which is abnormally low amplitude. This would be classified as an abnormal background.

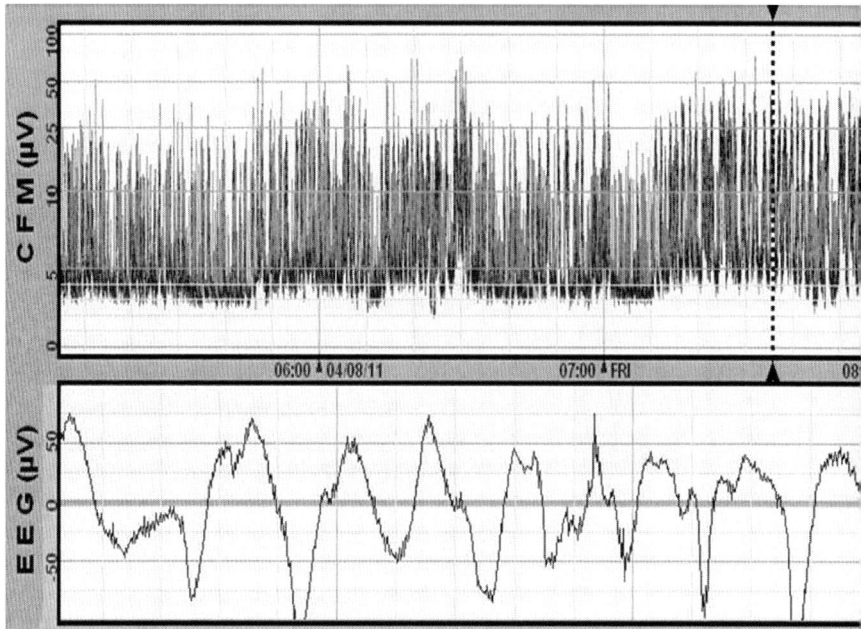

FIGURE 12.3 aEEG tracing from a newborn receiving hypothermia for HIE. The upper box shows the aEEG trend over 3 hours and the lower box shows 15 seconds of source EEG at the time marked by the cursor in the upper box. The upper box demonstrates several areas of increase in baseline amplitude characteristic of recurrent seizures on aEEG while the lower box demonstrates rhythmic activity of a single seizure on source EEG.

○ Artifacts and nonseizure movements are common in newborns with HIE, and must be distinguished from electrographic seizures. Clinical movements that mimic seizure can include shivering and myoclonus. In a neonate, myoclonus can last for minutes and may be mistaken for seizures.

B. Children Resuscitated From Cardiac Arrest

● Retrospective series of acutely ill children with nonconvulsive seizures have reported HIE as a common etiology (15–17).
● Electrographic seizures, mostly without any clinical correlate, are common in children resuscitated from cardiac arrest undergoing TH.
  ○ Nineteen consecutive children resuscitated from cardiac arrest and treated with TH underwent cEEG during hypothermia (24 hours), re-warming (12–24 hours), and an additional 24 hours of normothermia.
    ● Electrographic seizures occurred in 47%, status epilepticus occurred in 32%.
    ● Seizures were subclinical in 67%.
    ● Seizures began during the first half of hypothermia in one patient, the second half of hypothermia in four, and during re-warming in four patients (Figures 12.4 and 12.5).

- Seizures occurred in all eight patients with a severely abnormal background, and in only one patient with a mild-to-moderately abnormal background. (Severe background abnormalities included excessive discontinuity, burst suppression, or highly attenuated tracings.) (18).
- The impact of clinical and electrographic seizures on neurodevelopmental outcome is unknown.

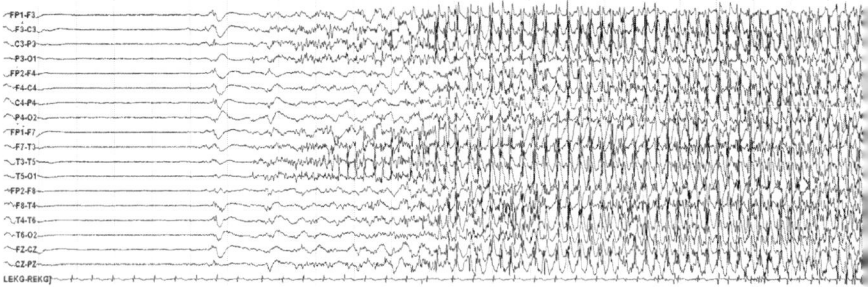

FIGURE 12.4 A child resuscitated from cardiac arrest and treated with TH had an attenuated and discontinuous record during hypothermia and then developed multifocal nonconvulsive seizures during return to normothermia. This seizure had focal onset in the left hemisphere and then generalized. There was no clinical correlate even though the patient was not receiving paralytics.

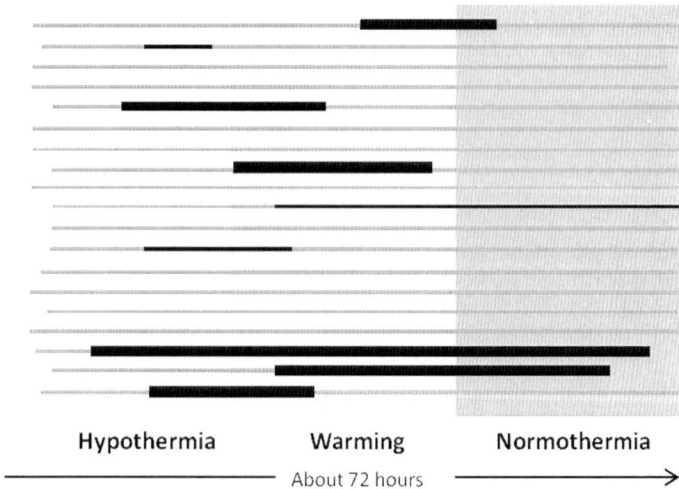

FIGURE 12.5 Seizures during and following therapeutic hypothermia in children resuscitated from cardiac arrest. Each horizontal gray line represents a single patient's continuous EEG recording. Thin black bars represent periods with electrographic seizures and thick black bars represent status epilepticus. Image based on Abend NS. *Neurology*, 2009.

- cEEG may provide prognostic information in children resuscitated from cardiac arrest.
  - Prior to the introduction of TH, some EEG features including severe attenuation, burst suppression, status epilepticus (especially myoclonic status epilepticus), and possibly periodic epileptiform discharges were associated with unfavorable outcome following pediatric cardiac arrest.
  - If TH is neuroprotective, then the predictive value of these EEG features and the time after arrest when they are most predictive may be altered.
  - EEGs were scored in 35 consecutive children treated with TH following cardiac arrest
    - During both hypothermia and normothermia, children with EEGs that were either continuous and unreactive or excessively discontinuous (including excess discontinuity, burst suppression, or lack of cerebral activity) were more likely to have an unfavorable short-term outcome than children with EEGs that were continuous (Table 12.1) (19).

TABLE 12.1   EEG Category Short-Term Outcome

EEG CATEGORY	PPV FOR UNFAVORABLE OUTCOME (95% CI)	
	HYPOTHERMIC	NORMOTHERMIC
Continuous and reactive	27%(12–42%)	31%(15–46%)
Continuous and unreactive	80%(67–93%)	92%(83–100%)
Discontinuous and/or suppressed	93%(84–100%)	89%(78–99%)
Continuous and unreactive or Discontinuous and/or suppressed	88%(77–98%)	91%(81–100%)

Source: Based on Kessler S, *Neurocrit Care*, 2011.

CI, confidence interval; PPV, positive predictive value.

C. Children With Traumatic Brain Injury (TBI)

- About one-quarter of children with moderate-to-severe TBI have been noted to experience electrographic seizures.
- In adults with TBI, electrographic seizures may be associated with increased intracranial pressure and metabolic dysfunction. The impact of electrographic seizures in children is unknown.

III. FURTHER CONSIDERATIONS/REMAINING QUESTIONS

A. Neonates With HIE

- Although seizures are known to occur in neonates with HIE, and are often subclinical (thus requiring EEG monitoring for identification), further research is required to establish whether seizures have a causal impact on neurodevelopmental outcome and to determine the optimal management of neonatal seizures.

B. Children Resuscitated From Cardiac Arrest

- Data are needed to determine whether TH improves outcome after cardiac arrest in children.
- While seizures are known to occur in children following cardiac arrest, and are often subclinical (thus requiring EEG monitoring for identification), further research is required to establish whether seizures have a causal impact on neurodevelopmental outcome and to establish the optimal management for seizures following cardiac arrest.

C. Children With TBI

- Studies are ongoing to further explore whether TH has benefit for some children with TBI.
- Data are needed to better define which children with TBI experience seizures, whether these have a causal impact on neurodevelopmental outcome, and the optimal management of seizures following TBI.

REFERENCES

1. Murray DM, Boylan GB, Ali I, et al. Defining the gap between electrographic seizure burden, clinical expression and staff recognition of neonatal seizures. *Arch Dis Child Fetal Neonatal Ed.* 2008;93:F187–F191.

2. Clancy RR, Legido A, Lewis D. Occult neonatal seizures. *Epilepsia.* 1988;29:256–261.

3. Scher MS, Alvin J, Gaus L, et al. Uncoupling of EEG-clinical neonatal seizures after antiepileptic drug use. *Pediatr Neurol.* 2003;28:277–280.

4. Gluckman PD, Wyatt JS, Azzopardi D, et al. Selective head cooling with mild systemic hypothermia after neonatal encephalopathy: Multicentre randomised trial. *Lancet.* 2005;365:663–670.

5. Shankaran S, Laptook AR, Ehrenkranz RA, et al. Whole-body hypothermia for neonates with hypoxic-ischemic encephalopathy. *N Engl J Med.* 2005;353:1574–1584.

6. Azzopardi DV, Strohm B, Edwards AD, et al. Moderate hypothermia to treat perinatal asphyxial encephalopathy. *N Engl J Med.* 2009;361:1349–1358.

7. Hutchison JS, Ward RE, Lacroix J, et al. Hypothermia therapy after traumatic brain injury in children. *N Engl J Med.* 2008;358:2447–2456.

8. Nash KB, Bonifacio SL, Glass HC, et al. Video-EEG monitoring in newborns with hypoxic–ischemic encephalopathy treated with hypothermia. *Neurology.* 2011;76: 556–562.

9. Wusthoff CJ, Dlugos D, Guteirrez-Colina AM, et al. Incidence of electrographic seizures during therapeutic hypothermia for neonatal encephalopathy. *J Child Neurol.* 2011;26: 724–728.

10. Low E, Boylan GB, Mathieson SR, et al. Cooling and seizure burden in term neonates: An observational study. *Arch Dis Child Fetal Neonatal Ed.* 2012;97:F267–272.

11. Glass HC, Glidden D, Jeremy RJ, et al. Clinical neonatal seizures are independently associated with outcome in infants at risk for hypoxic–ischemic brain injury. *J Pediatr.* 2009;155:318–323.

12. Shellhaas RA, Gallagher PR, Clancy RR. Assessment of neonatal electroencephalography (EEG) background by conventional and two amplitude-integrated EEG classification systems. *J Pediatr.* 2008;153:369–374.

13. Wusthoff CJ, Shellhaas RA, Clancy RR. Limitations of single-channel EEG on the forehead for neonatal seizure detection. *J Perinatol.* 2009;29:237–242.

14. van Rooij LG, Toet MC, van Huffelen AC, et al. Effect of treatment of subclinical neonatal seizures detected with aEEG: Randomized, controlled trial. *Pediatrics.* 2010;125: e358–e366.

15. Abend NS, Dlugos DJ. Nonconvulsive status epilepticus in a pediatric intensive care unit. *Pediatr Neurol.* 2007;37:165–170.

16. Tay SK, Hirsch LJ, Leary L, et al. Nonconvulsive status epilepticus in children: Clinical and EEG characteristics. *Epilepsia.* 2006;47:1504–1509.

17. Jette N, Claassen J, Emerson RG, Hirsch LJ. Frequency and predictors of nonconvulsive seizures during continuous electroencephalographic monitoring in critically ill children. *Arch Neurol.* 2006;63:1750–1755.

18. Abend NS, Topjian A, Ichord R, et al. Electroencephalographic monitoring during hypothermia after pediatric cardiac arrest. *Neurology.* 2009;72:1931–1940.

19. Kessler S, Topjian AA, Guterrez-Colina AM, et al. Short-term outcome prediction by electroencephalographic features in children treated with therapeutic hypothermia after cardiac arrest. *Neurocrit Care.* 2011;14:37–43.

THIRTEEN

Prognosis

Leslie Rudzinski

KEY POINTS

- Although continuous EEG monitoring (cEEG) has greatly improved our ability to detect electrographic seizures and nonconvulsive status epilepticus (NSCE) it is unclear whether treatment of electrographic seizures and NCSE leads to improved neurological outcome.
- Prior to the era of therapeutic hypothermia (TH), the presence of burst suppression or generalized periodic discharges were useful predictors of poor outcome in comatose survivors after cardiac arrest.
- Although less is known about the utility of EEG in determining prognosis in cardiac arrest patients following TH, some studies have shown that lack of EEG reactivity correlates with poor neurological outcome. However, large prospective studies correlating specific EEG findings with neurological outcome following TH are needed.

I. BACKGROUND

A. Distinct EEG patterns may be associated with poor neurological outcomes in specific clinical settings.
  - Studies have evaluated the utility of EEG for prediction of prognosis in the following settings: cardiac arrest both with and without hypothermia, intracranial hemorrhage (ICH), subarachnoid hemorrhage (SAH), and nonconvulsive status epilepticus (NCSE) (Table 13.1).

B. Prognosis in comatose survivors after cardiopulmonary resuscitation (CPR) cannot be determined by EEG in isolation. However, specific EEG findings in association with other clinical findings, and data from somatosensory evoked potentials (SSEPs) help increase the positive predictive value of poor functional outcomes.

II. BASICS (TABLE 13.1)

A. EEG and Prognosis After ICH

- Seizures following ICH have been associated with worsening neurological function (measured by NIH stroke scale), progressive midline shift, and a trend toward worse outcome (1).
- Another study, described many features of ICH that are associated with seizures and periodic discharges. However, this single center study failed to demonstrate an association between seizures in patients with ICH and worse outcome (2).
  - Patients with expanding hemorrhages experience nonconvulsive seizures (NCS) twice as often as those with static hemorrhages.
  - Proximity of the hemorrhage to the cortical surface was a predictor of the presence of periodic discharges (PDs) as well as NCS.
    - 23% of patients with lobar hemorrhage experienced NCS versus 11% of patients with deep hemorrhages.
    - 29% of patients with hemorrhage within 1 mm of the cortex demonstrated PDs versus 8% with hemorrhages 1 mm or deeper.
  - Periodic discharges (PDs) were seen more frequently in patients with hemorrhages greater than 60 mL on head CT.
  - Poor outcome in patients with ICH was associated with any PDs, lateralized periodic discharges (LPDs), and focal stimulus-induced rhythmic, periodic, or ictal discharges (SIRPIDs) but there was no association between seizures and poor outcome.

TABLE 13.1   EEG Patterns Associated With Outcome

	POOR OUTCOME	GOOD OUTCOME
Intracranial hemorrhage	PDs, LPDs, SIRPIDs (2)	–
Subarachnoid hemorrhage	No reactivity, no state change first 24 hr, NCSE within 24 hr, GPDs, BIPDs (3)	Presence of sleep architecture, state changes, reactivity, absence of PDs (3)
Nonconvulsive status epilepticus	Generalized SE, burst-suppression, LPDs, ictal discharges after control of SE (5,6,7)	Focal SE, normalization of EEG background (5,6,7)
Cardiac arrest (without therapeutic hypothermia)	Myoclonic SE within the first 24 hr, generalized suppression less than 20 μV/mm, burst-suppression pattern, GPDs on flat background, alpha/theta/spindle coma without reactivity (8,9)	Presence of reactivity (9)
Cardiac arrest after therapeutic hypothermia	No reactivity, early myoclonus, burst-suppression, generalized suppression, SE (9,10,12)	Continuous EEG background with generalized slow-wave activity, reactivity (11,12)

BIPDs, bilateral independent periodic discharges; B-S, burst suppression; GPDs, generalized periodic discharges; NCSE, nonconvulsive status epilepticus; PDs, periodic discharges; LPDs, lateralized periodic discharges; SE, status epilepticus; SIRPIDs, stimulus-induced rhythmic, periodic, or ictal discharges.

B. EEG and Prognosis in Poor-Grade SAH

- A single center study evaluated 116 patients with SAH who underwent cEEG. 88% had a Hunt & Hess grade of 3 or worse on admission. Functional outcome was assessed at 3 months using the modified Rankin Scale (3).
- Poor outcome was associated with:
  - Absence of sleep architecture during the first 24 hours of cEEG hook up (OR 10.4, 95% CI 1.4–78.1) or at any time of the hospital stay (OR 4.3., 95% CI 1.1–17.2).
  - Presence of LPDs at any time (OR 18.8, 95% CI 1.6–214.6).
  - Presence of any type of PDs, even after controlling for age, Hunt & Hess grade, and IVH (OR 9.0, 95% CI 1.7–49.0).
- Poor outcome at 3 months was seen in all patients with the following characteristics:
  - No EEG reactivity.
  - No state changes within the first 24 hours.
  - NCSE within 24 hours.
  - Generalized periodic discharges (GPDs).
  - Bilateral independent periodic discharges (BIPD).
  - Each of these factors had a positive predictive value (PPV) of 100%, but findings should be interpreted with caution due to the small number of patients with these factors (2%–4%).
- There was no relationship between SIRPIDs and outcome in this cohort.
- In general, the presence of sleep architecture, state changes, reactivity to external stimuli, and the absence of periodic discharges on EEG were associated with better outcomes (3).

C. EEG and Prognosis Following NCSE

- NCSE has been defined as an epileptic state lasting greater than 30 minutes; clinically evident alteration in mental status or behavior from baseline; and seizure activity on the EEG (4).
- Outcomes in NCSE are difficult to determine because patients with widely heterogeneous clinical features and etiologies have been reported. Studies evaluating NCSE and outcome have included patients described as anywhere from lightly obtunded ("the wandering confused") to deeply comatose (4).
- Some studies have shown that absence or complex partial SE in the noncomatose patient, is rarely associated with permanent neurological injury (4).
- The etiology of SE remains the primary determinant of outcome (5).
  - The clinical course and outcome of 119 adult patients with clinical and electrographic SE were reviewed.
  - Generalized SE (OR 8.50, 95% CI 1.7–43.7) and coma on presentation (OR 152, 95% CI 18.6 –> 1000) were predictive of poor outcome.
  - Patients with anoxia/hypoxia as an etiology had poor outcomes (OR 19.0, 95% CI 2.47–146) (5).
  - SE caused by epilepsy as an etiology (OR 0.002, 95% CI 0–0.04) and focal SE (vs. generalized) were predictors of better outcome.
  - Neither overall duration of SE, nor SE duration greater than 10 hours was predictive of outcome.

- In patients with SE, normalization of the cEEG findings correlated with good outcome, whereas burst suppression, ictal discharges after control of SE, and LPDs were associated with poor outcome (6,7).

D. EEG and Prognosis in Coma After Cardiac Arrest

- The American Academy of Neurology (AAN) developed a Practice Parameter in 2006 titled "Prediction of outcome in comatose survivors after cardiopulmonary resuscitation" (8).
  - Clinical factors associated with poor outcome included:
    - Absent pupillary or corneal reflexes after 3 days (level A evidence).
    - Absent or extensor motor responses after 3 days (level A evidence).
    - Myoclonic SE within the first 24 hours in patients with primary circulatory arrest; defined as spontaneous, repetitive, generalized multifocal myoclonus involving the face, limbs, and axial musculature in comatose patients (level B evidence).
  - Biochemical markers associated with poor outcome (level B evidence):
    - Serum NSE level greater than 33 µg/L at days 1 to 3 post-CPR
  - Electrophysiological factors associated with poor outcome include (level B evidence):
    - Bilateral absent cortical somatosensory evoked potential (SSEP) responses recorded 3 days after CPR.
  - EEG findings associated with poor outcome included (level C evidence):
    - Generalized suppression to ≤20 µV
    - Burst-suppression pattern with generalized epileptiform activity
    - Generalized periodic complexes on a flat background
    - It is important to note that the above EEG findings were strongly but not invariably associated with poor outcome.
- It is important to note that the AAN practice parameter guidelines were developed prior to routine utilization of TH and since that time, few studies have evaluated the impact of TH on EEG findings and prognosis.
- One retrospective study evaluated 29 adult patients following cardiac arrest, with or without treatment with mild hypothermia (9).
  - The presence of reactivity was a relatively favorable EEG feature (sensitivity 90%, specificity 94%).
  - Generalized suppression (less than 20 µV) or generalized epileptiform activity, both without reactivity, were associated with a lack of recovery of awareness.
  - In addition, EEG patterns were classified as benign versus malignant to evaluate if additional EEG findings could aid in determination of outcome (recovery of awareness before hospital discharge).
    - Benign pattern = delta/theta greater than 50% of the recording (not theta coma), with or without reactivity.
    - Malignant patterns = triphasic waves, burst-suppression pattern (with or without epileptiform activity), alpha/theta/spindle coma pattern (no reactivity), or generalized suppression.
  - The use of the "benign vs. malignant" EEG classification for determination of prognosis had a sensitivity of 94%, however, the specificity was low (63%). Specifically, four patients with a malignant EEG pattern recovered awareness.

- A larger prospective study evaluated 111 adult survivors of cardiac arrest who underwent treatment with TH (10). The association of EEG, SSEP, and clinical exam findings were correlated with outcome, both alone and in combination.
  - An unreactive EEG background was a strong risk factor for mortality and poor long-term neurological recovery (false-positive rate of 7%).
  - The presence of a combination of two or more of the following variables (bilaterally absent N20s on SSEP, unreactive EEG background, early myoclonus, and incomplete recovery of brainstem reflexes) yielded a very high positive predictive value (PPV) for poor functional outcome (specificity 1.00, PPV 1.00).
  - Motor response to pain, had a high false-positive rate (24%).
  - These data suggest that clinical exam alone should not be used in isolation to prognosticate after cardiac arrest; rather, a multimodal approach should be used. In addition, evaluation of EEG reactivity significantly improved prognostication.

III. FURTHER CONSIDERATIONS/REMAINING QUESTIONS

A. ICH and SAH
- Does seizure type and/or duration affect outcome?
- Does treatment or prevention of seizures with AEDs affect short-term or long-term outcomes?
- Does treatment or prevention of PDs affect short-term or long-term outcomes?
- Does the evolution of the EEG pattern over time using cEEG monitoring more accurately predict outcome?

B. NCSE
- A new classification scheme for patients with NCSE depicting the depth of coma and underlying etiology may allow homogenization of patient populations and studies that better predict prognosis (4).
- Large prospective studies are needed with well-defined and stratified patient populations addressing whether the treatment of NCSE with AEDs or anesthetic agents improves outcome or causes greater morbidity.

C. Anoxic–Hypoxic Injury After Cardiac Arrest
- Future studies should avoid the "self-fulfilling prophecy" of withdrawing care in patients given no hope of recovery. Allowing weeks rather than days for potential recovery may avoid this confounder. Exact causes of death, the role of withdrawal of care, and long-term outcomes of survivors (at least one year) need to be documented (8,10).
- More prospective studies and better clinical guidelines are needed assessing EEG features associated with outcomes in cardiac arrest survivors who have received TH.
- There is need for a prospective study on comatose survivors of cardiac arrest with established stimulation protocols to determine whether specific types of reactivity (slowing vs. accelerating EEG) are more predictive of outcome (9).

- Prospective and systematic studies of specific "malignant" EEG patterns using a standardized classification system may provide better prognostic information.

REFERENCES

1. Vespa PM, O'Phelan K, Shah M, et al. Acute seizures after intracerebral hemorrhage: A factor in progressive midline shift and outcome. *Neurology.* May 13, 2003;60(9):1441–1446.
2. Claassen J, Jette N, Chum F, et al. Electrographic seizures and periodic discharges after intracerebral hemorrhage. *Neurology.* Sep 25, 2007;69(13):1356–1365.
3. Claassen J, Hirsch LJ, Frontera JA, et al. Prognostic significance of continuous EEG monitoring in patients with poor-grade subarachnoid hemorrhage. *Neurocrit Care.* 2006;4(2):103–112.
4. Kaplan PW. Assessing the outcomes in patients with nonconvulsive status epilepticus: Nonconvulsive status epilepticus is underdiagnosed, potentially overtreated, and confounded by comorbidity. *J Clin Neurophysiol.* Jul 1999;16(4):341–352; discussion 353.
5. Drislane FW, Blum AS, Lopez MR, Gautam S, Schomer DL. Duration of refractory status epilepticus and outcome: Loss of prognostic utility after several hours. *Epilepsia.* Jun 2009;50(6):1566–1571.
6. DeLorenzo RJ, Waterhouse EJ, Towne AR, et al. Persistent nonconvulsive status epilepticus after the control of convulsive status epilepticus. *Epilepsia.* Aug 1998;39(8):833–840.
7. Jaitly R, Sgro JA, Towne AR, Ko D, DeLorenzo RJ. Prognostic value of EEG monitoring after status epilepticus: A prospective adult study. *J Clin Neurophysiol.* Jul 1997; 14(4):326–334.
8. Wijdicks EF, Hijdra A, Young GB, Bassetti CL, Wiebe S. Practice parameter: Prediction of outcome in comatose survivors after cardiopulmonary resuscitation (an evidence-based review): Report of the Quality Standards Subcommittee of the American Academy of Neurology. *Neurology.* Jul 25 2006;67(2):203–210.
9. Thenayan EA, Savard M, Sharpe MD, Norton L, Young B. Electroencephalogram for prognosis after cardiac arrest. *J Crit Care.* Jun 2010;25(2):300–304.
10. Rossetti AO, Oddo M, Logroscino G, Kaplan PW. Prognostication after cardiac arrest and hypothermia: A prospective study. *Ann Neurol.* Mar 2010;67(3):301–307.
11. Kawai M, Thapalia U, Verma A. Outcome from therapeutic hypothermia and EEG. *J Clin Neurophysiol.* Oct 2011;28(5):483–488.
12. Fugate JE, Wijdicks EF, Mandrekar J, et al. Predictors of neurologic outcome in hypothermia after cardiac arrest. *Ann Neurol.* Dec 2010;68:907–914.

ADDITIONAL READING

Bauer G, Trinka E. Nonconvulsive status epilepticus and coma. *Epilepsia.* Feb 2010;51(2):177–190.

Fugate JE, Wijdicks EF, Mandrekar J, et al. Predictors of neurologic outcome in hypothermia after cardiac arrest. *Ann Neurol.* Dec 2010;68(6):907–914.

FOURTEEN

EEG Monitoring Outside of the Neuro ICU

Stephen Hantus

KEY POINTS

- Altered mental status has been associated with nonconvulsive seizures in critically ill patients with a primary neurologic injury, but less is known about the incidence of seizures in patients with altered mental status outside of the neurological ICU.
- In the medical ICU (MICU), altered mental status is common and linked to a variety of etiologies, with sepsis being the most common.
- On the basis of retrospective studies, sepsis is an independent risk factor for electrographic seizures in the MICU (1), but prospective analyses are needed to assess this risk better.
- Continuous EEG (cEEG) monitoring outside of the neurological ICU can provide important diagnostic and prognostic information regarding cerebral function, yet it is under-utilized in these settings.

I. BACKGROUND

A. Nonconvulsive seizures (NCS) have been reported in 8% to 37% of critically ill patients undergoing continuous EEG monitoring (cEEG) (2–4).

- Most patients in these series presented with altered mental status and/or primary neurologic injury.
- In the largest series of 570 patients, NCS was found in 19%.
- A higher proportion of NCS (37% of 198 patients) was seen in patients who underwent emergency EEGs for altered mental status and clinically suspected status epilepticus (SE) (5).
- Studies that attempted to eliminate bias by prospectively performing EEGs on all comatose patients (excluding those with clinical signs of seizures) found that 8% of 236 patients in coma were experiencing either NCS or NCSE (4).

B. Altered mental status outside of the neuro ICU is common and is often associated with seizures (Figure 14.1).
- There are many etiologies of altered mental status in this population and the exact cause is often never discovered.
- These patients always undergo continuous cardiac and respiratory monitoring but cerebral function monitoring (with cEEG) is rare.
- Estimates of altered mental status in the MICU range from 40% to 60% of patients (6).
- Common etiologies of altered mental status in the MICU:
  - Sepsis is the most frequent etiology.
    - Sepsis-related encephalopathy has been associated with neuronal damage, mitochondrial and endothelial injury, and disturbances in neurotransmission (7).
  - Metabolic encephalopathy often stems from liver or renal dysfunction.
  - Other primary systemic diseases can present as altered mental status from secondary neurologic injury and are also associated with seizures.
    - Posterior-reversible leukoencephalopathy (PRES), secondary to malignant hypertension, medications (cyclosporine, tacrolimus), eclampsia, or metabolic disturbances (hypercalcemia, uremia).
    - Embolic cerebral infarcts or mycotic aneurysms from endocarditis.
    - CNS vasculitis from an underlying autoimmune disease such as polyarteritis nodosa, systemic lupus erythematosus, and Sjorgren's syndrome.
    - Paraneoplastic syndromes; limbic encephalitis.
  - Because seizures are often associated with these entities, EEG monitoring should be considered in any MICU patient with altered mental status.
- Anoxic brain injury is a common cause of severe encephalopathy as well as seizures in the cardiac ICU (see Chapters 11, 12, 24).
  - Causes include cardiac arrest with or without therapeutic hypothermia as well as respiratory arrest.
- Transplant patients in the post-surgical ICU are another population at risk for altered mental status and seizures.
  - Causes of seizures include severe metabolic derangements, toxicity from immunosuppressive therapy, and post-operative complications.
- Recently, there have been reports of both clinical and subclinical seizures in the cardio-thoracic surgical ICU.

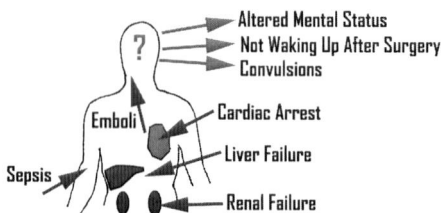

FIGURE 14.1 Causes of encephalopathy and seizures outside of the neuro ICU.

○ In a single center review of 74 patients in the cardio-thoracic surgical ICU undergoing cEEG, 22% experienced electrographic seizures during monitoring, the majority of which were subclinical.

II. BASICS

A. A retrospective study by Oddo et al evaluated the risk of seizures in the MICU of a university hospital (1). Patients with a primary neurologic injury were excluded from the study.

- 10% of 201 patients who had cEEG monitoring experienced seizures.
- Sepsis on ICU admission was the only independent predictor of seizures (1) (Table 14.1).
  ○ 60% of patients were septic and 48% were comatose at the time of the cEEG.
  ○ Seizures detected on cEEG were without clinical signs in 67% of patients.
  ○ Electrographic seizures or periodic discharges (PDs) were found in 22% of patients.
  ○ The presence of PDs was associated with a higher incidence of death or severe disability at hospital discharge.
  ○ The clinical significance of PDs is controversial.
    - Unresolved issues include whether they represent a metabolic encephalopathy (triphasic morphology), an ictal or potentially ictal pattern, their association with acute structural injury, and how they should be treated (or not).
  ○ Despite controversy over the appropriate management of PDs, their appearance in MICU patients appears to be associated with a negative prognosis.

TABLE 14.1   Number of Consecutive MICU Patients Who Experienced Nonconvulsive Seizures

MICU ADMITTING DIAGNOSIS	ESZ OR PDs	ESZs ONLY	PDs ONLY	ESZs AND PDs
Sepsis, $n = 120$	38 (32%)	11/120 (9%)	19 (16%)	8 (7%)
No sepsis $n = 81$	7 (9%)	0 (0%)	5 (6%)	2 (2%)

ESZ = clinically silent electrographic seizure.
PD = periodic discharge.
Source: Oddo M, Carrera E, Claassen J, Mayer SA, Hirsch LJ. Continuous electroencephalography in the medical intensive care unit*. *Crit Care Med* 2009;37:2051–2056.

B. cEEG monitoring has additional uses for assessing cerebral function outside of seizure detection.

- cEEG can be used to characterize encephalopathy, detect early ischemia, and changes in cerebral blood flow (CBF) as well as alert physicians to the possibility of impending cerebral herniation (8–10).
- Important to note: Not all presumed alterations in mental status are cerebral in origin.

○ Patients with inability to follow commands and normal EEG should alert clinicians for the possibility of severe neuromuscular dysfunction (critical illness neuropathy/myopathy), brain-stem pathology (locked-in syndrome), neuroleptic malignant syndrome, or psychiatric illness (catatonia).
- Patients with encephalopathy have some characteristic EEG findings, but with wide variation.
  ○ Diffuse delta or theta-slowing is often associated with encephalopathy but may also be iatrogenic (from sedative medications).
  ○ Periodic discharges with triphasic morphology may be associated with an array of toxic or metabolic factors.
- cEEG has been used to detect changes in CBF predominantly in the neurocritical care setting in patients with vasospasm secondary to subarachnoid hemorrhage (SAH) (8,9).
  ○ Although patients with SAH are not often cared for in the MICU, the fact that cEEG changes correlate with changes in CBF from vasospasm suggests its potential value for monitoring alterations in CBF from other disease states.
    - Example: patients with septic shock being maintained on vasopressors who are at risk for diffuse cerebral hypoxia.

C. Technical considerations for cEEG monitoring outside of the neuro ICU.
- Video is important to identify sources of artifact and must be correctly repositioned when the nursing staff moves either the patient or the bedside EEG acquisition unit.
- Sweating and scalp breakdown are common in patients with fevers, sepsis, and prolonged systemic disease requiring frequent electrode changes.
- Routine ICU care such as compressive chest therapy, suctioning, and oral care can create rhythmic artifacts that mimic electrographic seizures but are easily identified with video analysis.
- Electrical noise from intravenous pumps, electrical beds, dialysis machines, and other medical devices can obscure the EEG recording and requires proper identification and trouble shooting.

III. FURTHER CONSIDERATIONS/REMAINING QUESTIONS

A. Although preliminary studies suggest that cEEG monitoring is useful for diagnosis of NCS, evaluation of encephalopathy, detection of evolving ischemia, and determination of prognosis, very little data are available outside of the neuro ICU population.
- At present, only a small fraction of MICU patients are selected for cEEG monitoring.
- Criteria for monitoring MICU patients are not clearly defined.
- Prospective studies on the utility of cEEG in the MICU are needed to address this paucity of information.

B. Resources for cEEG monitoring outside of the neuro ICU are limited, despite likely benefits in this population.

- Improving EEG monitoring efficiency would increase impact of cEEG by monitoring more patients, particularly outside of the neurological ICU, with utilization of fewer resources.
- Identifying high-risk patients that would benefit most from cEEG would also be useful.
  - At present, sepsis is the most common underlying medical condition that prompts cEEG monitoring, but this still represents a very large patient population for which EEG monitoring resources are limited.

C. Future prospective studies of cEEG outside of the neuro ICU will need to address the association of encephalopathy and seizures in this patient population.

REFERENCES

1. Oddo M, Carrera E, Claassen J, et al. Continuous electroencephalography in the medical intensive care unit *. *Crit Care Med.* 2009;37:2051–2056.
2. Kurtz P, Hanafy KA, Claassen J. Continuous EEG monitoring: Is it ready for prime time? *Curr Opin Crit Care.* 2009;15:99–109.
3. Claassen J, Mayer SA, Kowalski RG, et al. Detection of electrographic seizures with continuous EEG monitoring in critically ill patients. *Neurology.* 2004;62:1743–1748.
4. Towne AR, Waterhouse EJ, Boggs JG, et al. Prevalence of nonconvulsive status epilepticus in comatose patients. *Neurology.* 2000;54:340–340.
5. Privitera M, Hoffman M, Moore JL, Jester D. EEG detection of nontonic–clonic status epilepticus in patients with altered consciousness. *Epilepsy Res.* 1994;18:155–166.
6. van den Boogaard M, Schoonhoven L, van der Hoeven JG, et al. Incidence and short-term consequences of delirium in critically ill patients: A prospective observational cohort study. *Int J Nurs Stud.* http://www.ncbi.nlm.nih.gov/pubmed/22197051
7. Zampieri FG, Park M, Machado FS, Azevedo LC. Sepsis-associated encephalopathy: Not just delirium. *Clinics (Sao Paulo).* 2011;66:1825–1831.
8. Vespa PM, Nuwer MR, Juhász C, et al. Early detection of vasospasm after acute subarachnoid hemorrhage using continuous EEG ICU monitoring. *Electroencephalogr Clin Neurophysiol.* 1997;103:607–615.
9. Claassen J, Hirsch LJ, Kreiter KT, et al. Quantitative continuous EEG for detecting delayed cerebral ischemia in patients with poor-grade subarachnoid hemorrhage. *Clin Neurophysiol.* 2004;115:2699–2710.
10. Newey C, Sarwal A, Hantus S. Continuous electroencephalography (cEEG) changes precede clinical changes in a case of progressive cerebral edema. *Neurocrit Care.* Nov 2011, epub ahead of print. 1–5.

FIFTEEN

EEG Monitoring in the Pediatric ICU

Cecil D. Hahn

KEY POINTS

- Seizures are common in certain groups of critically ill children, and are usually nonconvulsive requiring EEG for detection.
- Risk factors for nonconvulsive seizures include clinical seizures prior to the onset of continuous EEG monitoring (cEEG), interictal epileptiform discharges, younger age, and acute structural brain injury.
- Common indications for cEEG monitoring in the pediatric population include status epilepticus (SE), altered mental status with suspicion of seizures, characterization of clinical events suspected to represent seizures, and during use of neuromuscular blockade.
- The duration of cEEG monitoring depends on the clinical scenario; however, when screening for nonconvulsive seizures, 24 hours of monitoring is generally sufficient in most pediatric patients.

I. BACKGROUND

A. Continuous EEG Monitoring in the Pediatric ICU

- Historically, EEG monitoring has been mainly used for children with refractory SE.
- In children with refractory SE, the purpose of EEG monitoring was to guide titration of high-dose anesthetic therapy to an end point of either seizure suppression or burst suppression.
- Increasing awareness of nonconvulsive seizures (NCS) in critically ill children has led to wider use of cEEG monitoring, paralleling the experience in the adult ICU population.
- The prevalence of NCS in critically ill children is similar to that in adults; although some evidence suggests that prevalence is even higher in children.
- Risk factors for NCS in critically ill children are similar to those in adults.
  - ○ Children with an acute structural brain injury or acute presentation of clinical seizures are at highest risk.

TABLE 15.1   Reported Prevalence of Nonconvulsive Seizures and Nonconvulsive SE in Critically Ill Children

AUTHOR, YEAR	STUDY DESIGN	POPULATION	INDICATION FOR CONTINUOUS EEG MONITORING	SEIZURE PREVALENCE	
				NONCONVULSIVE SEIZURES	NONCONVULSIVE SE
Jette, 2006	Retrospective cohort, clinical EEG monitoring	117 children and neonates	Detection of subclinical seizures or unexplained diminished consciousness	39%	23%
Hyllienmark, 2007	Retrospective cohort, clinical EEG monitoring	42 children	Seizures or suspected seizures	–	9.5%
Shahwan, 2010	Prospective cohort, research EEG monitoring	100 children	Comatose children (GCS < 8)	7%	0%
Abend, 2010	Prospective cohort, clinical EEG monitoring	100 children	Per clinical protocol for altered mental status ± prior convulsions	46%	19%
Williams, 2011	Retrospective cohort, clinical EEG monitoring	122 children and neonates	Per clinical protocol for patients considered at risk for seizures	28% (1st 24 hours)	8%
McCoy, 2011	Retrospective cohort, clinical EEG monitoring	112 children and neonates	Per clinical protocol for patients considered at risk for seizures	29%	–

B. Epidemiology of Seizures Among Critically Ill Children
- Reported prevalence of seizures in critically ill children varies from 7% to 46% (Table 15.1).
  - This considerable variability is likely due to differences in study population as well as study design.
  - Reports of children with cEEG monitoring ordered because of high clinical suspicion of seizures are likely describing a subset of patients at higher risk for seizures than the broader ICU population.
    - Studies of cEEG ordered based on a high clinical suspicion of seizures found NCS in 28% to 46%.
    - In contrast, one prospective study of cEEG monitoring in a series of children with persistent coma of any etiology found NCS in only 7%.
- NCS are far more common than convulsive seizures in children (1–4).
- Prevalence rates for nonconvulsive and convulsive seizures have been reported as follows:
  - NCS only: 49% to 75%.
  - Nonconvulsive and convulsive seizures: 16% to 34%.
  - Convulsive seizures only: 0% to 17%.

C. Seizure prevalence has been evaluated in two specific pediatric patient populations.
- Infants undergoing cardiac surgery for congenital heart disease.
  - NCS occurred in 1.5% to 20% of infants undergoing cEEG monitoring for 48 to 72 hours following surgery (5,6).
  - Pre- and intra-operative seizures were not seen.
- Infants and children following cardiac arrest receiving therapeutic hypothermia.
  - Seizures occurred in 47%, and SE in 32% (7).
  - The timing of seizure onset was delayed, with most seizures during the late hypothermic and rewarming phases.

II. BASICS

A. Clinical and EEG Risk Factors for Seizures in Critically Ill Children (Table 15.2)
- Clinical characteristics associated with NCS:
  - Clinical seizures preceding cEEG monitoring (3).
  - Younger age (4 years vs. 7 years) (2).
  - Specific etiologies as a risk factor (3):
    - Acute presentation of epilepsy (50% prevalence).
    - Acute structural brain injury (40% prevalence).
    - Acute nonstructural etiology (14% prevalence).
- EEG characteristics associated with NCS:
  - Interictal epileptiform discharges, as well as lateralized periodic discharges (LPDs) (1,3).
  - Absence of sleep architecture (1).
  - Absence of reactivity to stimulation (1).

TABLE 15.2   Risk Factors for Nonconvulsive Seizures in Critically Ill Children

Clinical characteristics associated with nonconvulsive seizures
  Clinical seizures prior to cEEG monitoring
  Younger age
  Acute structural brain injury
  Acute presentation of epilepsy
EEG characteristics associated with nonconvulsive seizures
  Interictal epileptiform discharges, as well as LPDs
  Absence of sleep architecture
  Absence of reactivity to stimulation

B. Indications for cEEG Monitoring

- Protocols identifying indications that are appropriate for cEEG have been developed at many pediatric institutions.
- These indications may be based on particular clinical scenarios or specific diagnoses, in which case cEEG monitoring may be included as part of a clinical pathway (Table 15.3).
- Specific clinical scenarios for cEEG include the following.
  - ○ Therapeutic cEEG monitoring: purpose is primarily to guide treatment.
    - Refractory SE: to guide titration of high-dose anesthetic therapy to specific electrographic targets (eg, burst suppression).
    - Management of elevated intracranial pressure: to guide titration of anesthetic therapy to induce burst suppression.
  - ○ Diagnostic cEEG monitoring: purpose is primarily to assist with diagnosis of seizures.
    - Altered mental status with a suspicion of NCS.
    - During neuromuscular blockade to monitor for seizures which would otherwise be undetectable.
    - Characterization of involuntary movements suspected to represent seizures.
  - ○ cEEG may be indicated for patients with specific medical or neurological conditions for seizure detection, prognosis, and evaluation of nonictal events such as ischemia.

TABLE 15.3   Indications for cEEG Monitoring in Children

Clinical scenarios warranting EEG monitoring
  Refractory SE
  Intracranial pressure management
  Altered mental status, with suspicion of nonconvulsive seizures
  Neuromuscular blockade, with suspicion of seizures
  Characterization of clinical events suspected to be seizures
Diagnoses where EEG monitoring should be considered
  Traumatic brain injury (accidental, nonaccidental)
  Hypoxic–ischemic brain injury (neonatal, cardiac arrest, near drowning)
  Extracorporeal membrane oxygenation (ECMO) therapy
  Acute ischemic or hemorrhagic stroke
  Post-cardiac surgery
  Post-neurosurgery
  Acute metabolic encephalopathy (hepatic, renal, septic)

- Traumatic brain injury (accidental, nonaccidental)
- Hypoxic–ischemic brain injury (neonatal, cardiac arrest, near drowning)
- Extracorporeal membrane oxygenation (ECMO) therapy
- Acute ischemic or hemorrhagic stroke
- Post-cardiac surgery
- Post-neurosurgery
- Acute metabolic encephalopathy (hepatic, renal, septic)

C. Duration of cEEG Monitoring

- During of monitoring depends on indication diagnosis, EEG findings, and level of consciousness.
  - For clinical events suspected to be seizures, cEEG monitoring can usually be discontinued once typical events have been captured.
  - In refractory SE, cEEG monitoring can usually be discontinued 24 hours after high-dose anesthetic therapy has been tapered off if seizures have not recurred.
  - When screening for seizures in at-risk children, 24 hours of monitoring is probably sufficient (1–3).
    - More than 80% of children with seizures have their first seizure within the first 24 hours of monitoring.
    - However, seizures are identified in only 38% to 50% of children within the first hour of recording.
- After sustained improvement in mental status, and discontinuation of neuromuscular blockade, cEEG monitoring may be discontinued because any further seizures (even subtle or NCS) should be detected clinically.
- Children post-cardiac arrest may warrant a longer duration of cEEG monitoring because of the known risk for delayed seizures (see above).
- The presence of epileptiform discharges, as well as periodic patterns, may justify longer cEEG monitoring because of their association with seizures.

III. FURTHER CONSIDERATIONS/REMAINING QUESTIONS

A. The prevalence of seizures in the broad pediatric ICU population with altered mental status remains unknown.

- In particular, the prevalence of seizures among patients who do not routinely undergo cEEG monitoring (eg, those with encephalopathy due to acute respiratory disease or sepsis) requires further study.

B. The impact of NCS and SE on short- and long-term outcomes remains unknown.

- Data on the deleterious effects of NCS are required to justify the considerable resources that must be devoted to cEEG monitoring and to inform treatment decisions.
- How aggressively to treat children with NCS remains controversial and a wide range of approaches are reported by clinicians (8).

C. Further study is required to define which treatment approaches are the most effective at aborting seizures with the fewest side effects.

REFERENCES

1. Jette N, Claassen J, Emerson RG, Hirsch LJ. Frequency and predictors of nonconvulsive seizures during continuous electroencephalographic monitoring in critically ill children. *Arch Neurol.* Dec 2006;63(12):1750–1755.
2. Abend NS, Gutierrez-Colina AM, Topjian AA, et al. Nonconvulsive seizures are common in critically ill children. *Neurology.* Mar 22 2011;76(12):1071–1077.
3. McCoy B, Sharma R, Ochi A, et al. Predictors of nonconvulsive seizures among critically ill children. *Epilepsia.* Nov 2011;52(11):1973–1978.
4. Williams K, Jarrar R, Buchhalter J. Continuous video-EEG monitoring in pediatric intensive care units. *Epilepsia.* Jun 2011;52(6):1130–1136.
5. Clancy RR, Sharif U, Ichord R, et al. Electrographic neonatal seizures after infant heart surgery. *Epilepsia.* Jan 2005;46(1):84–90.
6. Helmers SL, Wypij D, Constantinou JE, et al. Perioperative electroencephalographic seizures in infants undergoing repair of complex congenital cardiac defects. *Electroencephalogr Clin Neurophysiol.* Jan 1997;102(1):27–36.
7. Abend NS, Topjian A, Ichord R, et al. Electroencephalographic monitoring during hypothermia after pediatric cardiac arrest. *Neurology.* Jun 2 2009;72(22):1931–1940.
8. Abend NS, Dlugos DJ, Hahn CD, Hirsch LJ, Herman ST. Use of EEG monitoring and management of nonconvulsive seizures in critically ill patients: A survey of neurologists. *Neurocrit Care.* Jun 2010;12(3):382–389.

SIXTEEN

Special Considerations for Neonatal Patients

Tammy N. Tsuchida

KEY POINTS

- Neonatal EEG monitoring is essential for accurate detection and treatment of seizures.
- Continuous EEG recording or serial routine EEG can be useful for predicting outcomes after injury, particularly hypoxic–ischemic injury.
- Amplitude integrated EEG (aEEG) is a useful adjunctive monitoring tool.
- Neonatal EEGs are typically performed utilizing a reduced montage and different EEG machine settings.
- Video can be useful for distinguishing artifact from seizure.
- The American Clinical Neurophysiology Society has published "Guidelines on Continuous EEG Monitoring in Neonates" which are highly recommended for further reference (see Additional Reading).

I. BACKGROUND

A. EEG Monitoring and Seizures

- Owing to concern that neonatal seizures contribute to cerebral injury, there is a trend toward aggressive seizure management.
- Studies suggest that early treatment of seizures may improve outcome.
- Since most seizures in neonates have no clinical manifestations, continuous EEG provides the most accurate method for seizure detection.
- EEG monitoring also helps avoid treating clinical events that have no EEG correlate.
- Current recommendations are to screen neonates at high risk for seizures with at least 24 hours of EEG monitoring.
- If seizures are detected, EEG recording should be continued until the patient is seizure-free for at least 24 hours.

B. EEG Monitoring and Prognosis
- EEG background patterns are predictive of mortality and neurodevelopmental outcome in premature and full-term (FT) infants with a variety of different diagnoses.
- The ability to prognosticate is affected by the time between brain injury and the EEG recording with serial recordings improving prognostic ability.
- EEG is less predictive of death and neurologic disability in infants with hypoxic–ischemic encephalopathy (HIE) who undergo hypothermia compared to those who do not receive hypothermia.

C. aEEG
- aEEG is a quantitative EEG (QEEG) trend generated from a single channel (usually P3–P4) or two-channel (C3–P3 and C4–P4) EEG recording which is filtered to exclude frequencies beyond 2 to 15 Hz and then displayed on a compressed time scale of 6 hours per page.
- Two-channel aEEG with concurrent raw EEG review has been shown to have a higher rate of seizure detection compared to aEEG review alone.
- aEEG is helpful in predicting outcomes following HIE.
- To ensure the most accurate seizure detection and background interpretation, aEEG interpretation should include analysis of both the QEEG display and raw EEG recording.

II. BASICS

A. EEG and Seizure Detection
- Detection of seizures on EEG is important because neonates with electrographic and electroclinical seizures have worse outcomes (1–3) compared to neonates with clinical seizures and no EEG correlate (4).
- Infants at high risk for seizures include those with HIE, stroke, congenital heart defects requiring surgery, severe respiratory conditions requiring ECMO, CNS trauma, intracranial hemorrhage, inborn errors of metabolism, hydrocephalus, intracranial infection, and preterm (PT) infants with intraventricular hemorrhage or encephalopathy.
- Seizures that occur in FT infants are mostly nonconvulsive (NCS).
- Up to 11% to 30% of FT and PT infants have exclusively subclinical seizures.
- Infants may experience NCS for several hours before they are clinically recognized (5,6).
- Continuous EEG is more sensitive for seizure detection than routine EEG since seizures can be intermittent in infants (7,8).
- Most seizures are detected within 24 hours of instituting EEG monitoring.
- Most infants undergoing hypothermia for suspected HIE have seizure onset within 24 to 48 hours of life (9,10).

B. EEG and Seizure Treatment
- After a seizure medication is initiated, up to 58% of FT and PT infants will experience purely NCS (11).

- Up to 27% of high-risk infants undergoing prolonged EEG recording experience status epilepticus, defined as greater than or equal to 50% of the record containing seizures (7–10,12).
- Certain types of clinical seizures in neonates have no EEG correlate and carry far less risk for adverse outcome than seizures that are electroclinical.
- Since seizure medications may cause neuronal injury in the neonate and older infant, seizures should be confirmed on EEG before exposing these patients to medication (13–15).
- EEG monitoring may be important for improving outcomes.
  - One study compared seizure characteristics and magnetic resonance imaging (MRI) injury for HIE patients treated for clinical or NCS (6).
  - Neonates treated only for clinical seizures had longer seizure duration and Neonates with longer total seizure duration had increased abnormalities seen on MRI.

C. EEG Can Predict Which Patients Will Have Seizures

- Neonates with a normal EEG are less likely to have seizures.
- Infants with focal or frequent sharp-wave discharges on EEG are more likely to have seizures.
- Therefore, initial EEG findings can help determine which neonates are at high risk for seizures and guide how long EEG monitoring should be continued.

D. EEG Background Features Can Predict Outcome in Both FT and PT Infants

- Normal EEG findings are associated with normal outcomes or only mild neurodevelopmental deficits.
- Several EEG features are predictive of poor outcome.
  - Low voltage, burst suppression, or inactivity (16,17)
  - High seizure burden and absent state changes (7)
  - Status epilepticus (18)
- FT infants with HIE (17)
  - A normal or mildly abnormal EEG at 2 to 7 days of life is associated with a normal outcome.
  - EEG patterns that are inactive (<5 μV), low-voltage invariant (≤ 15 μV), or burst suppression at greater than 12 to 24 hours of life are highly associated with death or significant disability.
  - The time between EEG recording and the cerebral insult affect the ability to prognosticate.
    - A normal EEG obtained 24 hours after HIE is more predictive of good outcome than normal EEG findings obtained earlier or after 1 week of age (19–24).
    - An inactive EEG obtained at greater than 12 hours of life is more predictive of poor outcome than an inactive EEG obtained earlier (19,20,24,25).
  - Serial EEG evaluations improve the ability to prognosticate.
    - Less than 24 hours after a cerebral insult, the EEG may be normal or moderately abnormal but can worsen by 24 to 48 hours and exhibit abnormalities associated with poor outcome.
    - In contrast, moderate-to-severe EEG abnormalities can improve over the first 24 to 48 hours and resolve 1 to 2 weeks after an insult (17,23,24,26).

- An inactive EEG within 12 hours of life that normalizes by 24 hours is associated with a good outcome (24,25).
- Infants undergoing hypothermia for HIE.
  - A normal or mildly abnormal EEG in the first 24 hours of life is associated with normal outcome (9,27).
  - An EEG with an inactive or burst suppression pattern obtained in the first 24 hours of life is not always predictive of death or neurologic impairment. However, seeing these same patterns after 24 hours of life are highly predictive of death or neurologic impairment (9,27).

E. aEEG for Seizure Detection
- Single-channel aEEG using bicentral (C3–C4) electrodes has been shown to detect 12% to 38% of seizures (28) while biparietal (P3–P4) aEEG recording has been shown to detect 31% to 54% of seizures (29,30).
- The highest sensitivity for seizure detection using aEEG has been shown using two-channel aEEG (C3–P3, C4–P4) and concurrent review of the raw EEG with detection of 76% of seizures (31).
- Since rhythmic artifact can be mistaken for seizures, the raw EEG should always be reviewed.
- Despite limitations, monitoring with aEEG is better than not being able to detect seizures at all.
  - Infants with seizures detected on aEEG and treated have been shown to have lower rates of developing epilepsy than historical controls (32).
  - In a study evaluating treatment of seizures based on clinical versus aEEG detection, seizure duration was shorter in the aEEG group and shorter seizure duration was associated with less MRI injury (6).

F. aEEG for Prediction of Outcome
- There is good correlation between aEEG and raw EEG for background patterns that are continuous, burst suppressed, or inactive but not for other patterns (30,33,34).
- To have the most accurate assessment of prognosis, serial studies should be obtained at similar times as one would obtain raw EEG recordings.
- Early aEEG is not always the best reflection of injury severity (35).
  - Resolution of abnormal aEEG patterns within 24 hours is associated with a better outcome (36,37).
  - As with raw EEG, hypothermia alters the predictive value of aEEG. Resolution of low voltage, burst suppression, or inactive patterns by 48 hours is associated with better outcomes (38,39).

G. Technical Issues Unique to Neonatal Recording
- Age is critical to proper interpretation of the recording-postmenstrual age (PMA) = gestational age (GA) measured from the time of last menstrual period + chronological age.
- Electrodes
  - Reduced neonatal montage is frequently used (Figure 16.1).
    - Advantage—Using a neonatal montage decreases the duration of manipulation and extent of skin manipulation. This can be especially important in unstable premature infants.

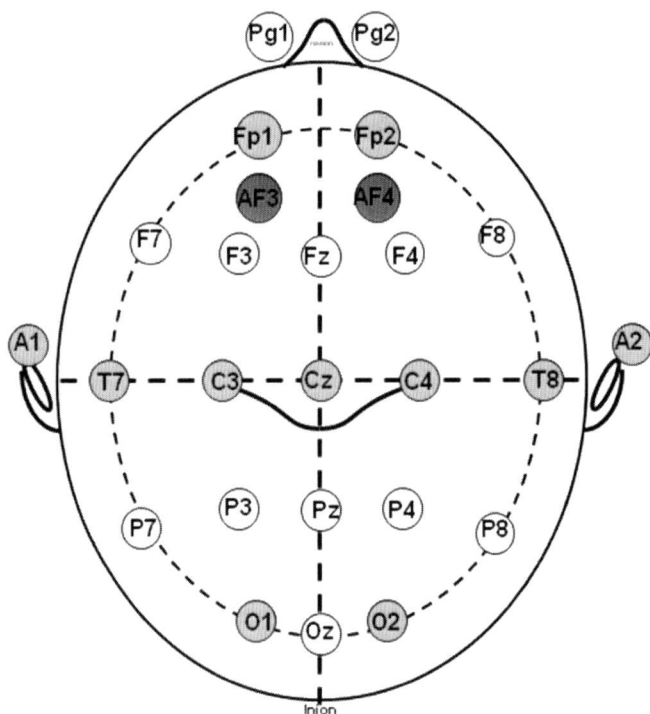

FIGURE 16.1 Scalp electrodes using the 10-10 system. Reduced neonatal electrodes in light gray. The dark gray electrodes (AF3, AF4) are in alternate frontal electrode positions due to the reduced size of the frontal region in some neonates.

- Disadvantage—reduced spatial coverage.
  - For background assessment, the neonatal montage has similar sensitivity and specificity to the full montage.
  - For seizure detection, the neonatal montage has 89% sensitivity for seizure detection compared to the full montage.
- Consider additional electrode placement.
  - Adding P3 and P4 electrodes results in electrode placement that allows a more direct comparison to aEEG recordings.
  - The improved spatial coverage may increase the sensitivity for seizure detection.
  - Noncephalic electrodes
    - EKG is necessary
    - A respiration monitor assists with identification of active and quiet sleep.
    - To perform polysomnography, electrodes for electrooculogram and electromyogram are added to accurately characterize sleep.
- Electrode type
  - Cup electrode is the most common.

- ○ Subdermal (needle or wire) electrodes are used in some European centers.
- ○ MRI and computed tomography (CT)-compatible electrodes are being used in some U.S. centers.
- Electrode application
  - ○ Use a mild abrasive gel to minimize breakdown of delicate skin, especially in premature infants.
  - ○ Impedances as high as 5 to 10 kΩ are tolerated to minimize skin breakdown.
  - ○ Technique to secure electrodes
    - Collodion may not be used due to lack of adequate ventilation.
    - To minimize impedances for as long as possible, place gauze or a cotton ball on top of each cup electrode, then wrap a stretch bandage around the head and wires (grouped in one bundle to minimize the artifact).
- Infant preparation to shorten the time to fall asleep.
  - ○ Have the bedside nurse change the diaper, feed the infant, and position the infant for greatest level of comfort just prior to recording to induce sleep.
- Instrument settings
  - ○ Low-frequency filter 0.3 to 0.6 Hz (time constant 0.27–0.53 second)
  - ○ Sensitivity
    - Typically 7 to 15 μV/mm
    - If low-amplitude recording, 5 μV/mm is useful to detect low-amplitude seizures.
  - ○ Paper speed
    - 15 mm/sec
      - – Often better for seizure detection since many seizures are low frequency.
      - – Can enhance the ability to detect changes in continuity that occur with state changes.
    - 10 mm/sec
      - – May be more helpful for assessing normal background since 15 mm/sec causes background features to have a sharper appearance.
  - ○ Aspect ratio
    - To detect low-amplitude seizures and enhance sharp features in rhythmic activity, have time scale and amplitude proportional to each other.
- Video
  - ○ Use an overhead warmer or heating pad to keep the infant warm while keeping face, head, and extremities visible.
  - ○ It can be more difficult to visualize premature infants since low light levels are preferred to reduce agitation and the isolette may distort the image.

H. Difficulties With Interpretation
- Artifacts can mimic seizure or rhythmic slowing.
  - ○ Be alert for the potential of artifact from chewing or sucking (temporal electrodes) and fontanelle pulsation (vertex electrode).
- EEG interpretation in premature infants.
  - ○ A discontinuous EEG can be normal for a particular CA and state. It is very helpful to refer to an atlas of normal neonatal EEG to determine if the background features are appropriate for age (Figure 16.2A).

(A)

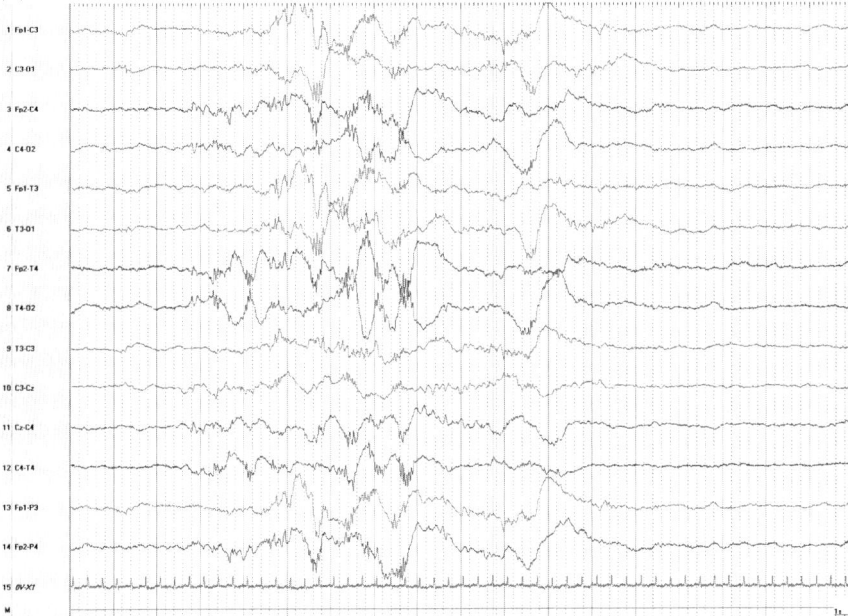

FIGURE 16.2A   A 35-week conceptional age infant in quiet sleep. A normal discontinuous pattern of tracé discontinu with delta brushes in the left occipital and right temporal regions.

- An excessively discontinuous EEG has prolonged interburst intervals and abnormal activity within the bursts such as excessive slowing or sharp activity (Figure 16.2B).
- Burst suppression can be identified by the lack of any normal activity and no change in the background pattern either spontaneously or due to stimulation (reactivity).
- Seizures can be more focal in neonates (single electrode) and have atypical morphology.

III. FURTHER CONSIDERATIONS/REMAINING QUESTIONS

A. Cost-effective electrode sets that are MRI and CT compatible and can be rapidly applied by ICU staff would enable early EEG monitoring for seizure detection and background assessment.

B. More studies are needed to determine whether intermediate degrees of EEG abnormalities can accurately predict outcomes after neonatal hypoxia–ischemia or seizures.

(B)

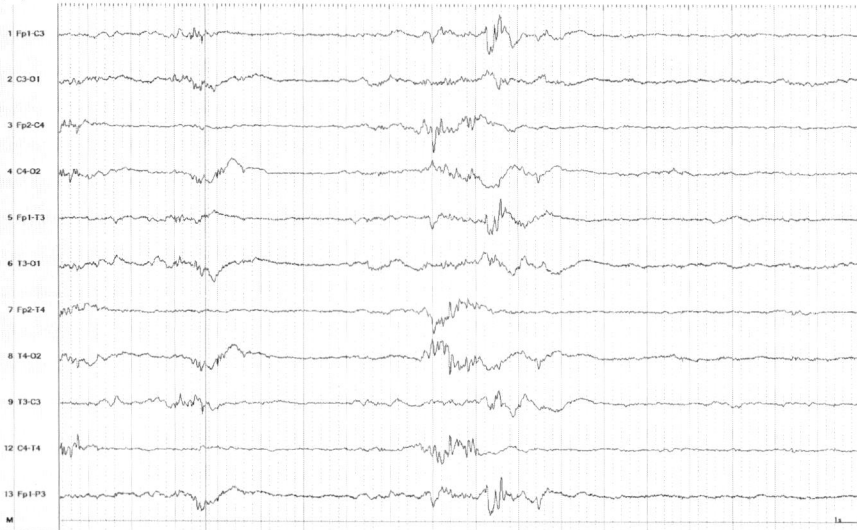

FIGURE 16.2B A 34-week conceptional age infant with tuberous sclerosis. A mildly abnormal tracing that is excessively discontinuous. On the left, activity is decreased in amplitude. This page also demonstrates a decrease in complexity.

C. Better resource utilization is needed.
- Are there ways to direct EEG resources to those infants at highest risk for seizures?
- Are there EEG features that predict who is more likely to have a seizure?
- Does EEG detection of seizures change management compared to aEEG detection of seizures?
- Are serial EEGs adequate for treating seizures?
- Does the use of EEG monitoring to treat seizures and monitor for significant background changes result in improved outcomes?

D. Standardized background and seizure terminology is needed to facilitate multicenter collaboration.

REFERENCES

1. Legido A, Clancy RR, Berman PH. Neurologic outcome after electroencephalographically proven neonatal seizures. *Pediatrics.* Sep 1991;88(3):583–596.
2. Boylan GB, Pressler RM, Rennie JM, et al. Outcome of electroclinical, electrographic, and clinical seizures in the newborn infant. *Dev Med Child Neurol.* Dec 1999;41(12):819–825.
3. Bye AM, Cunningham CA, Chee KY, Flanagan D. Outcome of neonates with electrographically identified seizures, or at risk of seizures. *Pediatr Neurol.* Apr 1997;16(3):225–231.

4. Holden KR, Mellits ED, Freeman JM, Neonatal seizures I. Correlation of prenatal and perinatal events with outcomes. *Pediatrics.* Aug 1982;70(2):165–176.

5. Helmers SL, Wypij D, Constantinou JE, et al. Perioperative electroencephalographic seizures in infants undergoing repair of complex congenital cardiac defects. *Electroencephalogr Clin Neurophysiol.* Jan 1997;102(1):27–36.

6. van Rooij LG, Toet MC, van Huffelen AC, et al. Effect of treatment of subclinical neonatal seizures detected with aEEG: Randomized, controlled trial. *Pediatrics.* Feb 2010;125(2): e358–e366.

7. McBride MC, Laroia N, Guillet R. Electrographic seizures in neonates correlate with poor neurodevelopmental outcome. *Neurology.* Aug 2000;55(4):506–513.

8. Bye AM, Flanagan D. Spatial and temporal characteristics of neonatal seizures. *Epilepsia.* Oct 1995;36(10):1009–1016.

9. Nash KB, Bonifacio SL, Glass HC, et al. Video-EEG monitoring in newborns with hypoxic–ischemic encephalopathy treated with hypothermia. *Neurology.* Feb 8 2011;76(6):556–562.

10. Wusthoff CJ, Dlugos DJ, Gutierrez-Colina A, et al. Electrographic seizures during therapeutic hypothermia for neonatal hypoxic–ischemic encephalopathy. *J Child Neurol.* Jun 2011;26(6):724–728.

11. Scher MS, Alvin J, Gaus L, Minnigh B, Painter MJ. Uncoupling of EEG-clinical neonatal seizures after antiepileptic drug use. *Pediatr Neurol.* Apr 2003;28(4):277–280.

12. Low E, Boylan GB, Mathieson SR, et al. Cooling and seizure burden in term neonates: An observational study. *Arch Dis Child Fetal Neonatal Ed.* 2012; Published Online First: 23 January 2012.

13. Bittigau P, Sifringer M, Genz K, et al. Antiepileptic drugs and apoptotic neurodegeneration in the developing brain. *Proc Natl Acad Sci USA.* Nov 12, 2002;99(23):15089–15094.

14. Glier C, Dzietko M, Bittigau P, et al. Therapeutic doses of topiramate are not toxic to the developing rat brain. *Exp Neurol.* Jun 2004;187(2):403–409.

15. Manthey D, Asimiadou S, Stefovska V, et al. Sulthiame but not levetiracetam exerts neurotoxic effect in the developing rat brain. *Exp Neurol.* Jun 2005;193(2):497–503.

16. Tharp BR, Cukier F, Monod N. The prognostic value of the electroencephalogram in premature infants. *Electroencephalogr Clin Neurophysiol.* Mar 1981;51(3):219–236.

17. Holmes GL, Lombroso CT. Prognostic value of background patterns in the neonatal EEG. *J Clin Neurophysiol.* Jul 1993;10(3):323–352.

18. Pisani F, Cerminara C, Fusco C, Sisti L. Neonatal status epilepticus vs recurrent neonatal seizures: Clinical findings and outcome. *Neurology.* Dec 4 2007;69(23): 2177–2185.

19. Tharp B. Use of the electroencephalogram in assessing acute brain damage in the newborn. In: DK Stevenson, P Sunshine, eds. *Fetal and neonatal brain injury: Mechanisms, management and the risks of practice.* New York: Oxford University Press; 1997:287–301.

20. Pezzani C, Radvanyi-Bouvet MF, Relier JP, Monod N. Neonatal electroencephalography during the first twenty-four hours of life in full-term newborn infants. *Neuropediatrics.* Feb 1986;17(1):11–18.

21. Watanabe K, Miyazaki S, Hara K, Hakamada S. Behavioral state cycles, background EEGs and prognosis of newborns with perinatal hypoxia. *Electroencephalogr Clin Neurophysiol.* Sep 1980;49(5–6):618–625.

22. Monod N, Pajot N, Guidasci S. The neonatal EEG: Statistical studies and prognostic value in full-term and pre-term babies. *Electroencephalogr Clin Neurophysiol.* May 1972; 32(5):529–544.

23. Takeuchi T, Watanabe K. The EEG evolution and neurological prognosis of neonates with perinatal hypoxia [corrected]. *Brain Dev.* 1989;11(2):115–120.

24. Murray DM, Boylan GB, Ryan CA, Connolly S. Early EEG findings in hypoxic-ischemic encephalopathy predict outcomes at 2 years. *Pediatrics.* Sep 2009;124(3): e459–467.

25. Pressler RM, Boylan GB, Morton M, et al. Early serial EEG in hypoxic ischaemic encephalopathy. *Clin Neurophysiol.* Jan 2001;112(1):31–37.
26. Sarnat HB, Sarnat MS. Neonatal encephalopathy following fetal distress. A clinical and electroencephalographic study. *Arch Neurol.* Oct 1976;33(10):696–705.
27. Hamelin S, Delnard N, Cneude F, Debillon T, Vercueil L. Influence of hypothermia on the prognostic value of early EEG in full-term neonates with hypoxic ischemic encephalopathy. *Neurophysiol Clin.* Feb 2010;41(1):19–27.
28. Shellhaas RA, Soaita AI, Clancy RR. Sensitivity of amplitude-integrated electroencephalography for neonatal seizure detection. *Pediatrics.* Oct 2007;120(4):770–777.
29. Rennie JM, Chorley G, Boylan GB, et al. Non-expert use of the cerebral function monitor for neonatal seizure detection. *Arch Dis Child Fetal Neonatal Ed.* Jan 2004;89(1):F37–40.
30. Hellstrom-Westas L. Comparison between tape-recorded and amplitude-integrated EEG monitoring in sick newborn infants. *Acta Paediatr.* Oct 1992;81(10):812–819.
31. Shah DK, Mackay MT, Lavery S, et al. Accuracy of bedside electroencephalographic monitoring in comparison with simultaneous continuous conventional electroencephalography for seizure detection in term infants. *Pediatrics.* Jun 2008;121(6):1146–1154.
32. Toet MC, Groenendaal F, Osredkar D, et al. Postneonatal epilepsy following amplitude-integrated EEG-detected neonatal seizures. *Pediatr Neurol.* Apr 2005;32(4): 241–247.
33. Toet MC, van der Meij W, de Vries LS, et al. Comparison between simultaneously recorded amplitude integrated electroencephalogram (cerebral function monitor) and standard electroencephalogram in neonates. *Pediatrics.* May 2002;109(5):772–779.
34. Clancy RR, Dicker L, Cho S, et al. Agreement between long-term neonatal background classification by conventional and amplitude-integrated EEG. *J Clin Neurophysiol.* Feb 2011;28(1):1–9.
35. Sarkar S, Barks JD, Donn SM. Should amplitude-integrated electroencephalography be used to identify infants suitable for hypothermic neuroprotection? *J Perinatol.* Feb 2008;28(2):117–122.
36. ter Horst HJ, Sommer C, Bergman KA, et al. Prognostic significance of amplitude-integrated EEG during the first 72 hours after birth in severely asphyxiated neonates. *Pediatr Res.* Jun 2004;55(6):1026–1033.
37. van Rooij LG, Toet MC, Osredkar D, et al. Recovery of amplitude integrated electroencephalographic background patterns within 24 hours of perinatal asphyxia. *Arch Dis Child Fetal Neonatal Ed.* May 2005;90(3):F245–F251.
38. Hallberg B, Grossmann K, Bartocci M, Blennow M. The prognostic value of early aEEG in asphyxiated infants undergoing systemic hypothermia treatment. *Acta Paediatr.* Apr 2010;99(4):531–536.
39. Thoresen M, Hellstrom-Westas L, Liu X, de Vries LS. Effect of hypothermia on amplitude-integrated electroencephalogram in infants with asphyxia. *Pediatrics.* Jul 2010;126(1):e131–e139.

ADDITIONAL READING

Shellhaas RA, et al. The American Clinical Neurophysiology Society's guideline on continuous electroencephalography monitoring in neonates. *J Clin Neurophysiol.* 2011;28(6): 611–617.
Clancy RR. Prolonged electroencephalogram monitoring for seizures and their treatment. *Clin Perinatol.* 2006;33(3):649–665.
Andre M, et al. Electroencephalography in premature and full-term infants. Developmental features and glossary. *Neurophysiol Clin* 2010;40(2):59–124.

SEVENTEEN

Standardized Critical Care EEG Terminology

Elizabeth Gerard

KEY POINTS

- Critical care EEG monitoring terminology was developed by the American Clinical Neurophysiology Society (ACNS) to standardize the description of rhythmic, periodic, and fluctuating patterns commonly encountered in the critically ill.
- The core nomenclature of the ACNS terminology includes two discrete main terms to describe the location and morphology of each pattern.
- **Main Term 1** describes the location of each pattern as Generalized, Lateralized, Bilateral-Independent (BI), or Multifocal (Mf). **Main Term 2** describes the morphology of each pattern as Periodic Discharges (PDs), Rhythmic Delta Activity (RDA), or Spike-wave (SW).
- Additional modifiers include descriptions of frequency, amplitude, persistence, duration, and polarity.
- Two studies have demonstrated that Main Terms 1 and 2 achieve good-to-excellent inter-rater reliability and modifiers of frequency and amplitude have moderate-to-good reliability. Further refinement of the terminology is still in process in order to optimize utility of some of the minor modifiers.

I. BACKGROUND

A. History
- In 2005, the Subcommittee on Research Terminology for continuous EEG monitoring of the ACNS proposed standardized terminology for EEG patterns frequently encountered in critically ill patients (1).
- The ACNS terminology has undergone several modifications since the original publication and is still being optimized for use (2). The terminology has been critically reviewed in two studies of inter-rater reliability (3,4).
- Although the terminology was originally developed for research purposes, it is now commonly used for clinical purposes at many academic medical centers utilizing continuous EEG (cEEG).

B. Rationale
- cEEG monitoring is an important tool for assessing neurologic function and is becoming the standard of care in many intensive care units (ICUs).
- There is no consensus on the EEG terms used to describe the many periodic and rhythmic patterns frequently seen in critically ill patients and which patterns are associated with neuronal injury and may require treatment.
- Many of the terms commonly used to describe EEG patterns in the critically ill carry clinical connotations that have not been validated, including the term "generalized periodic epileptiform discharges (GPEDs)" which implies that the pattern is epileptiform, and the term "triphasic waves" which typically implies a toxic or metabolic etiology.
- One of the main goals of the ACNS terminology is to create an objective EEG classification scheme using descriptive terms that are not biased regarding the clinical significance of a given pattern.
  - For example, under the ACNS terminology, the terms GPEDs (Generalized Periodic *Epileptiform* Discharges) and PLEDs (Periodic Lateralized *Epileptiform* Discharges) would be replaced by the terms GPDs (Generalized Periodic Discharges) and LPDs (Lateralized Periodic Discharges).
- The ACNS committee recognized that research regarding the clinical significance of these EEG patterns requires standardized terminology to allow for systematic, multicenter clinical trials, and for comparison of results between centers.

C. Concepts and Organization
- The terminology is designed to describe patterns of uncertain significance and specifically excludes patterns that most electroencephalographers consider as definite electrographic seizures.
- Therefore, the terminology excludes:
  - Generalized SW/sharp wave greater than or equal to 3 per second
  - Evolving discharges that reach greater than 4 per second
- However, the terminology does include some patterns that meet criteria for electrographic seizures based on evolution in field, morphology, or frequency, as long as the maximum frequency is less than 4 Hz. Generalized SW discharges at frequencies less than 3 Hz are also included.
- The terminology includes any rhythmic or periodic pattern that continues for at least six cycles (eg, 1 per second for 6 seconds, or 3 per second for 2 seconds).
- All patterns described by the terminology are assigned two main terms.
- Several modifiers also can be applied.

II. BASICS (TABLE 17.1)

A. Main Terms
- Main Term 1: The location of a given pattern. Each pattern should be assigned only one of the following terms:
  - Generalized (G)—any bilateral, symmetric, and synchronous pattern. The pattern may be frontally, midline or occipitally predominant but cannot be asymmetric.

TABLE 17.1 Main Terms and Some of the Modifiers Included in the ACNS Critical Care EEG Monitoring Research Terminology

TERM #1	TERM #2	PLUS MODIFIERS (ADD ONLY IF PRESENT WITH PATTERN AND NOT IN BACKGROUND)	
Generalized (G)	Periodic Discharges (PDs)	+ F	Superimposed FAST activity; use with PDs or RDA only
		+ R	Superimposed RHYTHMIC activity; use with PDs only
Lateralized (L)		+ FR	Use for PDs if both subtypes apply
	Rhythmic Delta Activity (RDA)	+ F	Superimposed FAST activity; use with PDs or RDA only
Bilateral Independent (BI)		+ S	Superimposed SHARP waves or Spikes; use with RDA only
		+ FS	Use for RDA if both subtypes apply
Multifocal (Mf)	Spike Wave (SW)	No + modifiers	

ADDITIONAL MODIFIERS

Prevalence (% of record)	Rare less than 1%	Occasional 1%–9%	Frequent 10%–49%	Abundant 50%–89%	Continuous ≥ 90%				
Duration	Very Brief < 10 seconds	Brief 10–59 seconds	Intermediate 1–4.9 min	Long 5–59 min	Very Long ≥1 hour				
Frequency: (cycles/sec)	< 0.5	0.5	1	1.5	2	2.5	3	3.5	≥4
Sharpness	Blunt	Sharply contoured	Sharp, 70–200 msec	Spiky, < 70 msec					
Polarity	Positive	Negative	Dipole, horizontal/ tangential	Unclear					
Absolute amplitude	Very Low, < 20 µV	Low, 20–49 µV	Medium, 50–199 µV	High, > 200 µV					
Stimulus induced	Stimulus induced (SI-)	Spontaneous (Sp-)	Unknown						

ACNS Standardized Critical Care EEG Terminology. Abbreviated version.

- ○ Lateralized (L)—unilateral hemispheric or focal patterns. This also includes patterns seen synchronously over both hemispheres but clearly more prominent on one side (bilateral asymmetric).
  - ○ BI—asynchronous hemispheric or focal patterns occurring independently over both hemispheres.
  - ○ Mf—patterns occurring in at least three discrete brain regions and involving both hemispheres (rare).
- Main Term 2: The morphology of the pattern or pattern type. Each pattern should have only one of the following terms applied (Figure 17.1):
  - ○ Periodic Discharges (PDs)
    - • Repeating waveforms or discharges with relatively uniform morphology and occurring at nearly regular intervals.
    - • Applies only to single discharges lasting less than 0.5 second and not bursts.
    - • Quantifiable interval between waveforms.
    - • Intervals in between discharges have less than 50% variation from one cycle to the next.
  - ○ Rhythmic Delta Activity (RDA)
    - • Repetition of a waveform with relatively uniform morphology and duration.
    - • No interval between consecutive waveforms.
  - ○ Spike Wave (SW)
    - • Spike or sharp wave consistently followed by a slow wave.
    - • Regularly repeating pattern (SW-SW-SW).
    - • Consistent relationship between the spike/sharp component and the slow wave.
- Each pattern is described by a combination of the most appropriate choice from Main Terms 1 and 2 (see Table 17.1). Examples:
  - ○ Lateralized Periodic Discharges (LPDs) (Figure 17.2)
  - ○ Generalized Periodic Discharges (GPDs) (Figure 17.3)
  - ○ Generalized Spike Wave (GSW) (Figure 17.4)
  - ○ Additional localizing information

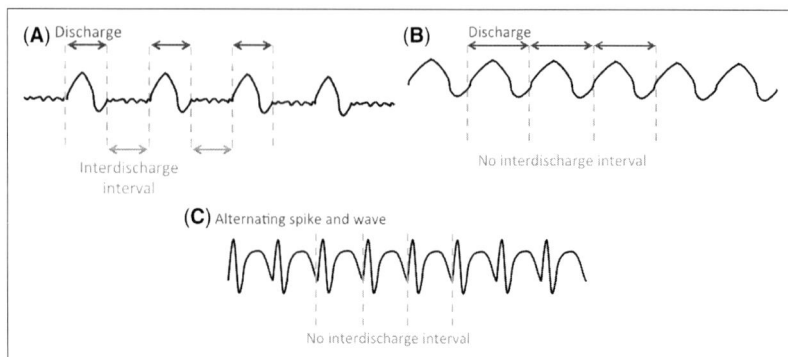

FIGURE 17.1 (A) Periodic discharges, (B) rhythmic delta activity, and (C) spike-wave.

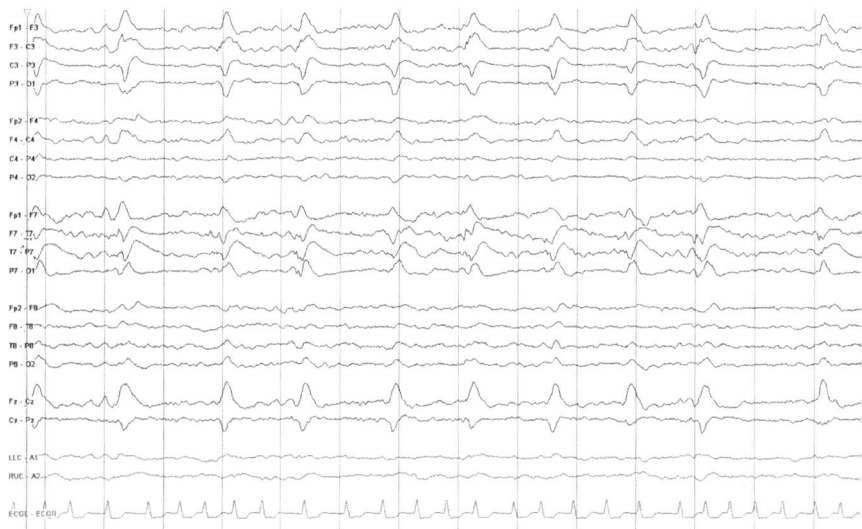

FIGURE 17.2   Lateralized periodic discharges (LPDs). Reproduced with permission of Lawrence J. Hirsch MD and Richard Brenner MD.

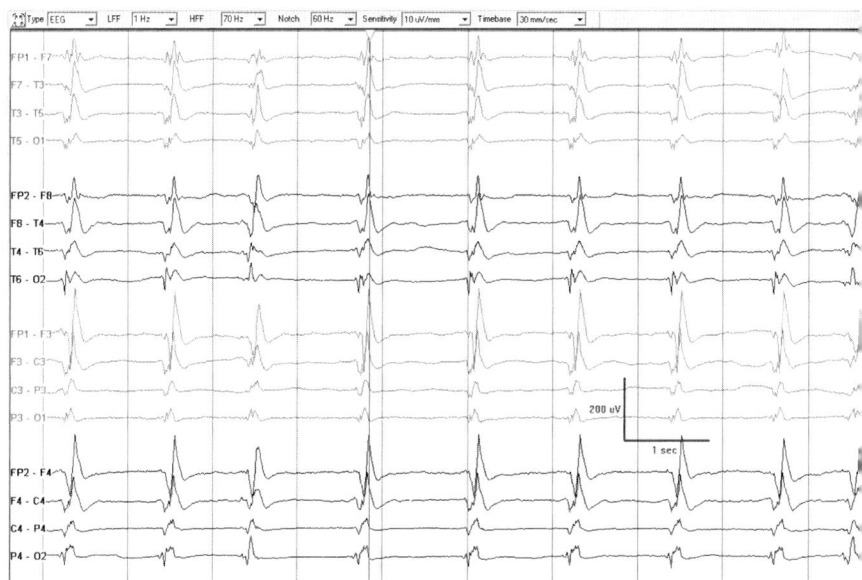

FIGURE 17.3   Generalized periodic discharges (GPDs). Reproduced with permission of Lawrence J. Hirsch MD and Richard Brenner MD.

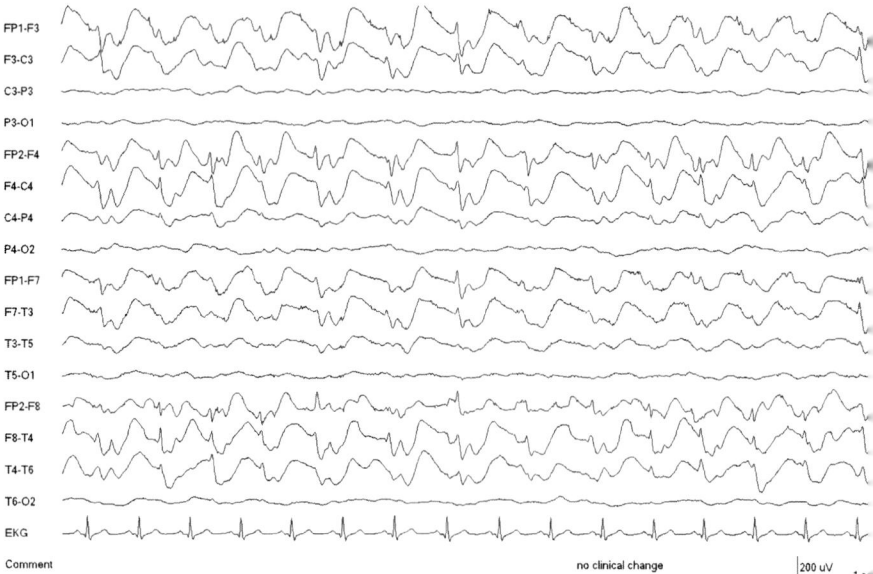

FIGURE 17.4 Generalized spike-wave (GSW). Reproduced with permission of Lawrence J. Hirsch MD and Richard Brenner MD.

- For G: Specify frontally, midline or occipitally predominant, versus "generalized, not otherwise specified."
- For L, BI, or Mf: Specify lobe(s) involved : Frontal (F), Parietal (P), Temporal (T), or Occipital (O).

B. Modifiers

- These provide further descriptive information and can be added to Main Terms 1 and 2. These include Frequency, Amplitude, Prevalence, Duration, Sharpness, Polarity, Stimulus-induced and the Plus (+) modifiers (Table 17.1).
- Frequency refers to the typical rate of repetition of a given pattern and should be categorized as: less than 0.5 per second, 0.5 per second, 1 per second, 1.5 per second, and so on, up to 4 per second.
- Amplitude refers to the absolute height of a pattern and should be measured in standard longitudinal bipolar 10–20 montage in the channel in which it is best seen, from peak to trough (ie, positive peak to negative peak; not peak to baseline).
  - ○ Very low = <20 μV
  - ○ Low = 20–49 μV
  - ○ Medium = 50–199 μV
  - ○ High = >200 μV
  - ○ For PDs, this refers to the highest amplitude component. For SW, this refers to the spike/sharp wave.

- Prevalence refers to percent of the record occupied by a pattern and should be categorized as:
  - Continuous = greater than 90% of record/epoch
  - Abundant = 50–89% of record/epoch
  - Frequent = 10–49% of record/epoch
  - Occasional = 1–9% of record/epoch
  - Rare = <1% of record/epoch
- Duration refers to the typical duration of a single occurrence of the pattern, regardless of whether the pattern occurs rarely or frequently.
  - Very long = >1 hour
  - Long = 5–59 minute
  - Intermediate = 1–4.9 minute
  - Brief = 10–59 seconds
  - Very brief = <10 seconds
- Sharpness (applies to PDs and SW only, not RDA)
  - Spiky = <70 msec
  - Sharp = 70–200 msec
  - Sharply contoured—used for theta or delta waves that are greater than 200 msec but have a sharp wave morphology (steep slope to one side of the wave).
  - Blunt
- Polarity of the predominant phase (applies to PDs and SW, not RDA).
  - Positive—downward deflection in referential montage
  - Negative—upward deflection in referential montage
  - Dipole (horizontal/tangential)
  - Unclear
- Stimulus Induced: Patterns that are reproducibly brought on by an alerting stimulus
  - Example: RDA that appears following stimulation by suctioning would be called SI-RDA (Figure 17.5).
- Evolving or Fluctuating: Patterns that change over time
  - Evolving: at least 2 unequivocal, sequential changes in frequency, morphology, or location.
  - Fluctuating: greater than or equal to 3 changes, not more than 1 minute apart, in frequency (by at least 0.5 per second), greater than or equal to 3 changes in morphology, or greater than or equal to 3 changes in location (by at least 1 standard inter-electrode distance), but *not qualifying as evolving*.
- Plus (+) Modifiers
  - The plus modifiers were designed to distinguish patterns that appear more ictal in morphology and may be associated more closely with seizures.
  - They include the following features that can be superimposed upon PDs or RDA (not used with SW).
    - +F (fast activity),+R (rhythmic activity), and +FR when they are present in combination can be added to the description of PDs.
    - +F (fast activity), +S (sharp, spike activity, or sharply contoured activity), or +FS when they are present in combination can be added to the description of RDA.

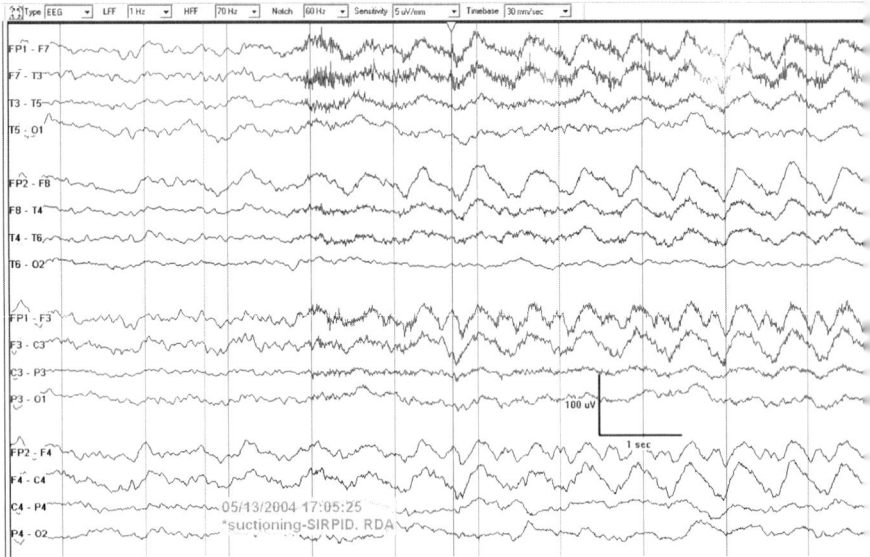

FIGURE 17.5 Stimulus-induced generalized rhythmic delta activity (SI-GRDA). In this case, the GRDA pattern was elicited by suctioning. Reproduced with permission of Lawrence J. Hirsch MD and Richard Brenner MD.

- Example: LPDs associated with high-frequency activity seen only in association with the LPDs and not in the background EEG would be called LPDs +F (Figure 17.6).
- Example: LRDA associated with superimposed sharply contoured activity would be called LRDA+S (Figure 17.7).

III. FURTHER CONSIDERATIONS/REMAINING QUESTIONS

A. What is the prognostic significance of periodic and rhythmic patterns encountered in the critically ill?
- Clarification is needed regarding which patterns and which clinical scenarios are associated with ongoing neuronal injury, in order to determine which require treatment and how aggressive.
- Large-scale multicenter studies are needed to achieve better understanding of these indeterminant patterns encountered in the critically ill.

B. What is the inter-rater reliability of the ACNS research terminology?
- In a single-center study, five board-certified readers evaluated the reliability of the ACNS terminology proposed in 2005 (3).
  - There was moderate inter-rater agreement (kappa = 0.49) for Main Term 1 and fair agreement for Main Term 2 (kappa = 0.39).

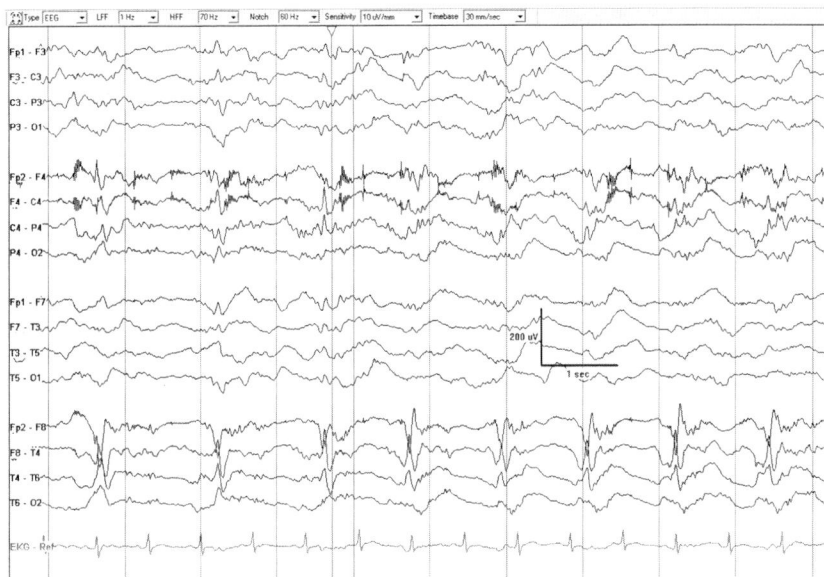

FIGURE 17.6   Lateralized periodic discharges plus fast activity (LPDs + F). Reproduced with permission of Lawrence J. Hirsch MD and Richard Brenner MD.

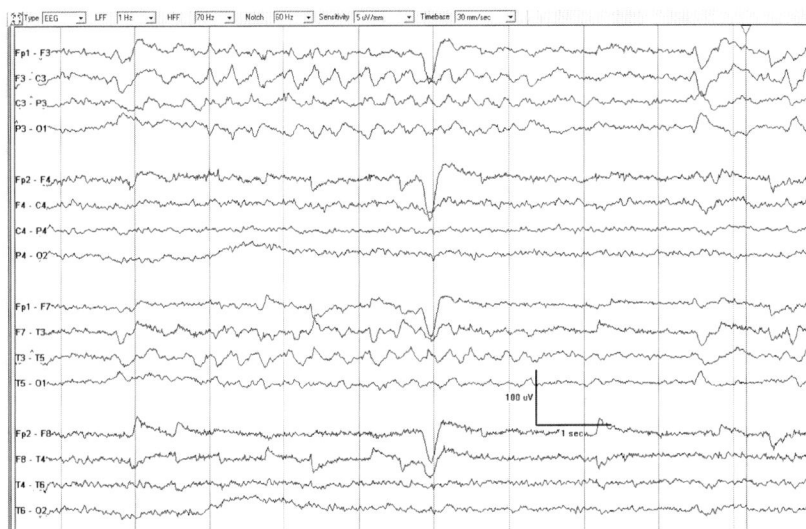

FIGURE 17.7   Lateralized rhythmic delta activity plus sharp activity (LRDA + S). Reproduced with permission of Lawrence J. Hirsch MD and Richard Brenner MD.

- ○ There was poor-to-fair agreement for modifiers.
- ○ Since this study, the ACNS terminology has been revised multiple times, and an online training module with certification test was created.
- • A recent multicenter study (4) evaluated the performance of 16 members of the Critical Care EEG Monitoring Research Consortium after utilizing the online training module. Test questions consisted of 10 seconds EEG samples.
  - ○ Main Terms 1 and 2 achieved "almost perfect" agreement (kappa values of 0.87 and 0.92, respectively).
  - ○ The modifier of amplitude showed good reliability, whereas frequency had moderate-to-fair reliability.
  - ○ For "plus +" modifiers there was considerable variability in inter-rater agreement: fast (+F) and rhythmic (+R) modifiers demonstrated moderate agreement while sharp/spike (+S) modifier showed only slight agreement.

C. What is the current status of the ACNS research terminology?

- • Studies suggest that Main Terms 1 and 2 of the ACNS research terminology are easy to use and achieve high inter-rater reliability, particularly when raters have been trained in their use. Modifiers of frequency and amplitude achieve moderate-to-good inter-rater agreement.
- • Future research must clarify whether some of the additional modifiers can achieve reasonable inter-rater reliability in order to be of practical use for research or clinical purposes.
- • Further research is also necessary to evaluate inter- and intra-rater reliability of prolonged EEG recordings as opposed to 10 seconds samples.

REFERENCES

1. Hirsch LJ, Brenner RP, Drislane FW, et al. The ACNS subcommittee on research terminology for continuous EEG monitoring: Proposed standardized terminology for rhythmic and periodic EEG patterns encountered in critically ill patients. *J Clin Neurophysiol.* 2005;22:128–135.
2. ACNS standardized research terminology and categorization for the investigation of rhythmic and periodic patterns encountered in critically ill patients: July 2009 version. In: LJ Hirsch and RP Brenner eds. *Atlas of EEG in Critical Care.* West Sussex: Wiley-Blackwell, 2010;315–321.
3. Gerber PA, Chapman KE, Chung SS, et al. Interobserver agreement in the interpretation of EEG patterns in critically ill adults. *J Clin Neurophysiol.* 2008;25:241–249.
4. Mani R, Arif H, Hirsch L, et al. Inter-rater reliability of ICU EEG research terminology. *J Clin Neurophysiol.* In Press.
5. Hirsch LJ, LaRoche SM, Gaspard N, et al. American Clinical Neurophysiology Society's standardized critical care EEG terminology. *J Clin Neurophysiol.* In Press.

EIGHTEEN

Encephalopathy and Coma

Daniel Friedman

KEY POINTS

- EEG in patients with altered levels of arousal can be used to assess depth of coma, provide prognostic information, and exclude nonconvulsive seizures.
- EEG patterns in encephalopathy and coma are often nonspecific, but some features can be suggestive of underlying etiology.
- Reactivity and spontaneous variability should be assessed during the EEG recording of all comatose patients.
- Continuous EEG monitoring is useful for determining the evolution of coma patterns and can provide useful prognostic information.

I. BACKGROUND

A. Alteration of consciousness occurs on a continuum (1).
- Delirium/mild encephalopathy
  - Patients may be agitated, confused, inattentive, drowsy, and/or have perceptual problems and hallucinations.
- Stupor/obtundation
  - Patients have a depressed level of consciousness but are arousable to vigorous stimulation and can interact with the environment in some way (follow simple commands).
- Coma
  - Patients are unresponsive with eyes closed; they do not respond appropriately to external stimuli. In lighter stages of coma, some evidence of processing of external stimuli can be seen such as withdrawal or grimace to pain.

B. Decreased levels of consciousness are due to dysfunction of cerebral hemispheres and/or the diencephalon or brainstem.

C. Etiologies may include a variety of primary brain disorders.
- Diffuse cerebral injury from trauma
- Anoxia/hypoxia

- Encephalitis/meningitis
- Structural lesions or ischemia involving the brainstem, thalamus, or both hemispheres.
- Insults that exert mass effect and raise intracranial pressure.

D. Systemic etiologies may include
- Systemic infection/sepsis
- Renal dysfunction
- Hepatic dysfunction
- Electrolyte abnormalities (especially sodium and calcium)
- Hyper- or hypoglycemia
- Endocrine dysfunction
- Nutritional deficiencies
- CNS toxins
- Hypercarbia

E. Continuous EEG monitoring can be used for a variety of purposes outside of the detection of electrographic seizures.
- Help determine the etiology of altered levels of consciousness
- Assess for changes in levels of cerebral dysfunction over time
- Provide prognostic information
- Help differentiate coma from other states of unresponsiveness:
  - Patients with the following causes of unresponsiveness will demonstrate a preserved and reactive posterior dominant rhythm.
    - Catatonia
    - Psychogenic coma
    - "Locked-in" syndrome secondary to ventral pontine lesions that spare arousal systems but disrupt descending motor systems.

II. BASICS

A. EEG typically demonstrates progressive slowing as the level of consciousness decreases. However, the EEG and clinical state are not always correlated (1, 2).
- Mild encephalopathy
  - Slowing of the posterior dominant rhythm to less than or equal to 8 Hz, diffuse theta activity, occasional delta activity.
- Moderate encephalopathy
  - Loss of posterior dominant rhythm, diffuse delta slowing but reactivity and state changes are still present.
- Severe encephalopathy
  - Predominantly delta: may be admixed with faster frequencies, variable periods of diffuse background attenuation, absence of reactivity, and state changes.
- Electrocerebral inactivity (ECI)
  - Absence of EEG activity greater than 2 μV
  - Typically signifies brain death when the appropriate technical standards for EEG recording are met including normothermia and the absence of sedative medications.

○ ECI can be seen in cases of anesthetic/sedative intoxication or severe hypothermia.

B. Technical Aspects of Recording
- Recordings in comatose patients should include stimulation by the technologist to test for reactivity.
- Stimulation should be graded.
  ○ Start with auditory stimulation, calling patient's name.
  ○ Progress to more noxious stimulation if no response is seen: cotton-tip applicator in patient's nose or nail bed pressure.
- Recordings should also include quiet periods where there is no stimulation to assess for spontaneous variability.
- In cases where ECI is suspected, efforts should be made to limit electrical and extracerebral artifacts arising from ICU equipment such as monitors, IV pumps, and respirators.

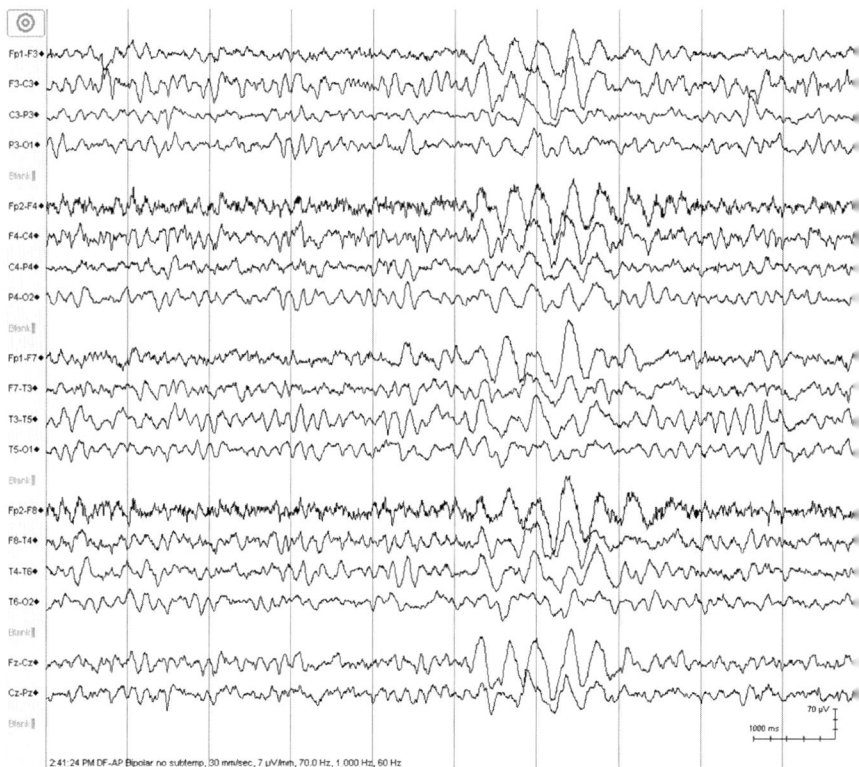

FIGURE 18.1 Frontal intermittent rhythmic delta activity (FIRDA) in a 52-year-old woman with sepsis and altered mental status.

C. Specific EEG Patterns in Encephalopathy and Coma (9)

- Intermittent rhythmic delta activity (IRDA)
  - 2 to 3 Hz bisynchronous, monomorphic activity
    - Frontally predominant (FIRDA) typically seen in adults (Figure 18.1)
    - Occipitally predominant (OIRDA) more commonly seen in children
  - IRDA in a generalized distribution (GIRDA) is a nonspecific pattern commonly seen in comatose patients.
  - IRDA is most commonly seen in toxic/metabolic encephalopathy but can also represent subcortical and cortical structural lesions, or hydrocephalus.
  - OIRDA can also be seen in idiopathic generalized epilepsies.
- Triphasic waves (Figure 18.2)
  - Moderately high-amplitude, typically frontally predominant generalized discharges.
  - Morphology consists of a brief, low-amplitude negative phase then a longer duration positive phase which usually has the highest amplitude followed by a final negative phase that is most often the phase of the longest duration.
  - An anterior–posterior "lag" can be seen in many cases.
  - Often repeat in a periodic fashion and considered by many to be a "subset" of generalized periodic discharges (GPDs) but also may occur in runs of 1.5 to 2.5 Hz.

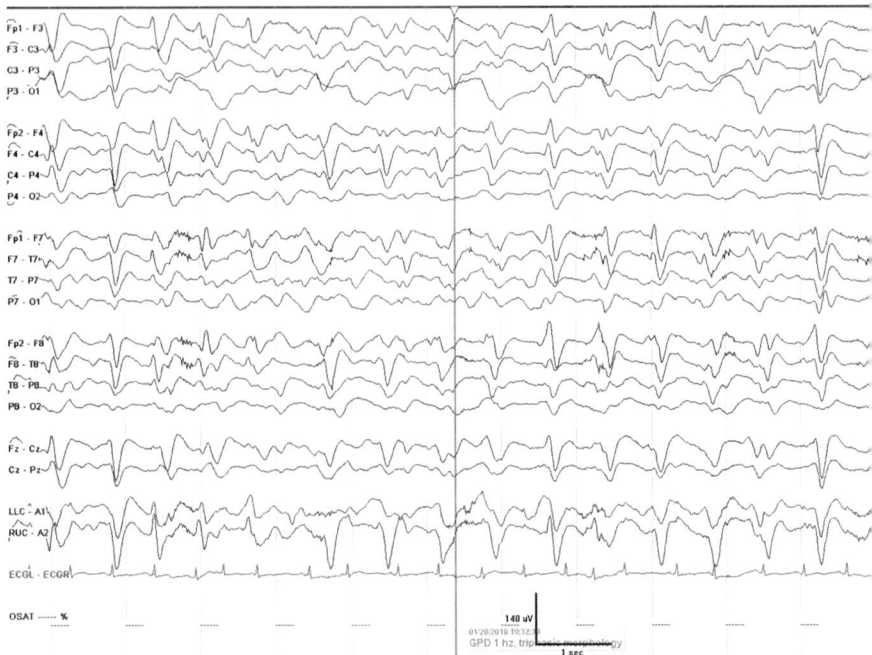

FIGURE 18.2   Triphasic waves in a 62-year-old man with coma and renal failure.

- ○ According to ACNS Critical Care EEG terminology, this pattern would typically be described as periodic discharges with additional modifier of "triphasic morphology".
- ○ Typically seen with toxic or metabolic encephalopathies such as hepatic and uremic encephalopathy, sepsis, hypercalcemia, or hyperosmolarity, but have also been associated with seizures.
- ○ In some cases, may be difficult to reliably distinguish from epileptiform patterns.
- Low-voltage, slow, nonreactive EEG
  - ○ Theta and delta activity less than 20 μV that is invariant to stimulation
  - ○ Often seen with diffuse cortical and subcortical injury such as traumatic brain injury or anoxia
  - ○ Can also be seen in severe hypothyroidism
- Excess beta frequency activity (8)
  - ○ Often seen in encephalopathies due to benzodiazepine or barbiturate ingestion as well as patients on anesthetic/sedative medications such as midazolam or propofol
- Spindle coma (Figure 18.3) (3)
  - ○ Predominantly less than 8 Hz, low-voltage background with bursts of symmetric 11 to 14 Hz spindle-like discharges.
  - ○ Other sleep transients also can be seen (K complex, vertex waves).

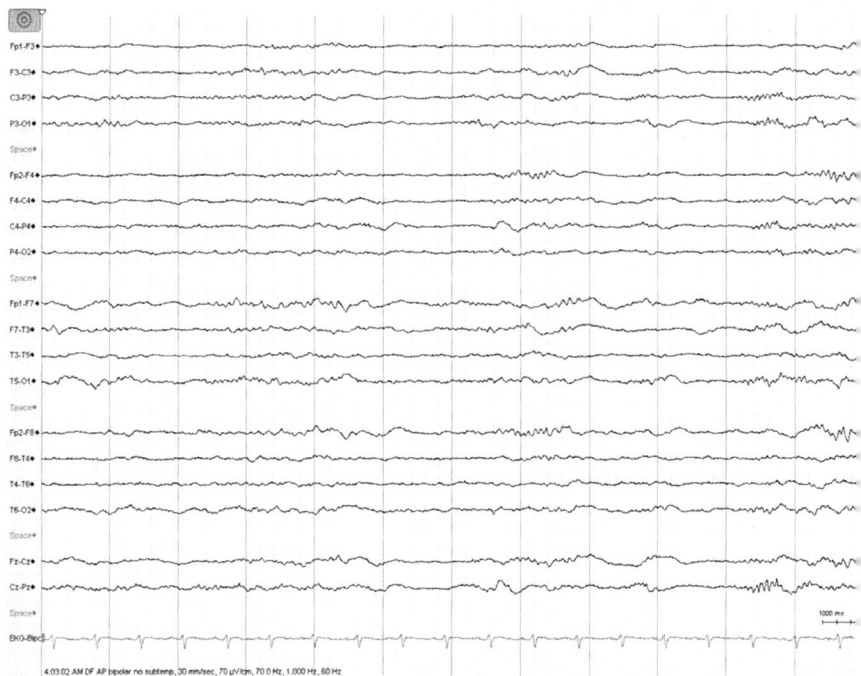

FIGURE 18.3 Spindle coma in a woman with severe hepatic failure and renal failure.

- ○ Nonspecific as to etiology but suggests predominant dysfunction caudal to the thalamus (ie, pons or midbrain), which is required to generate spindles.
  - ○ Prognosis is often favorable if there is no structural lesion and reactivity is present.
- • Alpha coma (Figure 18.4) (4, 5)
  - ○ Nonreactive alpha frequency rhythms (8 to 12 Hz)
  - ○ In anoxic brain injury, often anteriorly predominant and of moderate voltage
  - ○ Invariant and does not change with stimulation
  - ○ Prognosis is usually poor when seen in association with cardiac arrest, although meaningful recovery has been reported.
  - ○ Alpha frequency activity intermixed with beta frequencies is also commonly. seen in comatose patients on sedative medications (midazolam or propofol).
  - ○ Alpha frequency activity in a seemingly comatose patient with typical posterior prominence should raise the possibility that the patient is in a "locked-in state."
    - • EEG in these patients demonstrates variability and reactivity as well as the presence of sleep architecture.
- • Alpha/theta coma (5)
  - ○ Coma after anoxic injury may sometimes be associated with mixed alpha and theta frequencies, often anteriorly predominant.
  - ○ Like alpha coma, this pattern is often associated with poor prognosis in the setting of cardiac arrest.

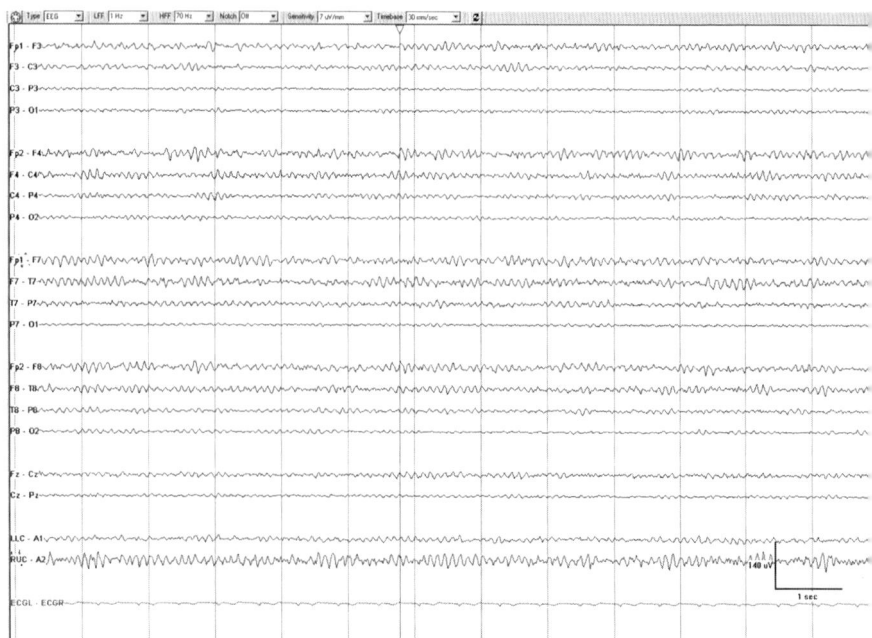

FIGURE 18.4 Alpha coma in a 56-year-old man following cardiac arrest.

- Burst suppression
  - ○ Bursts of high-amplitude mixed-frequency activity alternating with diffuse attenuation of the background (less than 10 μV).
  - ○ Duration of suppression can be variable but is often correlated with degree of cerebral dysfunction.
  - ○ Reversible in the cases of anesthetic/sedative-induced coma or severe hypothermia.
  - ○ In anoxic brain injury, it is associated with poor neurological outcome.
    - Generalized or lateralized periodic discharges (GPDs or LPDs) are often seen within the bursts and may be associated with clinical myoclonus (Figure 18.5).

III. FURTHER CONSIDERATIONS/REMAINING QUESTIONS

A. **What is the utility of continuous EEG monitoring (compared to routine EEG) for assessment of encephalopathy and coma?**
- The EEG of coma is dynamic—factors associated with favorable prognosis such as variability, reactivity, and presence of sleep architecture may be missed on routine EEGs.
- Routine EEG may also miss nonconvulsive seizures that may be a contributing factor to altered levels of arousal.

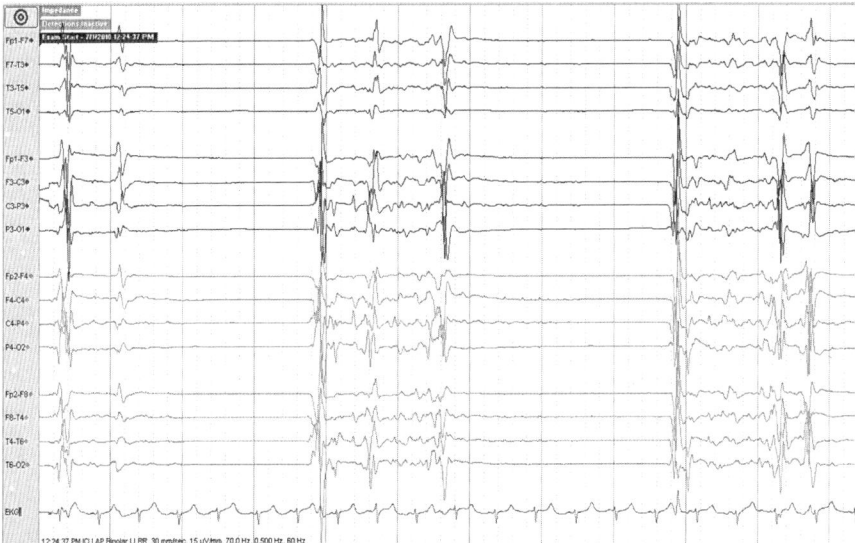

FIGURE 18.5 Burst suppression in a 65-year-old woman with frequent myoclonic jerks following cardiac arrest (post-anoxic myoclonus).

- The prognostic utility of routine EEGs, including serial routine EEGs, versus cEEG monitoring in coma and encephalopathy requires further study.

B. What is the prognostic value of certain EEG coma patterns in anoxic brain injury following cardiac arrest following hypothermia?
- Hypothermia protocols are now becoming routine practice after cardiac arrest.
- Complete neurological recovery has been reported in post-arrest patients with myoclonic status epilepticus, a pattern previously associated with universally poor outcomes (6).
- Absence of reactivity on EEG performed 36 to 72 hours post-arrest was a strong predictor of poor outcome in one prospective study (7).
- Further studies are needed to determine if patterns such as alpha coma, alpha/theta coma, and burst suppression continue to portend poor neurological outcome in patients who have been treated with hypothermia.

REFERENCES

1. Husain AM. Electroencephalographic assessment of coma. *J Clin Neurophysiol.* 2006;23(3):208–220.
2. Young GB. The EEG in coma. *J Clin Neurophysiol.* 2000;17(5):473–485.
3. Britt CW. Nontraumatic "spindle coma": Clinical, EEG, and prognostic features. *Neurology.* 1981;31(4):393–397.
4. Kaplan PW, Genoud D, Ho TW, Jallon P. Etiology, neurologic correlations, and prognosis in alpha coma. *Clin Neurophysiol.* 1999;110(2):205–213.
5. Young GB, Blume WT, Campbell VM, et al. Alpha, theta and alpha-theta coma: A clinical outcome study utilizing serial recordings. *Electroencephalogr Clin Neurophysiol.* 1994;91(2):93–99.
6. Rossetti AO, Oddo M, Liaudet L, Kaplan PW. Predictors of awakening from postanoxic status epilepticus after therapeutic hypothermia. *Neurology.* 2009;72:744–749.
7. Rossetti AO, Oddo M, Logroscino G, Kaplan PW. Prognostication after cardiac arrest and hypothermia: A prospective study. *Annals of Neurol.* 2010;67:301–307.
8. Van Cott AC, Brenner RB. Drug effects and toxic encephalopathies. In: JS Ebersole, TA Pedley eds. *Current Practice of Clinical Electroencephalography*. Philadelphia: Lippincott Williams & Wilkins, 2003:463–481.
9. Kaplan PW. The EEG in metabolic encephalopathy and coma. *J Clin Neurophysiol.* 2004;21(5):307–318.

ADDITIONAL READING

Brenner RP. The interpretation of the EEG in stupor and coma. *The Neurologist.* 2005;11(5):271–284.
Kaplan PW. The EEG in metabolic encephalopathy and coma. *J Clin Neurophysiol.* 2004;21(5):307–318.

NINETEEN

Lateralized Periodic Discharges

Elizabeth Gerard

KEY POINTS

- Lateralized Periodic Discharges (LPDs) are stereotyped repetitive discharges that occur at regular intervals and maximally involve one hemisphere.
- LPDs are classically associated with viral encephalitis, particularly herpes encephalitis, but their most common etiology is ischemic stroke.
- LPDs are associated with an increased risk for seizures.
- LPDs may represent an ictal or interictal pattern.
- The clinical significance and management of LPDs are controversial, particularly in comatose patients. Many experts regard LPDs as a pattern on the "ictal–interictal continuum," representing an unstable, potentially epileptogenic state.

I. BACKGROUND

A. Epidemiology and Natural History

- On the basis of several retrospective series, the frequency of LPDs formally known as periodic lateralized epileptiform discharges (PLEDs), on routine EEG recordings ranged between 0.4% and 1% (1).
- Within a selected population of neurological and neurosurgical intensive care patients, the prevalence of LPDs was as high as 20% (2).
- LPDs are most commonly seen in patients with focal neurologic deficits but also associated with varying degrees of altered consciousness with or without a focal deficit.
- In three large series, 10% to 35% of patients with LPDs were comatose (3–5).

B. Etiology

- LPDs are most commonly associated with an acute, destructive, structural lesion involving the cortex.
- Ischemic stroke is the most common etiology associated with LPDs in adult patients (1,3–5). Other common etiologies include viral encephalitis (including,

but not limited to herpes encephalitis), brain tumors, intracranial hemorrhage, and anoxic encephalopathy.

- An infectious etiology may be more common than stroke in the pediatric population, with the exception of neonates, in whom stroke and hypoxic–ischemic encephalopathy (HIE) are commonly associated with LPDs (6).
- LPDs have been described less frequently in the setting of Creutzfeldt–Jakob disease (CJD), demyelinating diseases, posterior reversible encephalopathy syndrome (PRES), migraine, and mitochondrial encephalopathy with lactic acidosis and stroke-like episodes (MELAS).
- Metabolic disturbances in combination with structural lesions may have a role in the genesis of LPDs, but are not a requirement.
  - Uremia, electrolyte disturbances, and a history of alcohol abuse were seen more commonly in early studies of LPDs (3), but have not been reported in more recent, larger series (1,7).
- LPDs are typically regarded as a transient phenomenon following an acute neurologic insult.
  - LPDs are most commonly encountered within the first days of an acute brain insult and usually resolve within days to weeks (1).
  - Chronic LPDs have also been reported in patients with preexisting structural lesions and localization related epilepsy (1,5).
  - Most patients presenting with LPDs do not have a prior history of epilepsy. Epilepsy has been reported in only 5% to 22% of patients found to have LPDs (4,5,7).

II. BASICS

A. EEG Characteristics
- LPDs are discrete repetitive discharges with a consistent morphology that recur *periodically,* typically at regular intervals of 0.5 up to 3 Hz (1,3) (Figure 19.1).
  - Simultaneous electrocardiographic recording (ECG) is important to distinguish LPDs from EKG or pulse artifact.
- LPDs are predominantly *lateralized* to one hemisphere.
  - LPDs may be maximal in any focal brain region (3).
  - The field of individual discharges is typically broad, including the parasagittal and temporal chains of the ipsilateral hemisphere, but it can be more restricted.
  - The field of the discharges can involve the contralateral hemisphere, particularly if the discharges are maximal in the frontal or occipital regions. Typically, however, they remain higher in amplitude over one hemisphere (3).
  - LPDs are usually associated with additional evidence of ipsilateral–cerebral dysfunction (focal slowing, loss of posterior dominant rhythm).
  - The contralateral hemisphere may be unaffected or may demonstrate evidence of encephalopathy, depending on the state of the patient.
- As classically described, the individual discharges in LPDs are usually *epileptiform* in appearance.
  - LPDs are typically sharp waves or sharp-wave complexes ranging from 50 to 300 μV in amplitude.

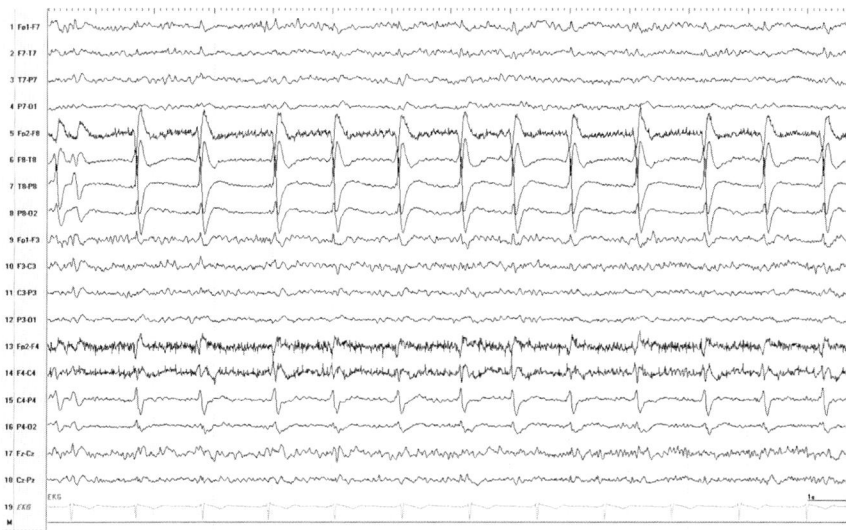

FIGURE 19.1   LPDs in a 69-year-old man with non-Hodgkin's lymphoma and a history of seizures following placement of a right frontal Omaya reservoir. Continuous EEG was obtained following a witnessed seizure and demonstrated persistent 1 Hz right hemisphere LPDs as well as frequent electrographic seizures from the same region. Seizures resolved following treatment with lorazepam and phenytoin. Right hemisphere LPDs resolved over 4 days.

- The standardized critical care EEG terminology proposes that LPDs include all periodic discharges regardless of morphology (ie, blunt delta waves that recur in a stereotyped periodic fashion).

B. Neuroimaging
- LPDs are most commonly associated with cortical gray matter or subcortical gray and white matter lesions (64%) although they can also occur in the setting of subcortical white matter lesions alone, or rarely with isolated subcortical gray matter lesions (5,8).
- LPDs can be seen in the absence of a structural lesion.
  - Studies have shown that between one-quarter and one-third of patients with LPDs have no structural abnormality on neuroimaging (4,7).

C. Association With Seizures
- Clinical seizures
  - Clinical seizures occur in the majority of patients with LPDs.
    - Across 16 retrospective series of EEG recordings containing LPDs, clinical seizures were noted in 47% to 100% of patients (1). Since history of clinical seizures is a common indication for EEG, these numbers are affected by selection bias.

- In 1989, Snodgrass et al. reported clinical seizures in 90% of 147 patients with LPDs (7). In this study, seizures were most commonly noted prior to, or at the same time as, the detection of LPDs. In some cases, however, seizures occurred after initial identification of LPDs.
- In a more recent study involving 82 patients with LPDs, 70% had clinical seizures. In this series, seizures were more common in patients with LPDs associated with stroke and brain tumors and less common in patients with infection or other etiologies (5).
- A series of 130 patients with LPDs showed that 50% of patients experienced clinical seizures during the course of their acute illness, but the other half of the patients did not develop seizures. In this study, there was no correlation between the incidence of clinical seizures and the underlying etiology associated with the LPDs (4).
  - Focal motor seizures are the most common seizure type associated with LPDs (1,3,7).
- Nonconvulsive seizures (NCS)
  - LPDs are highly associated with nonconvulsive seizures on continuous EEG.
    - Claassen et al. documented a significant association between LPDs and NCS on prolonged EEG recordings. The authors found that in patients who had seizures identified during monitoring, 40% also had LPDs whereas only 11% of patients without seizures on cEEG demonstrated LPDs (9).
    - This study also demonstrated that the presence of LPDs was associated with seizures that occurred after the initial 24 hours of EEG recording. Therefore, EEG monitoring longer than 24 hours should be considered in patients with LPDs.

D. Prognosis
- Across several series, LPDs have been associated with a high-mortality rate ranging from 24% to 53% (1,5).
- In a series of 45 pediatric patients, LPDs were associated with death in 22.7% (6).
- A recent review of 79 patients with LPDs found that 21.5% returned to independent function but 54.4% were dependent and 24% died.
  - Patients with a neoplastic etiology of LPDs were more likely to have a poor outcome compared to patients with a vascular etiology.
  - The presence of clinical seizures in a patient with LPDs was associated with a better prognosis than LPDs in the absence of clinical seizures (5), although this was not observed in an earlier series (4).
- LPDs have been shown to be independent predictors of poor outcome (moderate-to-severe disability or death) in patients with subarachnoid hemorrhage (10), intracranial hemorrhage (11), and patients in the medical intensive care unit (12).
- Adults with a prior history of epilepsy or children with acute infections tend to have a better prognosis than patients with LPDs from other etiologies.
- LPDs and subsequent epilepsy
  - In two small series of adult patients, 6/9 (13) and 4/9 (14) patients who presented with LPDs and an acute seizure later developed epilepsy (follow-up period 3–50 months).

E. Subtypes of LPDs

- LPDs Plus
  - The term LPDs Plus was originally proposed by Reiher et al. to describe LPDs associated with superimposed rhythmic discharges (usually low-voltage fast activity) (15).
    - LPDs Plus were present in 50 of 84 patients with LPDs and were more likely to be associated with clinical or electrographic seizures than LPDs alone (74% vs. 6%).
    - EEG recordings typically showed an evolution from LPDs to LPDs Plus culminating in seizures followed by a reverse transition to more "benign," less persistent LPDs following resolution of seizures.
  - Current EEG monitoring research terminology defines LPDs Plus as LPDs with superimposed fast activity (F), rhythmic activity (R), or both (FR) (Figure 19.2).
- BIPDs (Bilateral independent periodic discharges)
  - Asynchronous periodic discharges that occur independently over both hemispheres (Figure 19.3).
  - BIPDs are much less common than LPDs; thus, data on their significance are limited.
  - BIPDs are associated with similar etiologies as LPDs (stroke, infection, tumor); however, metabolic abnormalities and bilateral lesions may be more common with BIPDs (5).

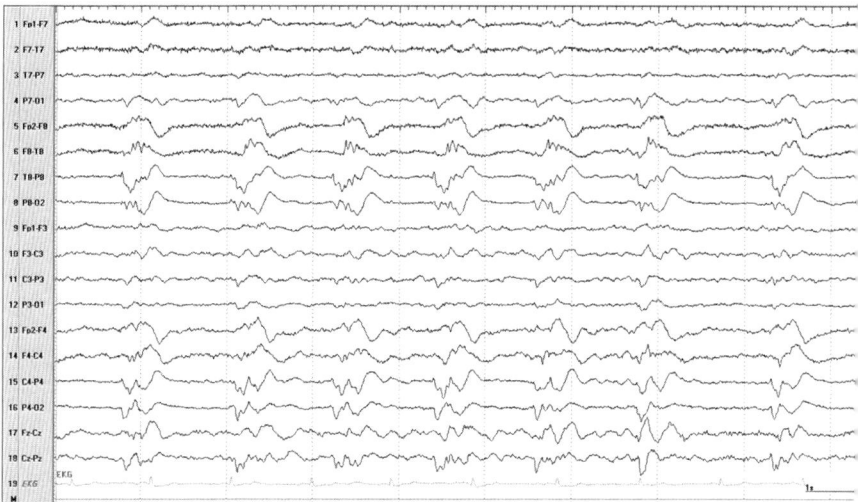

FIGURE 19.2 LPDs Plus in a 41-year-old man with HIV/AIDs and diffuse B-cell lymphoma with multiple brain metastases in the right occipital and frontal regions. Continuous EEG after two convulsive seizures demonstrated 1 Hz right hemispheric LPDs with fast activity (LPDs Plus F) as well as frequent electrographic seizures. Seizures resolved following treatment with lorazepam, levetiracetam, and lacosamide. LPDs persisted for over 2 weeks.

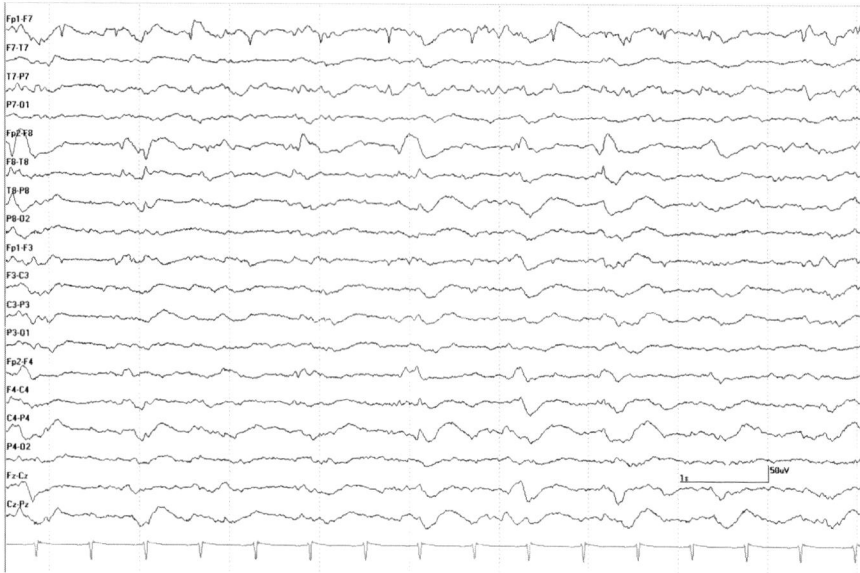

FIGURE 19.3 BIPDs in a 45-year-old woman with limbic encephalitis. The patient presented in complex partial status epilepticus with seizures arising from the left and right temporal regions. On emergence from pentobarbital-induced coma, continuous EEG demonstrated BIPDs, best seen over the temporal derivations. Electrographic and clinical seizures ultimately returned requiring prolonged pharmacological coma.

- ○ Coma is more commonly associated with BIPDs than with LPDs (47.8% vs. 14%) (5).
- ○ Seizures may be less common in patients with BIPDs compared to patients with LPDs (43% vs. 70%) (5).
  - • However, in a small series of patients with CNS infections, 4/4 (100%) with BIPDs had clinical or electrographic seizures whereas only 8/14 (57%) with LPDs experienced seizures (16).
- ○ In a single study which included 23 patients with BIPDs and 82 patients with LPDs, mortality was greater in patients with BIPDs (39% vs. 24% with LPDs), although there was no clear difference in functional outcomes (5).
- • Stimulus-induced LPDs
  - ○ Hirsch et al described the phenomena of stimulus-induced rhythmic, periodic, or ictal discharges (SIRPIDs) in 33 stuporous or comatose patients.
  - ○ Out of 33 patients, nine had stimulus-induced LPDs. Five (55%) of the patients with stimulus-induced LPDs had electrographic or clinical seizures or status epilepticus during their acute illness.
  - ○ Whether the pathological or prognostic significance of stimulus-induced LPDs is different from spontaneous LPDs is not clear.

III. FURTHER CONSIDERATIONS/REMAINING QUESTIONS

A. What is the incidence of LPDs in critically ill patients?

- Existing studies of LPDs are retrospective and based largely on intermittent recordings.
- The true prevalence of LPDs and their association with seizures and prognostic significance would be better defined in prospective studies using continuous EEG monitoring of unselected critically ill patients.

B. Do LPDs represent an ictal pattern?

- Debate exists over the pathophysiological significance of LPDs and how aggressively they should be managed.
- LPDs are generally considered an ictal pattern when they are associated with a clinical correlate.
  - Focal clonic seizures including epilepsia partialis continua (EPC) contralateral to LPDs are a common manifestation of ictal LPDs that is easy to recognize.
  - The pattern is considered ictal when individual discharges are time-locked to electromyographic (EMG) recordings showing clonic activity (Figure 19.4).

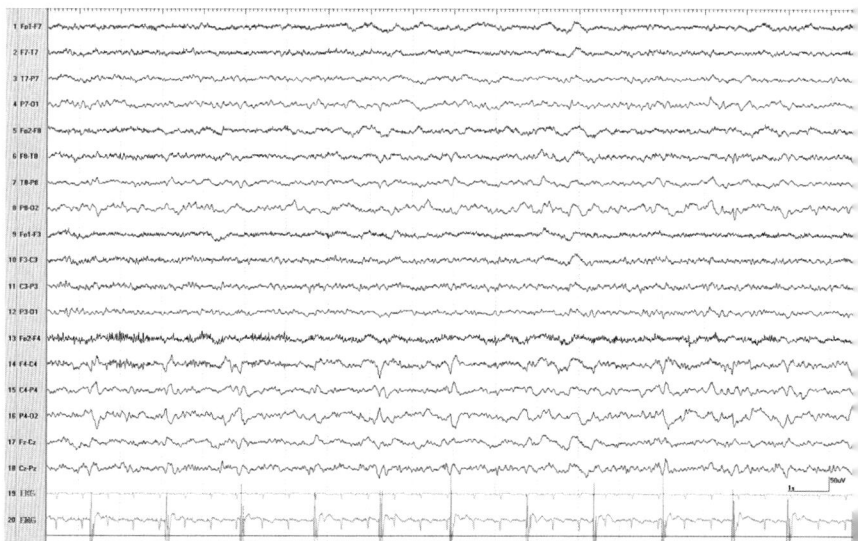

FIGURE 19.4 Ictal LPDs in a 70-year-old woman with breast cancer metastatic to the right frontal lobe and associated radiation necrosis following gamma knife treatment. The patient presented with persistent left arm clonic movements. Continuous EEG demonstrated right hemisphere LPDs maximal over the right central region that were time locked to EMG evidence of left arm clonic movements (bottom channel).

- In patients with altered mental status or coma, discerning a clinical correlate of LPDs can be difficult, particularly if they are located in noneloquent cortex (parietal, occipital, or fronto-polar).
  - In such patients, LPDs may be associated with subtle or subjective clinical correlates such as eye deviation, hemiparesis, aphasia, hemianopia, or sensory disturbances.
  - One case series described seven elderly patients with recurrent confusional states including speech disturbance and visual hallucinations that were temporally associated with LPDs (17). LPDs tended to be maximal over the posterior hemispheres (temporo–parieto–occipital regions). Both LPDs and clinical symptoms resolved with antiepileptic drug (AED) treatment.
- LPDs have been associated with regional increases in glucose metabolism on positron emission tomography (PET) and increased cerebral perfusion on single-photon-emission computed tomography (SPECT; Figure 19.5) (18,19). Some have argued that these metabolic alterations indicate that LPDs are a form of partial status epilepticus, whereas others interpret this as an indication that

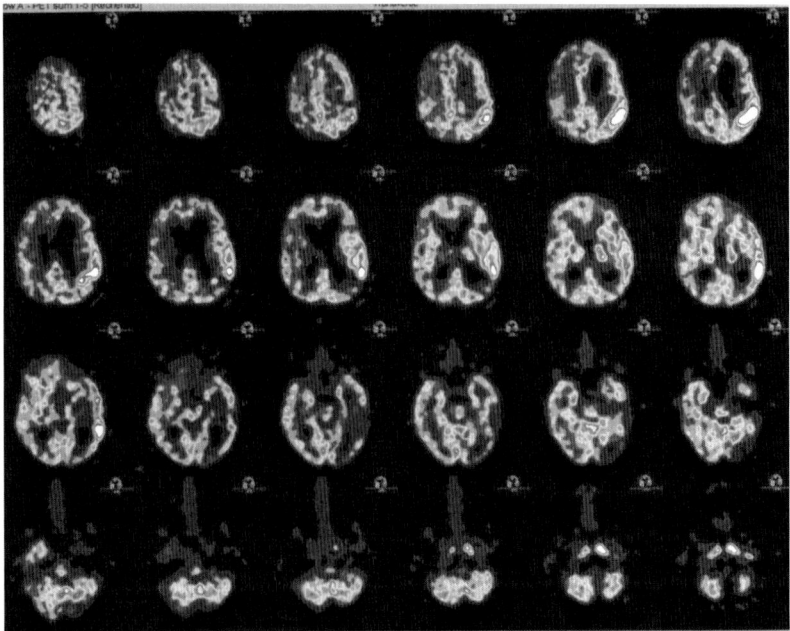

FIGURE 19.5 HMPAO–SPECT scan in a 78-year-old man with a remote history of a left parietal subdural hematoma who presented in complex partial status epilepticus. Clinical and electrographic seizures resolved with numerous antiepileptic medications including pentobarbital coma but left parietal LPDs persisted. SPECT scan demonstrated focal hyperperfusion corresponding to the distribution of the LPDs. (HMPAO: hexamethylpropylenamine oxide)

LPDs are markers of an unstable pathophysiological state on an "ictal–interictal continuum."

C. What is the appropriate management of patients with LPDs?

- No consensus exists on the appropriate management of LPDs, and there are no data to indicate whether intervention improves outcome in comatose patients with this electrographic pattern.
- LPDs may have different implications depending on the clinical scenario and this should be taken into account in determining a treatment plan.
- Neuroimaging should be performed in all patients with LPDs and metabolic or other reversible systemic conditions should be treated.
- Given the association between LPDs and subclinical seizures, prolonged EEG monitoring, ideally greater than 24 hours, is recommended in these patients.
- AED prophylaxis
  - Given the strong association between LPDs and seizures, most patients with LPDs should be treated with a prophylactic AED for at least the acute phase of their illness.
  - Since a percentage of patients presenting with LPDs and seizures will develop epilepsy, it may be worthwhile to continue antiepileptic medications for a period of time after hospitalization.
- Elimination of LPDs
  - Whether to escalate AED treatment with the goal of eliminating LPDs is controversial.
    - LPDs often resolve on their own over days to weeks without additional treatment which would support conservative management.
    - On the other hand, LPDs can be responsible for ongoing encephalopathy as well as focal changes in cerebral metabolism which would support more aggressive treatment.
  - The resolution of LPDs **in addition** to clinical symptoms (focal deficits or confusion) in response to a low-dose benzodiazepine or a loading dose of an AED suggests that LPDs represent an ictal state, and that further management with AEDs is necessary.
  - Evidence of regional hypermetabolism such as increased signal on PET or SPECT imaging during the time that LPDs are present may support more aggressive management.
  - Prospective controlled studies will be necessary to determine the correct approach to treating LPDs, particularly in comatose patients.

REFERENCES

1. Pohlmann-Eden B, Hoch DB, Cochius J, et al. Periodic lateralized epileptiform discharges—A critical review. *J Clin Neurophysiol.* 1996;13(6):519–530.
2. Pandian JD, Cascino GD, So EL, et al. Digital video-electroencephalographic monitoring in the neurological–neurosurgical intensive care unit: Clinical features and outcome. *Arch Neurol.* 2004;61(7):1090–1094.

3. Chatrian GE, Shaw CM, Leffman H. The significance of periodic lateralized epileptiform discharges in EEG: An electrographic, clinical and pathological study. *Electroencephalogr Clin Neurophysiol.* 1964;17:177–193.

4. García-Morales I, García MT, Galán-Dávila L, et al. Periodic lateralized epileptiform discharges: Etiology, clinical aspects, seizures, and evolution in 130 patients. *J Clin Neurophysiol.* 2002;19(2):172–177.

5. San Juan Orta D, Chiappa KH, Quiroz AZ, et al. Prognosis implications of periodic epileptiform discharges. *Arch Neurol.* 2009;66(8):985–991.

6. Chen KS, Kuo MF, Wang HS, et al. Periodic lateralized epileptiform discharges of pediatric patients in Taiwan. *Pediatr Neurol.* 2003;28(2):100–103.

7. Snodgrass SM, Tsuburaya K, Ajmone-Marsan C. Clinical significance of periodic lateralized epileptiform discharges: Relationship with status epilepticus. *J Clin Neurophysiol.* 1989;6:159–172.

8. Gurer G, Yemisci M, Saygi S, et al. Structural lesions in periodic lateralized epileptiform discharges (LPDs). *Clin EEG Neurosci.* 2004;35(2):88–93.

9. Claassen J, Mayer SA, Kowalski RG, et al. Detection of electrographic seizures with continuous EEG monitoring in critically ill patients. *Neurology.* 2004;62(10):1743–1748.

10. Claassen J, Hirsch LJ, Frontera JA, et al. Prognostic significance of continuous EEG monitoring in patients with poor-grade subarachnoid hemorrhage. *Neurocrit Care.* 2006;4(2):103–112.

11. Claassen J, Jetté N, Chum F, et al. Electrographic seizures and periodic discharges after intracerebral hemorrhage. *Neurology.* 2007;69(13):1356–1365.

12. Oddo M, Carrera E, Claassen J, et al. Continuous electroencephalography in the medical intensive care unit. *Crit Care Med.* 2009;37(6):2051–2056.

13. Schraeder PL, Singh N. Seizure disorders following periodic lateralized epileptiform discharges. *Epilepsia.* 1980;21:647–653.

14. Walsh JM, Brenner RP. Periodic lateralized discharges—long term outcome in adults. *Epilepsia.* 1987;28(5):533–536.

15. Reiher J, Rivest J, Grand'Maison F, Leduc CP. Periodic lateralized epileptiform discharges with transitional rhythmic discharges: Association with seizures. *Electroencephalogr Clin Neurophysiol.* 1991;78:12–17.

16. Carrera E, Claassen J, Oddo M. Continuous electroencephalographic monitoring in critically ill patients with central nervous system infections. *Arch Neurol.* 2008;65(12):1612–1618.

17. Terzano MG, Parrino L, Mazzucchi A, Moretti G. Confusional states with periodic lateralized epileptiform discharges (LPDs): A peculiar epileptic syndrome in the elderly. *Epilepsia.* 1986;27:446–457.

18. Handforth A, Cheng JT, Mandelkern MA, et al. Markedly increased mesiotemporal lobe metabolism in a case with LPDs: Further evidence that LPDs are a manifestation of partial status epilepticus. *Epilepsia.* 1994;35(4):876–881.

19. Assal F, Papazyan JP, Slosman DO, et al. SPECT in periodic lateralized epileptiform discharges (LPDs): A form of partial status epilepticus? *Seizure.* Jun 2001;10(4):260–265.

TWENTY

Generalized Periodic Discharges

Matthew H. Wong and Nathan B. Fountain

KEY POINTS

- Generalized periodic discharges (GPDs) were once a rarely recognized electrographic pattern, but are now being seen more frequently in the era of intensive EEG monitoring (cEEG).
- GPDs are associated with severe bihemispheric dysfunction with diverse functional or structural causes that include toxic–metabolic encephalopathy, hypoxic–ischemic encephalopathy, degenerative diseases such as Creutzfeldt–Jakob disease (CJD), and generalized convulsive status epilepticus in its terminal stages.
- In a small proportion of cases, GPDs may represent an ictal phenomenon. However, it is unknown whether antiepileptic treatment of GPDs in such cases alters overall outcome.
- GPDs have diverse electrographic morphologies. The morphology does not allow one to discern etiology. However, certain features of the clinical history, taken in combination with certain electrographic attributes, such as the degree of suppression of intervening activity, may correlate with prognosis.

I. BACKGROUND

A. GPDs were once an uncommon electrographic finding that now, in the age of continuous EEG (cEEG) monitoring, is being detected more often because more patients with severe brain injury are undergoing cEEG.

B. GPDs are never a normal finding and inevitably associated with a patient who is encephalopathic.

C. GPDs should be differentiated from lateralized periodic discharges (LPDs) and bilateral independent periodic discharges (BIPDs).

II. BASICS

A. The Electroencephalogram

- GPDs are periodic generalized synchronous discharges whose amplitude is relatively equal across homologous regions of the brain.
- GPDs usually have a frontocentral predominance but may also have a frontotemporal midline or occipital predominance (1).
- The discharges are usually spikes, polyspikes or sharp waves, (2) and typically have a negative polarity (1).
- The periodic discharge itself can be very short, such as the length of a spike discharge, or prolonged, up to 0.5 seconds.
- The period between the generalized discharges is usually not absolutely fixed, but rather varies from discharge to discharge, which some have termed quasi-periodic. The inter-discharge interval should not vary by more than 50%.
- The intervening activities between the periodic discharges can be composed of varying frequencies, but the most common patterns are diffuse delta activities or suppression. These activities are seen because they correlate with the severe bihemispheric dysfunction that typically accompanies GPDs.
- Some burst suppression patterns that are common in hypoxic–ischemic encephalopathies can be categorized as GPDs if the duration of the bursts is less than 0.5 seconds. According to ACNS critical care EEG terminology, periodic discharges are distinguished from "bursts" by having fewer than 4 phases and duration of 0.5 seconds or less.
- The discharges in GPDs may have a triphasic morphology. They can sometimes be distinguished from typical triphasic waves of metabolic encephalopathy by their periodic nature and more severely abnormal background activity, two features that do not typically accompany triphasic waves due to metabolic encephalopathy.
  - GPDs with triphasic wave morphology have been reported in degenerative diseases such as CJD as well as nonconvulsive status epilepticus.

B. GPDs and Seizures

- A study of 25 patients with GPDs (2)
  - 32% had evidence of seizures in the form of either clear electrographic seizures, generalized tonic–clonic seizures, or EEG plus clinical response to AEDs.
  - 40% had a past history of seizures.
- Another study of 37 patients with GPDs (3)
  - 89.2% had seizures within 48 hours of the EEG, with 35.2% having myoclonic seizures, 21.6% having generalized tonic clonic convulsions, and 32.4% having status epilepticus.
- These studies may have been biased by the fact that these patients were selected to undergo EEG monitoring and hence some suspicion of seizures was likely present. However, some think it prudent to continuously monitor any patient with GPDs for at least 48 hours to determine if there are associated electrographic or clinical seizures.
- It is unknown whether treating GPDs or the seizures associated with them will improve the prognosis, especially when the prognosis associated with the underlying disease is poor.

- However, if either electrographic or clinical seizures are detected during cEEG monitoring of a patient with GPDs, treatment of the seizures is prudent.

C. GPDs and Etiology

- In general, the electrographic morphology of GPDs does not allow one to determine their etiology.
- GPDs are seen in a diverse number of clinical settings: hypoxic–ischemic injury, drug intoxication, metabolic disorders such as hepatic encephalopathy, degenerative diseases, central nervous system infections, and as the terminal electrographic sign of generalized convulsive status epilepticus (GCSE).
- Hypoxic–ischemic encephalopathy secondary to cardiac arrest may manifest as GPDs (Figures 20.1A and 20.1B). The GPDs may be temporally associated with post-anoxic myoclonus which is typically seen in this disorder.
- Toxic and metabolic encephalopathies may be associated with GPDs with triphasic wave morphologies, with the most common cause being hepatic encephalopathy, followed by uremic encephalopathy.
  - One report found that of 50 patients with generalized discharges with triphasic morphology, 56% had hepatic encephalopathy and 20% had uremic encephalopathy (3).
  - However, triphasic waves can also be seen in CJD, anoxia, and, rarely, as a manifestation of nonconvulsive status epilepticus.
  - GPDs with triphasic morphology are often associated with an anterior–posterior lag if they are associated with a toxic metabolic encephalopathy. This anterior–posterior lag means that the wave comes slightly later in the posterior derivations than the anterior derivations (Figure 20.2).
- Most sporadic or iatrogenic Creutzfeldt–Jakob (sCJD or iCJD) disease develops GPDs during the course of their disease, usually within a month of presentation (4) (Figure 20.3).
  - In the setting of a subacute dementia, GPDs can be a very specific finding for CJD. The myoclonic jerks seen with CJD typically correlate with the periodic discharges.
  - Variant CJD does not usually manifest GPDs (5).
- Subacute sclerosing panencephalitis (SSPE) secondary to the measles virus is a common cause of GPDs in regions where measles is still prevalent.
  - In one study, 29.7% of 37 patients with GPDs had SSPE (6).
  - The interval between discharges is typically greater than 4 seconds (2).
  - Because this same pattern can be seen in toxic metabolic encephalopathies, the clinical history is important in determining its significance.
- GCSE is reported to have an electrographic progression (7), with GPDs typically seen in the last stage.
  - Whether the GPDs should be treated as ictal activity during this stage is unknown (Figures 20.4A and 20.4B).

D. GPDs and Prognosis

- Many studies have shown high mortality associated with GPDs (64% and 48.7% in two studies) (6).
- Prognosis is dependent on the underlying etiology. In hypoxic–ischemic encephalopathy the prognosis is usually dire, with a mortality of 90% in one study

(A)

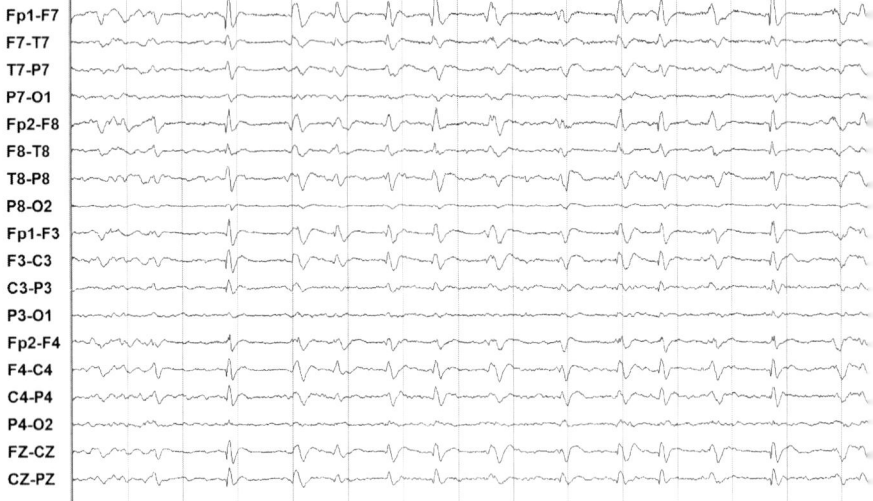

(B)

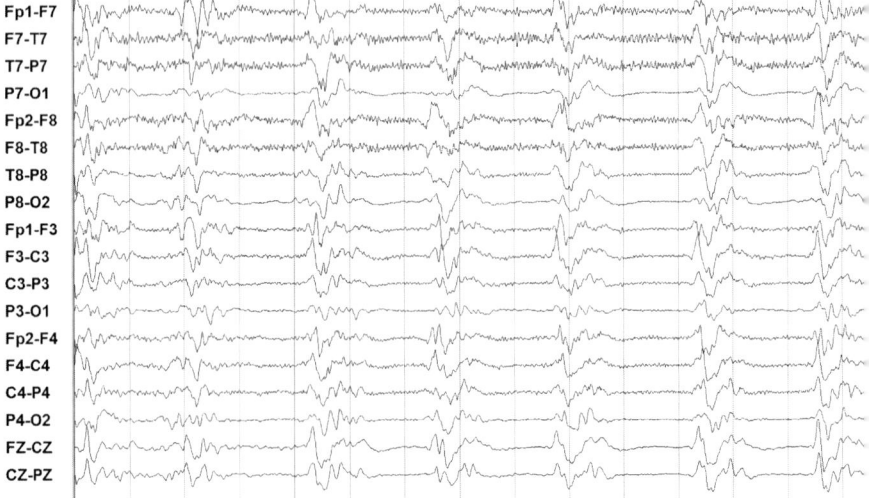

FIGURE 20.1 **(A)** GPDs in an 81-year-old woman after cardiac arrest demonstrating GPDs with simple sharp wave morphology. The GPDs have a periodicity of approximately 1 per second and are frontally dominant. Note that the morphology is not identical from discharge to discharge. **(B)** GPDs in a 77-year-old woman after cardiac arrest demonstrating GPDs with complex morphology. Myoclonic jerks occurred with the same periodicity as the GPDs. The complex GPD morphology is composed of multiple sharp waves superimposed on a slow wave (GPDs plus). The morphology of the GPDs has not been shown to be related to etiology, prognosis, or tendency toward seizures.

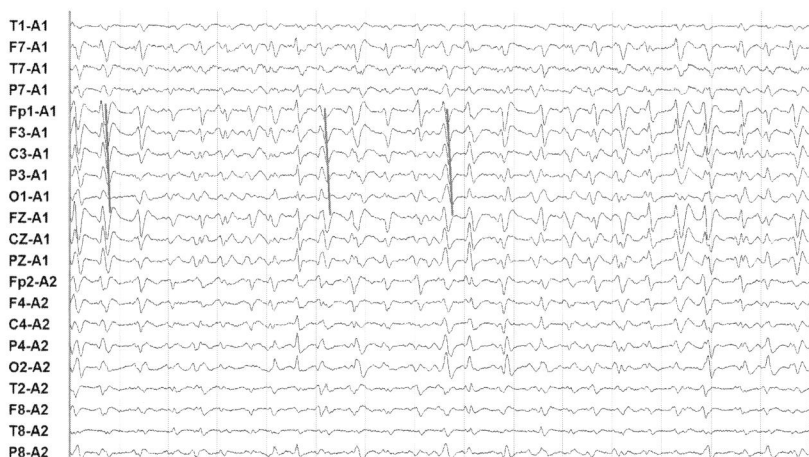

FIGURE 20.2 Triphasic waves in a 67-year-old woman with a right subdural empyema who presented with altered mental status and concern for nonconvulsive status epilepticus. The discharges improved after 2 mg of lorazepam but her clinical status did not (not shown). Because of the anterior–posterior lag (slanted vertical lines) and the rhythmicity of the discharges, these were diagnosed as triphasic waves of a metabolic or toxic etiology which are also known to improve with benzodiazepines without improvement in the clinical state of the patient.

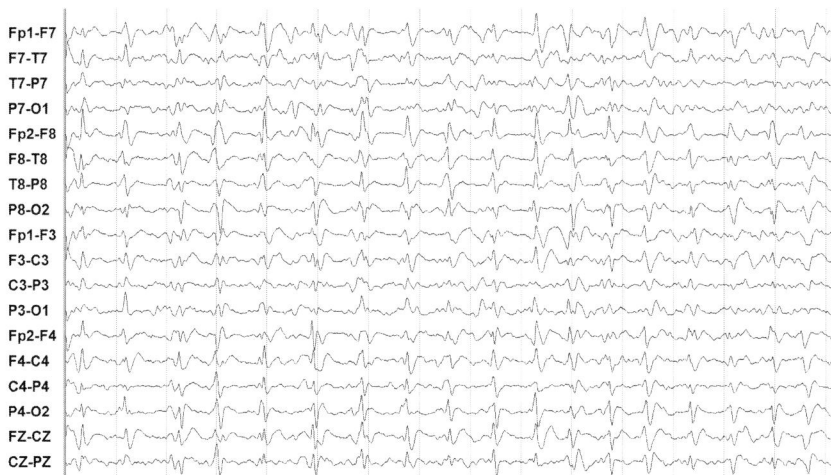

FIGURE 20.3 Generalized periodic discharges due to CJD in a 77-year-old woman with a 1-month history of subacute dementia and subtle myoclonic jerks. Note the high-amplitude initial negative component and relatively small positive component that distinguish these from typical triphasic waves. In this clinical setting the most likely diagnosis was CJD. She died 2 weeks later and sporadic CJD was confirmed at post-mortem.

(A)

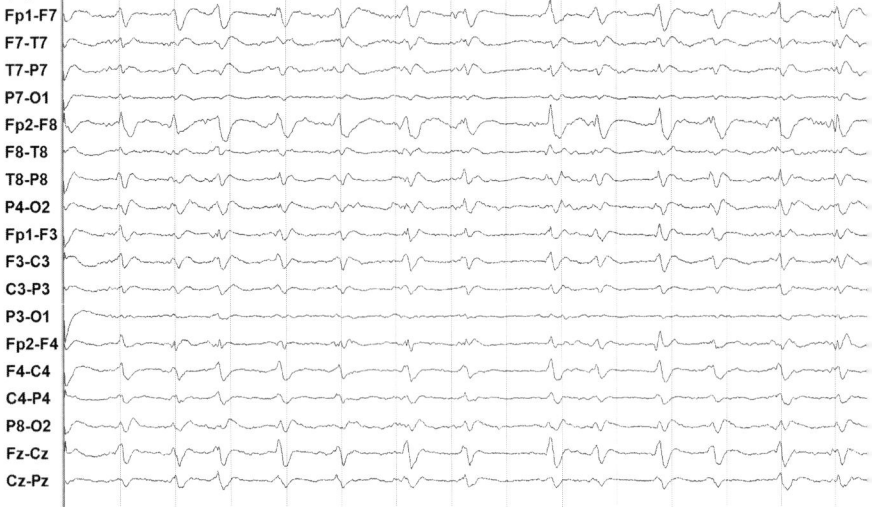

(B)

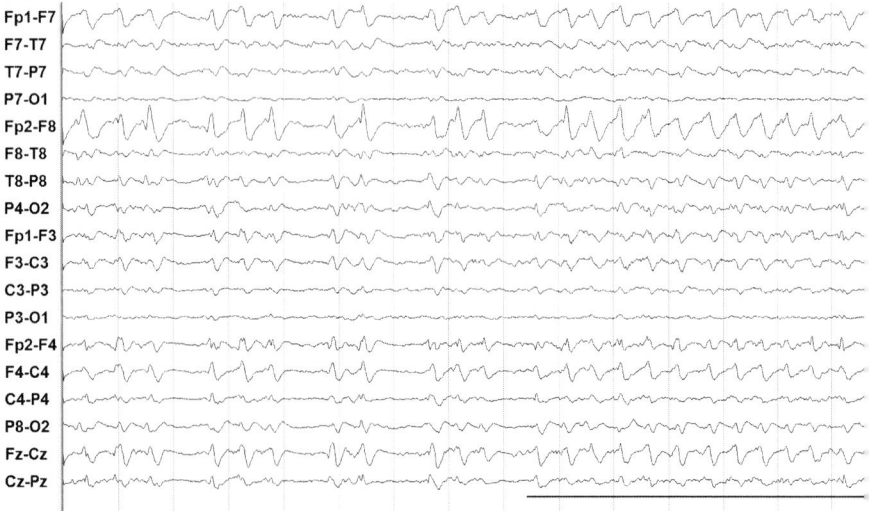

FIGURE 20.4 **(A)** GPDs in an 87-year-old woman with a history of epilepsy who presented with generalized convulsive status epilepticus. GPDs occurred after clinical evidence of status epilepticus resolved. **(B)** GPDs were shown to evolve and become rhythmic (underscored by black line), which was interpreted as an electrographic seizure. The seizure did not have a clinical accompaniment. The patient was treated aggressively for nonconvulsive status epilepticus and she returned to her pre-morbid function.

(remaining patients who survived required total care in a skilled nursing facility) (8). In another study, 100% of patients with anoxic–ischemic encephalopathy and GPDs died (1).

- GPDs associated with toxic-metabolic encephalopathies have a greater likelihood of survival (in another study 42.9% of survivors with GPDs had an underlying toxic or metabolic etiology) (8).
- Similarly, GPDs associated with status epilepticus seem to be associated with a higher chance of survival, with patients in one study showing a 44% survival rate (8).
  - ○ Higher inter-discharge amplitudes may also be associated with better prognosis.

III. FURTHER CONSIDERATIONS/REMAINING QUESTIONS

A. Do GPDs represent an ictal or an interictal phenomenon?
- It is likely that they can represent both depending on the etiology and the clinical setting.

B. In which, if any, clinical situations does treating GPDs as ictal activity alter the outcome?

C. Answers to the above questions would lead to the next logical step: determining optimal treatment.

REFERENCES

1. Orta DSJ, Chiappa KH, Quiroz AZ, et al. Prognostic implications of periodic epileptiform discharges. *Arch Neurol.* 2009;66:985–991.
2. Brenner RP, Schaul N. Periodic EEG patterns: Classification, clinical correlation, and pathophysiology. *J Clin Neurophysiol: Off Publ Am Electroencephalogr Soc.* 1990;7:249–267.
3. Karnaze DS, Bickford RG. Triphasic waves: A reassessment of their significance. *Electroencephalogr Clin Neurophysiol.* Mar 1984;57(3):193–198.
4. Wieser HG, Schwarz U, Blättler T, et al. Serial EEG findings in sporadic and iatrogenic Creutzfeldt–Jakob disease. *Clin Neurophysiol: Off J Int Federation Clin Neurophysiol.* 2004;115:2467–2478.
5. Zeidler M, Stewart GE, Barraclough CR, et al. New variant Creutzfeldt–Jakob disease: Neurological features and diagnostic tests. *Lancet.* 1997;350:903–907.
6. Yemisci M, Gurer G, Saygi S, Ciger A. Generalised periodic epileptiform discharges: Clinical features, neuroradiological evaluation and prognosis in 37 adult patients. *Seizure: J Br Epilepsy Assoc.* 2003;12:465–472.
7. Treiman DM, Walton NY, Kendrick C. A progressive sequence of electroencephalographic changes during generalized convulsive status epilepticus. *Epilepsy Res.* 1990;5:49–60.
8. Husain AM, Mebust KA, Radtke RA. Generalized periodic epileptiform discharges: Etiologies, relationship to status epilepticus, and prognosis. *J Clin Neurophysiol: Off Publ Am Electroencephalogr Soc.* 1999;16:51–58.

TWENTY-ONE

The Ictal–Interictal Continuum

Suzette M. LaRoche

KEY POINTS

- In critically ill patients, many EEG patterns lie along a "spectrum" ranging from nonictal to ictal in origin.
- Consensus is lacking on the definition and treatment approach to EEG patterns that fall along this spectrum.
- Treatment should be strongly considered in cases where decline in the patient's clinical or functional state coincides with the onset of the EEG pattern in question.
- Correlation of EEG patterns with other indicators of cerebral dysfunction including serum biomarkers, functional neuroimaging, and multimodality monitoring parameters such as tissue oxygenation and microdialysis can aid in determination of which patterns are more malignant and warrant treatment.

I. BACKGROUND

A. Definition

- Rhythmic and periodic patterns are common EEG presentations in critically ill patients.
- However, consensus is lacking on classification of patterns that lie somewhere between a definite electrographic seizure and nonictal activity.
- Agreement is also lacking on how aggressively to treat such patterns.
- To help determine which patterns should be considered ictal, criteria have been proposed for the definition of a nonconvulsive seizure (NCS) (1):
  - ○ Any pattern lasting 10 seconds or longer and meeting one of the following criteria:
    - Repetitive spikes, sharp waves, or spike and wave greater than 3 Hz.
    - Rhythmic discharges less than 3 Hz and incrementing onset, decrementing offset, and post-discharge slowing or voltage attenuation.
    - Repetitive spike, sharp waves, or spike and wave less than 3 Hz and significant improvement in EEG AND clinical state following administration of a rapidly acting antiepileptic drug (AED).

○ NOTE: Periodic epileptiform discharges (PDs) are often abolished by benzodiazepines without improvement in EEG background or clinical exam and does not confirm the activity as ictal.
- Most agree that patterns that meet the above criteria for an NCS would NOT fall along the ictal–interictal continuum.
- However, patterns outside of these strict criteria may, in fact, represent ictal activity.
  ○ Example: 2 Hz lateralized periodic discharges (LPDs) that are time-locked to clonic movements of the contralateral face and arm.

B. The Spectrum of EEG Activity (Figure 21.1)
- There are many periodic and rhythmic patterns commonly encountered in encephalopathic patients.
- By convention, some of these patterns are traditionally regarded as nonictal (frontally predominant intermittent rhythmic delta activity, aka FIRDA), whereas others are considered more likely to be ictal and have been named accordingly (periodic lateralized EPILEPTIFORM discharges, aka PLEDs).
- However, data on the association between many of these patterns and seizures is lacking, particularly since the introduction of continuous EEG (cEEG).
- In addition, these patterns often transition from one type into another making it difficult to establish associations between a single pattern and degree of "ictalness."
- It is often assumed that the degree of neuronal injury increases with EEG patterns that are more likely to be ictal, but cause–effect relationship between neuronal injury and these EEG patterns is not clear.

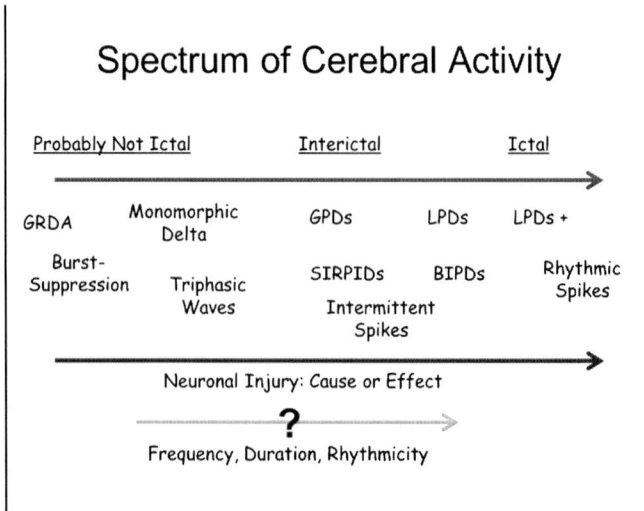

FIGURE 21.1   The spectrum of EEG activity commonly seen in critically ill patients ranges from nonictal to ictal in origin. Many questions remain as to whether these patterns are a cause or the effect of neuronal injury and what impact variations in frequency, duration, rhythmicity, and clinical correlate have on the potential for associated neuronal injury.

- The relationship between the frequency and duration of a pattern and extent of neuronal injury is also unknown (are faster frequency patterns that last longer associated with increased injury?).

C. **Clinical implications of "undertreating" an EEG pattern that may represent NCS/NCSE (nonconvulsive status epilepticus).**
- Mortality of patients experiencing NCS in published studies ranges from 27% to 100%, depending in part on the underlying etiology (2).
- NCS and NCSE following generalized convulsive status epilepticus (GCSE) is associated with marked increase in mortality compared to patients that do not experience NCS/NCSE (3).
  - NCSE after GCSE: 51% mortality
  - NCS after GCSE: 32% mortality
  - No seizures following GCSE: 13% mortality
- Patients with NCS of longer duration and greater delay to diagnosis have higher mortality (1).

D. **Clinical implications of "overtreating" an EEG pattern that does not represent NCS/NCSE.**
- Treatment may have no defined end point.
  - Should the pattern be treated until it resolves or until clinical improvement?
  - Underlying neurological condition and treatment with sedatives for other conditions such as elevated intracranial pressure (ICP) often make it difficult to establish these end points.
- Risk of treatment-related adverse effects, particularly in critically ill elderly patients, can be worse than the effect of seizures themselves (4).
  - 25 episodes of NCSE in the elderly were reviewed.
  - 13 patients died including 11 of 16 treated with IV benzodiazepines.

II. BASICS

A. **NCS and Evidence of Neuronal Injury**
- Intracerebral hemorrhage (ICH) (5)
  - A prospective study evaluated 63 patients undergoing cEEG for at least 72 hours.
  - NCS was seen in 18/63 (29%).
  - Patients experiencing NCS had poorer NIHSS scores and increase in midline shift independent of hemorrhage size.
- Traumatic brain injury (TBI) (6)
  - 10 TBI patients with NCS were compared with 10 TBI patients without NCS (matched by age, CT findings, and Glasgow Coma Score).
  - Increased ICP and lactate/pyruvate ratio (LPR) was seen in the group experiencing NCS.
- Relationship of neuron-specific enolase (NSE) to SE (7)
  - Elevated NSE levels have been associated with NCSE, even in the absence of an acute structural lesion.
  - Higher NSE levels have also been correlated with longer duration of SE.

B. Periodic Discharges as a MARKER of Neuronal Injury: Association With Poor Outcome
- Subarachnoid hemorrhage (SAH) (8)
  - 116 patients monitored with cEEG, were assessed with modified Rankin scale (mRS) at 3 months.
  - Independent predictors of poor outcome (mRS 4–6) included:
    - Any periodic discharges (PDs)
    - Generalized PDs (GPDs)
    - Bilateral independent periodic discharges (BIPDs)
    - NCSE in the first 24 hours.
- ICH (9)
  - 102 patients with nontraumatic ICH underwent cEEG for an average of 3 days
  - 17% of patients had PDs; more common with larger hemorrhages and hemorrhages within 1 mm of cortical surface.
  - Poor outcome was seen in greater than 50% of patients with any PDs, LPDs, or stimulus induced rhythmic, periodic, or ictal discharges (SIRPIDs).
  - Outcome was worse in patients with PDs compared to patients with documented NCS or NCSE.
- Emory University cohort (10)
  - 421 patients underwent cEEG in 2008.
  - 23% of patients had PDs.
  - Poor outcome (Glasgow Outcome Scale, GOS = 1 or 2) was associated with any type of PDs.
  - Higher incidence of poor outcome was seen in patients with PDs compared to patients with NCS/NCSE.
    - Perhaps a consequence of patients with NCS/NCSE being treated while patients with PDs were not treated but should have been?

C. Periodic Discharges as a CAUSE of Neuronal Injury: Functional Neuroimaging
- If the same functional neuroimaging findings that have been associated with clinical seizures are also seen concurrent with PDs, can an argument be made for PDs as a cause of neuronal injury?
- First report of correlation between changes in positron emission tomography (PET) and PDs was a single case report (11).
  - A 71-year-old patient with left thalamic ICH who presented with GCSE.
  - After resolution of GCSE, left temporal LPDs continued without clinical correlate.
  - PET hypermetabolism was seen in the left temporal region during LPDs and resolved after disappearance of LPDs.
- Subsequent series have shown similar findings of PET hypermetabolism corresponding to LPDs.
- LPDs and corresponding SPECT changes (12).
  - A focal area of increased cerebral blood flow corresponded to the region of LPDs in 17/18 patients.
  - Three patients received a follow-up SPECT scan after resolution of LPDs which showed normalization of cerebral blood flow.

- Conclusion: PDs can be associated with the same focal changes in cerebral metabolism and blood flow that are characteristically seen with seizures.

D. PD Subtypes
- GPDs
  - Studies suggesting GPDs are ictal:
    - Of 37 patients with GPDs on routine EEG, 89% experienced clinical seizures within 48 hours (13).
    - Another series showed that patients with GPDs were more likely to have seizures of any type, including NCS, as well as poor outcome (14).
    - GPDs of higher amplitude, greater duration, and higher amplitude background, have been associated with SE but also a better prognosis (15).
  - Studies suggesting GPDs are not ictal:
    - Patients with GPDs and underlying metabolic disturbance have been shown to have better outcome (16).
    - Long- and short-interval GPDs are commonly associated with subacute sclerosing panencephalitis (SSPE) and Creutzfeldt–Jakob disease (CJD) in the absence of clinical seizures.
  - Triphasic waves
    - Many consider to be a subtype of GPDs.
    - Highly associated with metabolic or toxic etiology and therefore less likely to represent an ictal pattern.
    - However, severe metabolic disease, particularly hepatic encephalopathy, is associated with increased risk of seizures.
- PDs plus
  - Originally referred to as LPDs with superimposed rhythmic discharges (either brief or prolonged) (17).
    - In a series of 84 patients with LPDs, 50/84 met criteria for LPDs plus.
    - Patients with LPDs plus had a much higher incidence of electrographic seizures compared to LPDs proper.
  - According to current ACNS terminology for EEG monitoring, plus modifier describes PDs with superimposed fast or rhythmic activity that render the pattern more "ictal-appearing."
  - More data regarding the association between PDs plus, seizures and outcome are needed.
- SIRPIDs
  - SIRPIDs were documented in 22% (33/150) of patients undergoing cEEG (18).
    - 50% experienced clinical or subclinical seizures; 33% had SE at some point.
    - Like PDs, SIRPIDs have been associated with seizures but it is unknown whether the pathophysiology is different from PDs that occur spontaneously and whether they should be treated

E. Approach to management of patterns that fall along the ictal–interictal continuum
- Clinical history and exam findings
  - Strongly consider treatment if:
    - Presence of myoclonic or clonic movements, nystagmus or rhythmic blinking that are time locked to the appearance of PDs (ie, ictal PDs).

- Decline in clinical or functional state that coincides with onset of the pattern in question (worsening mental status, increase in ICP or decline in other physiological parameters).
- History of any of the following:
  - Prior history of epilepsy or recent clinical seizure/SE.
  - Acute structural lesion associated with high risk of seizures (SAH, ICH, TBI).
  - Clinical symptoms such as aphasia, apraxia, or sensory disturbance can be harder to ascertain in comatose patients and therefore treatment implications less clear.
  - Example 1
    - A 24-year-old male patient with refractory SE on multiple AEDs and midazolam infusion who was transferred for further management including cEEG. (Figure 21.2A).
    - Based on history of confirmed SE, the patient was treated aggressively with additional AEDs.
    - Improvement was seen in the EEG and clinical exam following treatment (Figure 21.2B).
  - Example 2
    - A 69-year-old female patient underwent cEEG following coronary artery bypass graft because she was slow to return to baseline following surgery and propofol wean (Figure 21.3A).
    - Based on lack of prior seizures or evidence of any acute CNS lesion the EEG pattern was not treated.
    - She returned to clinical and EEG baseline within 24 hours (Figure 21.3B).
- Empiric medication trials
  - Benzodiazepine trial (19)
    - Sequential administration of small doses of a short-acting benzodiazepine.
    - Clinical and EEG assessment must be done between doses.
    - Monitor for respiratory depression or hypotension.
    - Test is positive for ictal pattern if EEG pattern resolves AND clinical improvement follows.
  - AED loading dose
    - Failure to respond to benzodiazepines does not prove that the pattern is not ictal.
    - If there is a strong clinical suspicion for seizure, follow negative benzodiazepine trial with an IV AED and assess for clinical and EEG changes.
  - Example
    - A 44-year-old female patient with acute left temporal contusion presented with aphasia, right hemiparesis, and EEG showing left hemisphere PDs with superimposed rhythmic activity, LPDs plus (Figure 21.4A).
    - Lorazepam was administered followed by transient resolution of LPDs but no clinical change.
    - Subsequent IV loading of fosphenytoin resulted in EEG improvement and return to clinical baseline (Figure 21.4B).
- Correlation with PET/SPECT findings
  - Hypermetabolism or increased blood flow in area correlating to the location of PDs can suggest the need for more aggressive treatment.
  - LPDs and SPECT (20)

(A)

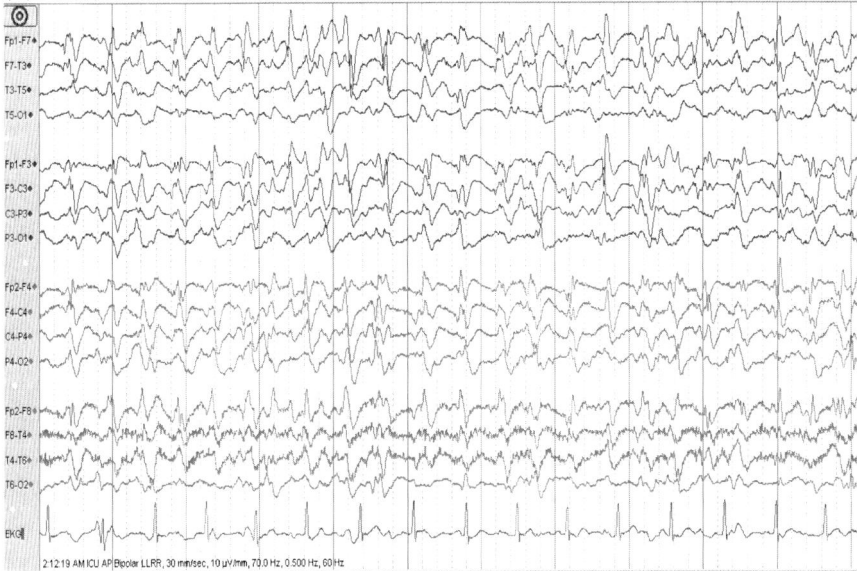

(B)

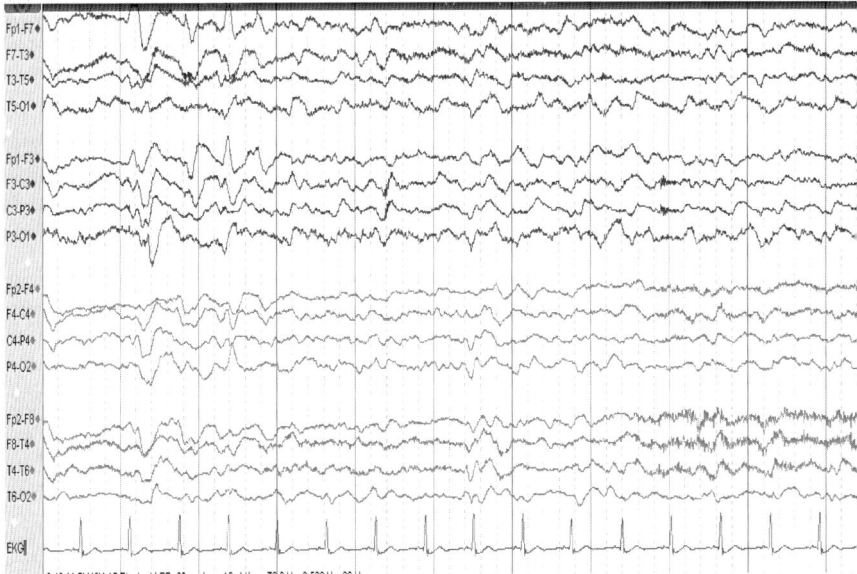

FIGURE 21.2 **(A)** Initial EEG recording of a 24-year-old male patient with history of refractory SE who was transferred for further management. The patient was being treated with fosphenytoin, phenobarbital, lacosamide, and continuous midazolam infusion. **(B)** EEG recording 24 hr later after more aggressive treatment with additional boluses of phenobarbital and addition of valproate.

(A)

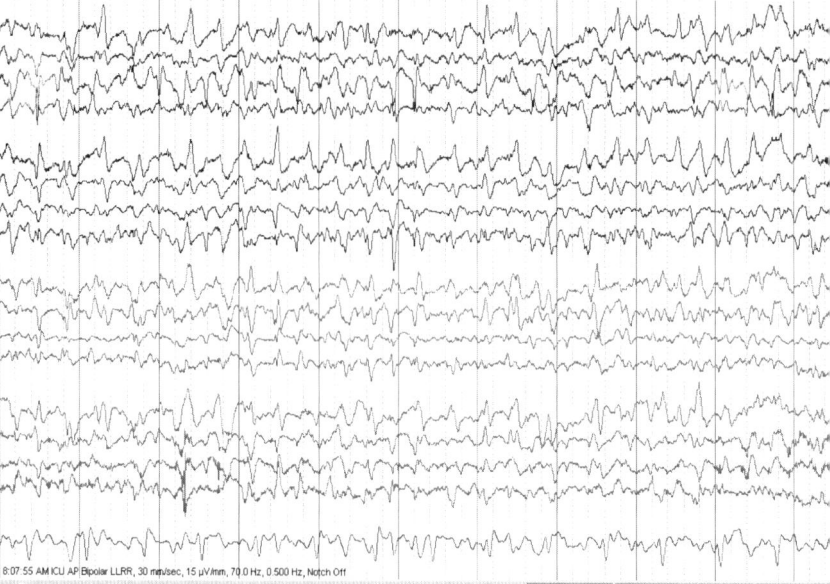

8:07:55 AM ICU AP Bipolar LLRR, 30 mm/sec, 15 µV/mm, 70.0 Hz, 0.500 Hz, Notch Off

(B)

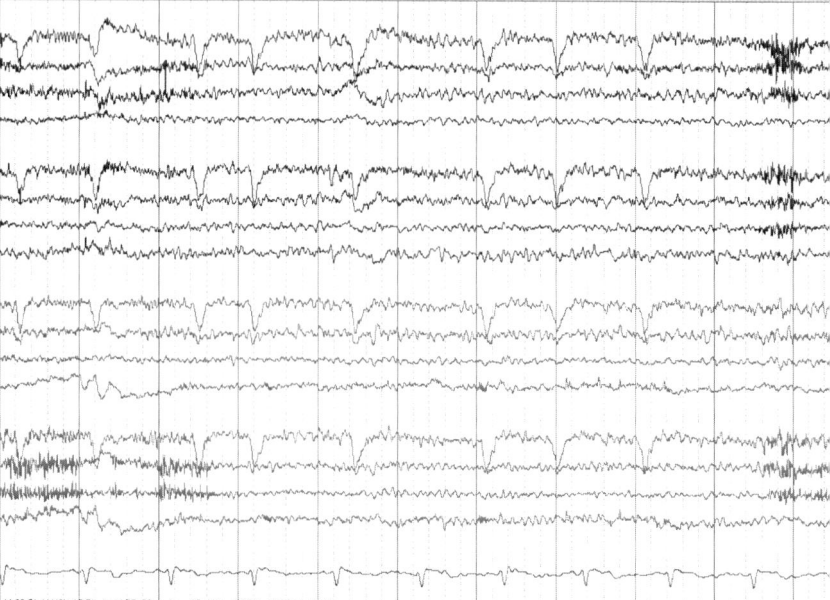

- A 69-year-old female patient presented with encephalopathy and right face twitching following right aneurysm clipping.
- Focal, clinical seizures resolved with treatment, but right hemisphere LPDs continued and she remained encephalopathic.
- SPECT scan during LPDs showed increased blood flow in the right hemisphere.
- This prompted more aggressive treatment, which was followed by clinical improvement and resolution of LPDs.
  ○ SIRPIDs and SPECT (21)
  - A 62-year-old patient with NCSE associated with aphasia and right hemiparesis.
  - NCSE resolved but aphasia and right hemiparesis continued and EEG revealed left temporal SIRPIDs.
  - SPECT revealed decreased blood flow in the corresponding left temporal region which led to less aggressive therapy.

III. FURTHER CONSIDERATIONS/REMAINING QUESTIONS

A. Correlation of questionable EEG patterns with other neurophysiological parameters can help determine if the pattern is malignant (see Chapter 31).

- Increased ICP in the absence of any other obvious cause could signify that an EEG pattern should be treated.
- Microdialysis findings such as elevated LPR and increased glutamate indicate abnormal cerebral metabolism and should prompt consideration of more aggressive management of an associated EEG pattern.
- Intracortical electrodes might reveal more obvious ictal patterns that are not visible on surface EEG monitoring and influence clinical decision making.

B. Multicenter Outcomes Studies

- Standardized terminology (see Chapter 17)
  ○ Widespread adoption of a standardized classification scheme for describing EEG patterns that represent both ictal phenomena as well as patterns that lie along the spectrum of ictal–interictal activity will allow for more widespread collaboration in identifying the clinical significance of these patterns.
  ○ The ACNS critical care EEG terminology has undergone multiple revisions as well as preliminary validation for use as such a research tool.
- Standardized treatment protocols
  ○ Developing an organized approach to the management of common EEG patterns encountered in the critically ill will enable a systematic evaluation of the utility of such treatment protocols.

FIGURE 21.3 (*opposite*) **(A)** A 69-year-old woman with recent coronary artery bypass graft who was noted to have persistent encephalopathy immediately following propofol wean. **(B)** EEG findings 24 hr later, no additional treatment or medications were added.

(A)

(B)

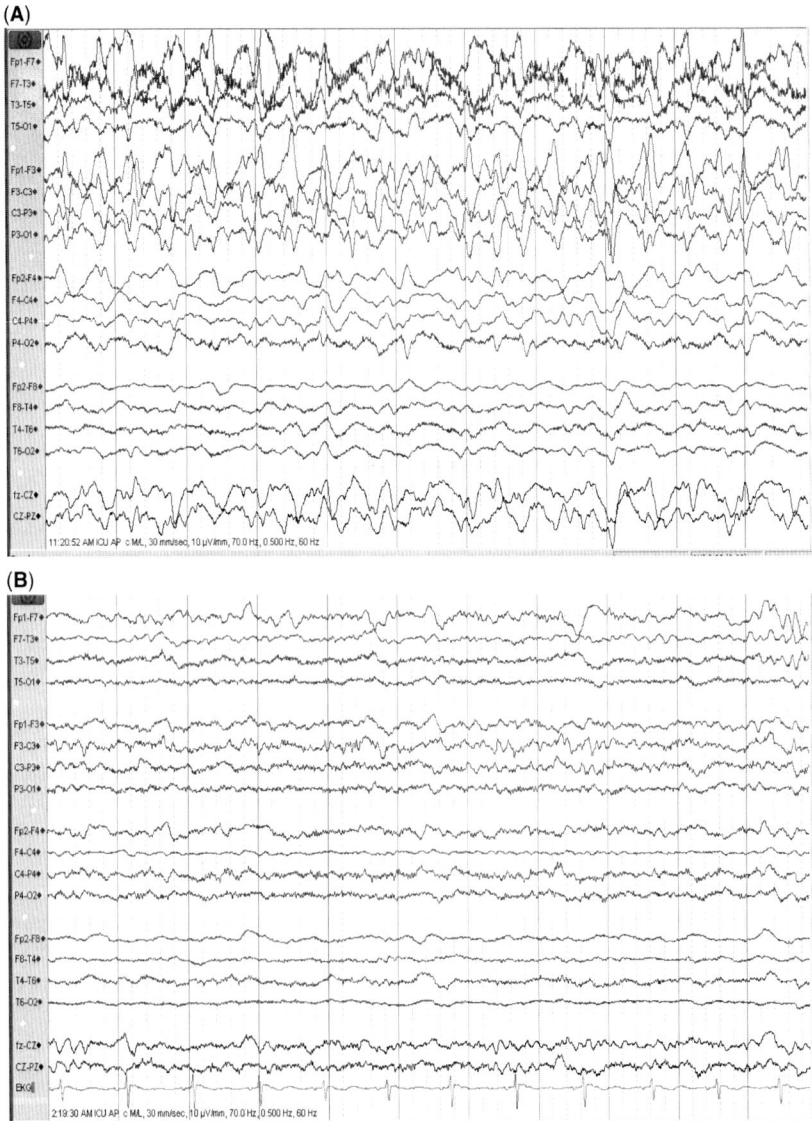

FIGURE 21.4 (**A**) A 44-year-old woman presented with aphasia and right hemiparesis following a left temporal contusion. EEG initially demonstrated lateralized periodic discharges over the left hemisphere with superimposed rhythmic activity (LPDs plus) which fluctuated in frequency from 2 to 3 Hz. Although the LPDs transiently resolved following administration of lorazepam, clinical exam did not improve. (**B**) Following administration of a fosphenytoin intravenous load, her clinical exam returned to baseline and EEG markedly improved.

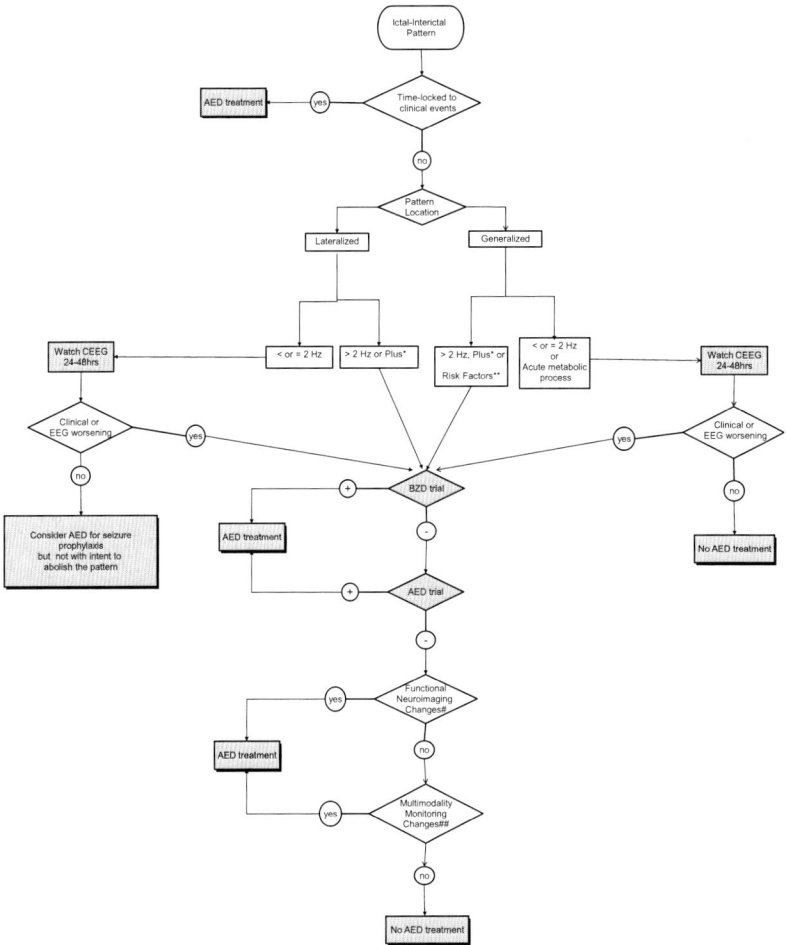

A proposed treatment algorithm to guide management of patients with EEG patterns that fall along the ictal–interictal continuum.

*Plus = superimposed fast or rhythmic features.
**Risk factors = Recent clinical seizure(s), history of epilepsy, acute CNS structural lesion.
#Evidence of regional hypermetabolism on PET or increase in cerebral blood flow on SPECT.
##Acute worsening of ICP, tissue oxygenation, cerebral blood flow, microdialysis parameters or elevated neuron-specific enolase. AED, antiepileptic drug; BZD, benzodiazepine.
Drs. Valia Rodriguez and Meghan Rodden contributed to the development of this algorithm.

- Multicenter database collection
  - A shared multicenter database format will allow for rapid collection of a variety of diverse EEG patterns in various patient populations and correlation with clinical outcomes.

REFERENCES

1. Young GB, Jordan KG, Doig GS. An assessment of nonconvulsive seizures in the intensive care unit using continuous EEG monitoring: An investigation of variables associated with mortality. *Neurology.* Jul 1996;47(1):83–89.
2. Drislane FW. *Nonconvulsive Status: Morbidity and Consequences.* Humana Press, New York, 2005.
3. DeLorenzo RJ, Waterhouse EJ, Towne AR, et al. Persistent nonconvulsive status epilepticus after the control of convulsive status epilepticus. *Epilepsia.* Aug 1998;39(8): 833–840.
4. Litt B, Wityk RJ, Hertz SH, et al. Nonconvulsive status epilepticus in the critically ill elderly. *Epilepsia.* Nov 1998;39(11):1194–1202.
5. Vespa PM, O'Phelan K, Shah M, et al. Acute seizures after intracerebral hemorrhage: A factor in progressive midline shift and outcome. *Neurology.* May 13, 2003;60(9): 1441–1446.
6. Vespa PM, Miller C, McArthur D, et al. Nonconvulsive electrographic seizures after traumatic brain injury result in a delayed, prolonged increase in intracranial pressure and metabolic crisis. *Crit Care Med.* Dec 2007;35(12):2830–2836.
7. DeGiorgio CM, Correale JD, Gott PS, et al. Serum neuron-specific enolase in human status epilepticus. *Neurology.* Jun 1995;45(6):1134–1137.
8. Claassen J, Hirsch LJ, Frontera JA, et al. Prognostic significance of continuous EEG monitoring in patients with poor-grade subarachnoid hemorrhage. *Neurocrit Care.* 2006; 4(2):103–112.
9. Claassen J, Jette N, Chum F, et al. Electrographic seizures and periodic discharges after intracerebral hemorrhage. *Neurology.* Sep 25, 2007;69(13):1356–1365.
10. Taylor D, Folami K, Wuu J, LaRoche S. Periodic patterns and their association to seizures and outcome in continuous EEG monitoring in the ICU. Poster presentation at the American Epilepsy Society Annual Meeting, Boston MA, December 2009.
11. Handforth A, Cheng JT, Mandelkern MA, Treiman DM. Markedly increased mesiotemporal lobe metabolism in a case with PLEDs: Further evidence that PLEDs are a manifestation of partial status epilepticus. *Epilepsia.* Jul–Aug 1994;35(4):876–881.
12. Assal F, Papazyan JP, Slosman DO, Jallon P, Goerres GW. SPECT in periodic lateralized epileptiform discharges (PLEDs): A form of partial status epilepticus? *Seizure: J Br Epilepsy Assoc.* Jun 2001;10(4):260–265.
13. Yemisci M, Gurer G, Saygi S, Ciger A. Generalised periodic epileptiform discharges: Clinical features, neuroradiological evaluation and prognosis in 37 adult patients. *Seizure: J Br Epilepsy Assoc.* Oct 2003;12(7):465–472.
14. Abou Khaled KJ, Hirsch LJ. Advances in the management of seizures and status epilepticus in critically ill patients. *Crit Care Clin.* Oct 2006;22(4):637–659; abstract viii.
15. Husain AM, Mebust KA, Radtke RA. Generalized periodic epileptiform discharges: Etiologies, relationship to status epilepticus, and prognosis. *J Clin Neurophysiol: Off Publ Am Electroencephalogr Soc.* Jan 1999;16(1):51–58.
16. Brenner RP, Schaul N. Periodic EEG patterns: Classification, clinical correlation, and pathophysiology. *J Clin Neurophysiol: Off Publ Am Electroencephalogr Soc.* Apr 1990;7(2):249–267.
17. Reiher J, Rivest J, Grand'Maison F, Leduc CP. Periodic lateralized epileptiform discharges with transitional rhythmic discharges: Association with seizures. *Electroencephalogr Clin Neurophysiol.* Jan 1991;78(1):12–17.

18. Hirsch LJ, Claassen J, Mayer SA, Emerson RG. Stimulus-induced rhythmic, periodic, or ictal discharges (SIRPIDs): A common EEG phenomenon in the critically ill. *Epilepsia.* Feb 2004;45(2):109–123.

19. Jirsch J, Hirsch LJ. Nonconvulsive seizures: Developing a rational approach to the diagnosis and management in the critically ill population. *Clin Neurophysiol: Off J Int Fed Clin Neurophysiol.* Aug 2007;118(8):1660–1670.

20. Claassen J. How I treat patients with EEG patterns on the ictal–interictal continuum in the neuro ICU. *Neurocrit Care.* Dec 2009;11(3):437–444.

21. Kaplan PW, Duckworth J. Confusion and SIRPIDs regress with parenteral lorazepam. *Epileptic Disord: Int Epilepsy J with Videotape.* Sep 2011;13(3):291–294.

TWENTY-TWO

Nonconvulsive Status Epilepticus

Frank W. Drislane

KEY POINTS

- Any patient who has not recovered from a seizure within 20 to 30 minutes should be considered to be in possible nonconvulsive status epilepticus (NCSE).
- NCSE should be suspected after strokes or other acute brain injuries when patients do not stabilize or improve as expected.
- EEG is crucial for diagnosis, but EEG findings in NCSE are varied, often controversial, and must be described precisely and interpreted in the clinical setting.
- EEG is necessary for diagnosis of NCSE and also to guide appropriate treatment and prevent, detect, and treat relapses.

I. BACKGROUND

A. Definitions
- Status epilepticus: "a condition characterized by an epileptic seizure that is sufficiently prolonged or repeated ... so as to produce an ... enduring epileptic condition" (International League Against Epilepsy).
- NCSE: greater than 30 minutes of epileptic seizures without convulsions. EEG is crucial for diagnosis but can be difficult to interpret or controversial (1).
- NCSE following generalized seizures and generalized convulsive status epilepticus (GCSE): GCSE continues in a more subtle form, and epileptiform discharges continue on EEG after convulsions cease. In this case, NCSE is considered a later stage of GCSE with regard to pathophysiology, clinical implications, and mandate for treatment.

B. Clinical Presentation
- Varied and often subtle.
- Includes impairment of mental status, cognition, or behavior; automatisms; change in sensory perception (auditory, visual, somatosensory, or psychic); amnesia; altered affect or language (mutism, paraphasic errors, aphasia); and confusion.

- NCSE may include minimal motor manifestations such as subtle facial or limb jerking, blinking, nystagmus, or perioral and eyelid myoclonus.

C. Etiology

- *Acute medical and neurologic illnesses*: infections, vascular disease, paraneoplastic syndromes, earlier seizures, or metabolic abnormalities, including electrolyte imbalance or hyperglycemia. Any of these conditions may cause or precipitate NCSE and also may obscure, or be mistaken for, the diagnosis due to the encephalopathy that can be associated with these conditions alone.
- *Associated chronic conditions*: dementia, mental retardation, psychiatric disorders. In the elderly, the "confusion" of NCSE may be mistaken for medication toxicity or dementia.
- *Medications*: neuroleptics, cephalosporins, radiologic contrast agents, GABA agonists (eg, baclofen, tiagabine).
- Diagnostic clues include a history of seizures or epilepsy, or risk factors for epilepsy.
- *Mimics*: migraine, postictal state, transient global amnesia (TGA), aphasia or other transient vascular syndromes; sleep disorders (eg, cataplexy); psychiatric disorders; cardiovascular disease; endocrine or autonomic dysfunction; limbic encephalitis (paraneoplastic or other antibody-mediated); encephalopathies, including from metabolic derangements and drugs, such as lithium, psychotropic medications, alcohol or other intoxications.

D. NCSE Diagnosis

- *Clinical symptoms*: altered responsiveness, cognition, behavior, or other neurologic deficit.
- *EEG findings*: Continuous or recurrent seizure activity or ictal discharges for greater than 30 minutes.
- The clinical and EEG response to antiepileptic drugs (AEDs) is often delayed.
- *AED challenge*: A rapid response to AEDs (eg, lorazepam) can be diagnostic if there is a prompt improvement in both the clinical state of the patient and the EEG pattern, (complete cessation of electrographic seizure activity and return of normal EEG background activity).
  - EEG improvement alone is not sufficient; benzodiazepines can abolish seizures but also suppress nonepileptic EEG patterns such as triphasic waves (TW).
  - Correspondingly, lack of prompt improvement after treatment with AEDs does NOT refute a diagnosis of NCSE; the response can be equivocal, delayed, or impaired by sedation.

II. BASICS

A. Types of NCSE
1. Simple Partial SE (SPSE)
- *Common causes*: Leading cause is stroke (ischemic or hemorrhagic). But also can be due to mass lesions, tumors, and encephalitis.

- *Rare causes*: vasculitis, multiple sclerosis, mitochondrial disorders, genetic "idiopathic" epilepsies (eg, Rolandic), trauma, and developmental abnormalities (heterotopias or other migration abnormalities).
- Motor, sensory, psychic, or autonomic symptoms, but no impairment of consciousness (as opposed to complex partial SE).
- Nonconvulsive forms include persistent sensory or autonomic disturbances, and cognitive deficits.
- Surface EEG (even during symptoms) has limited sensitivity for showing ictal discharges, as seizures may involve remote focus or a mall brain volume.
- Focal sensory NCSE
  - Includes hallucinations (most often, olfactory)
  - Cortical blindness or visual field loss can occur.
  - Autonomic symptoms are frequent, particularly in children.
  - Pure sensory SE is rare (especially in ICUs) and is often confused with TIAs.
  - Confers little or no morbidity
- "Transient epileptic amnesia" (TEA)
  - Pure amnesia (with preserved cognitive function otherwise) can be a manifestation of epileptic seizures and can persist greater than 30 minutes. Differential diagnosis includes transient global amnesia (TGA).
- Aphasic SE
  - Preserved responsiveness, without confusion; deficit restricted to language alone.

2. Complex Partial SE (CPSE)

- Recurrent or continuous complex partial seizures are the most common NCSE in adults who are ambulatory or not critically ill.
- CPSE begins with a focal-onset seizure and progresses to involve more of the brain such that responsiveness is impaired.
- Presentation consists of abnormal or fluctuating behavior, diminished responsiveness, confusion, automatisms, dystonic posturing, eye deviation, or fugue state.
- Most common causes include a history of chronic epilepsy, or vascular disease (acute or chronic), often with a precipitant of infection or metabolic derangement.
- Temporal CPSE may present with fear, anxiety, agitation, simple and complex automatisms, or unresponsiveness with motionless staring.
- Frontal CPSE
  - Can have continuous mood and behavioral disturbances or disinhibition, and subtle impairment of cognition.
  - Less often, there is greater impairment of consciousness, some with cyclic fluctuations and marked behavioral disturbance.
- EEG findings
  - Most CPSE is associated with discernible surface EEG changes, usually with repetitive focal seizures, and focal or lateralized background slowing between seizures (Figure 22.1).
  - CPSE arising from mesial temporal origins often begins with unilateral 5 to 7 Hz rhythmic activity.
  - CPSE arising from the frontal regions is often associated with bilateral, often asymmetric frontal discharges.

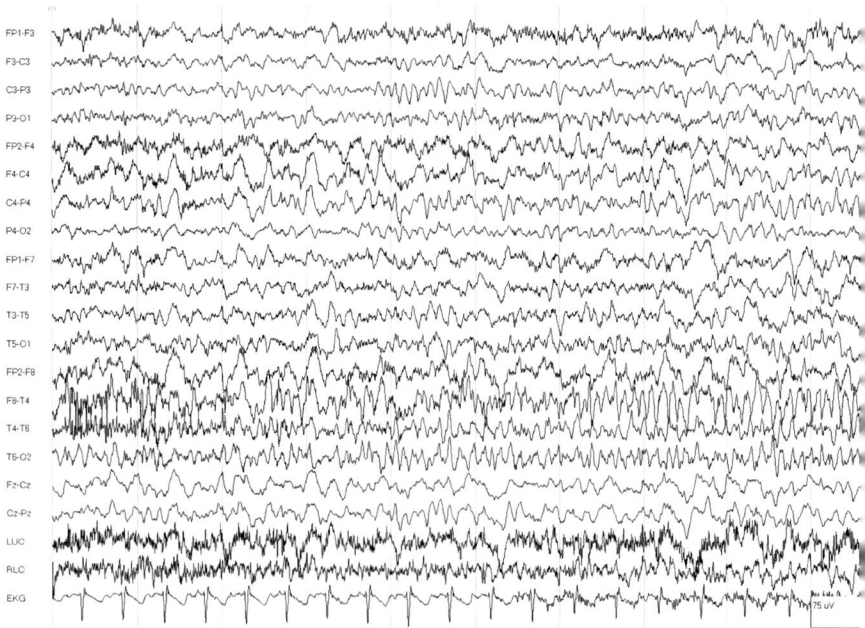

FIGURE 22.1 CPSE: "Psychic" status epilepticus in a 41-year-old woman with right mesial temporal sclerosis. She presented with mild confusion but could follow most commands. She did not answer questions and had bizarre speech, repeating "you are my Norm, you are my one true love". Complex partial seizures recurred without clinical recovery. With permission from Schomer DL, Lopes da Silva F, *Niedermeyer's Electroencephalography*, 6th edition, p. 608. Lippincott Williams & Wilkins, 2011.

- Treatment and outcome of CPSE
  - Immediately upon diagnosis (ie, *less than* 30 minutes), CPSE should be treated promptly with intravenous AEDs.
  - Owing to association with focal lesions and prior epilepsy, it is often difficult to treat.
  - In patients with a history of epilepsy, a less aggressive approach than for GCSE is often warranted.
  - Outcome depends mostly on etiology.
  - Morbidity often derives from complications of the underlying illness, for example, encephalitis or stroke.
  - Most patients return to normal or baseline cognitive function, but resolution can take weeks or months, and prolonged memory and other cognitive deficits can result.

3. **Absence SE**
   - "Pure" primary generalized epilepsy with clinical seizures greater than 30 minutes, usually in patients with idiopathic generalized epilepsy (IGEs), including typical childhood and juvenile absence epilepsy, juvenile myoclonic

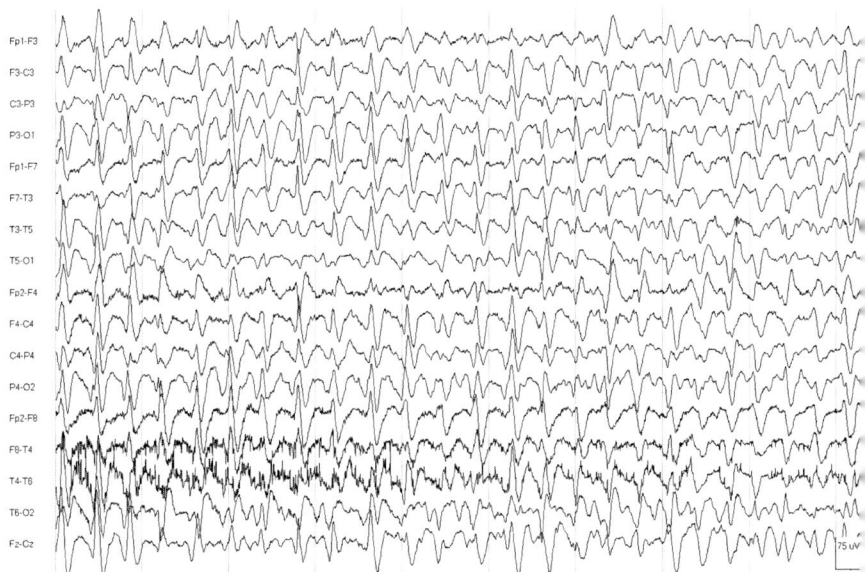

FIGURE 22.2 *De novo* absence status epilepticus: 58-year-old woman with no history of epilepsy, admitted with confusion. EEG shows generalized 2.5 Hz spike and slow-wave activity. A few minutes later (after 2 mg i.v. lorazapam), the EEG showed mild diffuse slowing with plentiful beta activity. The confusion improved concurrently with the EEG improvement, about 4 minutes after the lorazepam administration. With permission from Schomer DL, Lopes da Silva F, *Niedermeyer's Electroencephalography*, 6th edition, p. 617. Lippincott Williams & Wilkins, 2011.

epilepsy, and generalized convulsions upon awakening. A generalized convulsion may provoke or end an episode.

- *Clinical presentation*: confusion, blinking, occasional myoclonus; subtle change in responsiveness, with preserved alertness. Can last hours or days and is often recurrent.
- *Precipitants*: sleep deprivation, alcohol, metabolic abnormalities, intercurrent illnesses, and medications—(including withdrawal, ie, benzodiazepines).
- *EEG findings*: greater than 30 minutes of rhythmic, bilaterally symmetric spike-and-slow-wave discharges, up to 4 Hz at onset; sometimes with polyspikes. Maximal voltage is over frontal and central regions.
- *Treatment*: Absence SE may cease spontaneously or with treatment with low-dose benzodiazepines. It results in minimal or no morbidity.

4. *De novo* Absence SE

- Occasionally, somewhat older adults present with confusion, sometimes after using benzodiazepines (BDZs), including for sleep, and are found to be in NCSE with an EEG that appears very similar to that of absence SE (Figure 22.2). Some may have had primary generalized seizures earlier in life (or the genetic trait for that condition) and manifest the NCSE after some

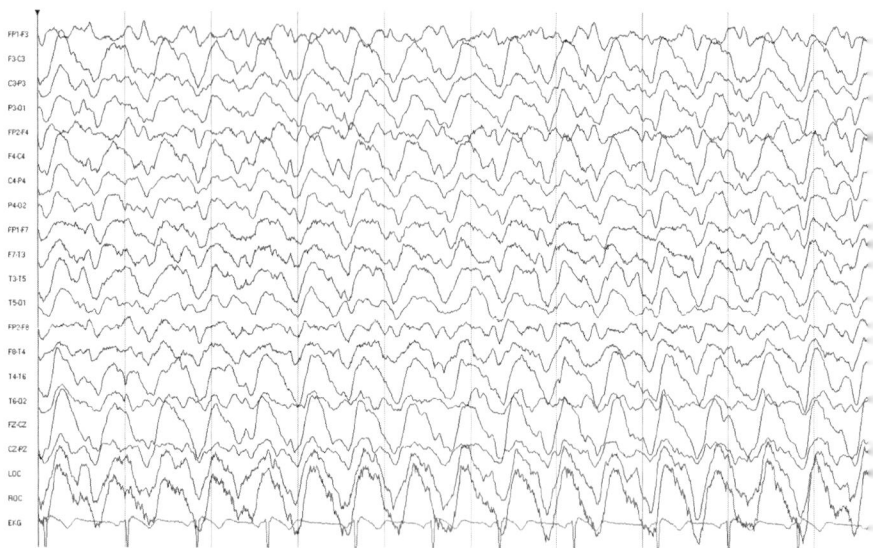

FIGURE 22.3   Secondarily generalized NCSE: A 31-year-old woman with metastatic colon cancer, admitted with catatonia. An earlier EEG showed rhythmic 1.5 to 2 Hz delta activity over the right hemisphere alone. Hours later, the EEG shows generalized sharp and slow-wave discharges at 1.5 Hz, suggesting generalized NCSE. With 4 mg i.v. lorazepam, the EEG showed resolution of all rhythmic and sharp activity, and the patient became more responsive clinically. With permission from Schomer DL, Lopes da Silva F, *Niedermeyer's Electroencephalography*, 6th edition, p. 621. Lippincott Williams & Wilkins, 2011.

physiologic stress. They are usually treated easily with low dose BDZs and often require no long term medication.

5. **Secondarily Generalized NCSE**
   - The most common NCSE in sick, hospitalized patients.
   - The diagnosis is often missed. Often occurs without prior history of seizures or epilepsy.
   - There is a frequent combination of a prior insult (vascular or epilepsy) and new precipitant (infection, metabolic disturbance, or drug). For example, renal failure and infection in an elderly patient with an old stroke.
   - Often manifested by a reduction in responsiveness or consciousness; sometimes accompanied by staring, facial twitching, or subtle myoclonus.
   - Generalized NCSE is seldom "absence SE." True absence SE occurs in patients with a history of IGE syndromes. Most "generalized" NCSE is *secondarily generalized*, although the EEG may show focal or generalized discharges at the onset (2) (Figure 22.3).
   - "Subtle SE" often characterizes the later stages of GCSE.
   - Urgency of treatment continues, especially after generalized convulsions, but abolition of electrographic seizures does not always lead to clinical improvement.

B. NCSE in the Intensive Care Unit
- Rhythmic, rapid epileptiform discharges typical for SE are seen on the EEG, often without obvious clinical seizures.
- Common in critically ill patients who are often confused, stuporous, or comatose.
- Many patients have had earlier clinical seizures or GCSE.
- Often seen in the setting of serious medical illness such as stroke, infection, hypoxia, or severe metabolic derangements.
- The underlying medical condition is the main determinant of outcome. For example, NCSE after anoxia is almost always fatal.
- NCSE is unsuspected in most and often discovered incidentally.
  - Following apparent control of clinical SE in 164 patients, 42% had continued seizure discharges and 14% were in NCSE.
  - In another study, 8% of 236 patients with coma of all causes (without clinical seizures) had NCSE (3).
  - With continuous EEG monitoring, 19% of patients in a neurologic ICU had seizures, 92% of which were strictly nonconvulsive.
  - In another cEEG study, NCSE was usually unsuspected—with a median delay to diagnosis of 48 hours.
- Main causes (In ICU patients, each of the following etiologies has been shown to have a 20%–30% incidence of NCS or NCSE in patients undergoing cEEG):
  - Acute neurologic injuries, especially intracerebral or subarachnoid hemorrhage.
  - CNS infection
  - Brain tumors
  - Severe head trauma
  - Following neurosurgery
- Risks for nonconvulsive seizures and NCSE in the ICU:
  - Highest risk includes patients who were in GCSE and thought to have been treated successfully but were not. A prolonged "post-ictal" state should raise concern for NCSE.
  - Coma (especially with unclear cause)
  - Recent generalized convulsions or history of epilepsy
  - Remote symptomatic CNS insults (eg, stroke, neurosurgery, tumor, etc), especially when the patient is encephalopathic.
  - Intercurrent electrolyte abnormalities
  - Infections such as pneumonia or UTI
  - Glucose dysregulation
- When to suspect NCSE in the ICU (4):
  - Prolonged "postictal state" after generalized convulsions
  - Diminished alertness in the post-operative period
  - After an acute neurologic insult such as a stroke when the patient "looks worse" than the deficit seen on neuroimaging.
  - Impaired mentation with myoclonus or nystagmus
  - Episodic staring, aphasia, automatisms, or perseveration
  - Aphasia without a structural lesion
  - Acutely altered behavior, without other explanation, especially in the elderly
- Mimics of NCSE in ICU patients
  - Severe toxic, metabolic, and infectious encephalopathies

○ Sedating medications
○ Post-ictal or post-operative encephalopathies (many due to medications)
○ Benzodiazepine withdrawal states or toxicity
○ Psychiatric illness
○ Hyperglycemia
○ Neuroleptic malignant and serotonin syndromes
○ Other systemic illnesses (which are often accompanied by abnormal EEGs, sometimes even with epileptiform features)

C. EEG in the Diagnosis of NCSE
1. EEG Criteria for Determination of an Electrographic Seizure
- Repetitive or rhythmic focal or generalized epileptiform discharges at greater than 3 Hz, and lasting longer than 10 seconds.
- Similar discharges at less than 3 Hz, with clear evolution in frequency (increase or decrease by greater than 1 Hz), location, waveform, or field (spread to greater than 2 adjacent electrodes) OR clinical motor manifestations (eg, limb or facial twitching).
- Clinical improvement and improvement or normalization of the EEG after acute administration of rapid-acting intravenous AEDs, typically benzodiazepines (5).
- Suspect NCSE if a patient returns rapidly to a baseline state (after AEDs, or spontaneously) and the EEG becomes normal.

2. Typical EEG Features Seen in NCSE
- Rhythmic, generalized, symmetric spike-and-waves or polyspikes and waves at 2 to 3.5 Hz
- Atypical spike and wave with lower frequency and less symmetry
- Multiple spike-and-wave
- High-voltage, repetitive, rhythmic (focal or generalized) delta activity with intermixed spikes, sharp waves, or sharp components (2)

3. Controversies
- Some NCSE EEG patterns are not "classic;" and show disorganized slowing (without rhythmicity or epileptiform abnormalities), more suggestive of encephalopathies.
- Current EEG criteria for determination of a an electrographic seizure were designed as research criteria so they are purposefully strict, but not all patients in NCSE meet them. "False negatives" occur.
- Criteria are also based on discrete electrographic seizures, not persistent conditions.
- EEG waveforms can be remarkably varied.
- Response to AEDs may be quite delayed (eg, after generalized convulsions, response may not be seen until 1 to 3 days).
- Well-established cases of NCSE demonstrated stereotypic spike-and-wave activity at greater than 3 Hz in only 7% of patients, whereas 61% were less than 2.5 Hz (2). These slow frequency rhythmic and sharp EEG patterns are still suggestive of seizures, especially after prior clinical seizures or SE.
- EEG terminology lacks consensus.

○ The American Clinical Neurophysiology Society (ACNS) has recommended standardization of terms for periodic and potentially epileptiform EEG findings to facilitate clinical research.

4. **Duration of cEEG for Detection of NCSE**
   - In one study, a routine 30-minute EEG identified seizures in 11% of critically ill patients; while subsequent cEEG monitoring detected seizures in 27%.
   - Half of all seizures seen occurred in the first hour.
   - After 24 hours of monitoring, 95% of seizures were seen in the noncomatose patients versus 80% in comatose patients.
   - After 48 hours of monitoring, 98% of seizures were detected in noncomatose patients versus 87% in comatose patients.
   - Thus, cEEG monitoring is appropriate for 24 hours in patients without coma and 48 hours for comatose patients, patients with periodic discharges, or during AED withdrawal (6).

III. FURTHER CONSIDERATIONS/REMAINING QUESTIONS

A. Controversial EEG Patterns
1. **Periodic Discharges (PDs)**
   - Sharp and rhythmic EEG features range from nonictal but "irritative" (post-, inter-, or pre-ictal) discharges to discharges that represent electrographic seizures. These findings fall along an "ictal–interictal continuum."
   - May be lateralized (LPDs), bilateral (BIPDs), or generalized (GPDs) in distribution.
   - Periodic discharges are more likely to be "ictal" when they are rapid (greater than 2 Hz) or show clear evolution in frequency or field..

2. **Lateralized Periodic Discharges (LPDs)**
   - Focal discharges, typically every 1 to 2 seconds
   - Relatively constant in an individual and typically slow and resolve over days to weeks.
   - Usually associated with structural lesions, especially stroke, tumor, abscess, and encephalitis.
   - Often associated with high mortality
   - Usually associated with clinical seizures before their appearance and chronic epilepsy later.
   - LPDs are generally not considered seizures by themselves; but some consider them to represent "the terminal phase of SE."
   - However, some LPDs DO represent seizures and SE, particularly those associated with subtle clinical signs. Consultation with ICU colleagues is advised.

3. **LPDs Plus**
   - LPDs admixed with fast, sharp, or rhythmic activity.
   - More likely to be associated with seizures than LPDs alone.

4. **Bilateral Independent Periodic Discharges (BIPDs)**
   - Asynchronous LPDs with two or more foci (at least one focus in each hemisphere).

- Discharges have different frequencies, voltage, and fields.
- Background activity is often attenuated.
- Causes include infection (28%), anoxia (28%), epilepsy (22%), or vascular etiology.
- Higher association with coma (72 vs. 24%) and mortality (61 vs. 29%) than LPDs, but lower association with seizures.

5. **Generalized Periodic Discharges (GPDs)**
   - Continuous generalized spikes, polyspikes, sharp-and-slow waves, or TW, often at ~1 Hz, usually on a diffusely slow or attenuated background.
   - Often seen in obtunded patients, typically after anoxia or other catastrophes or metabolic insults.
   - Associated with clinical seizures, but not necessarily indicative of seizures at the same time.
   - When associated with recent overt seizures, or in the late stages of GCSE (with "subtle" clinical features), they are considered continuing SE.
   - Prognosis depends on the underlying cause.

6. **"Stimulus-Induced Rhythmic, Periodic, or Ictal Discharges" (SIRPIDs)**
   - Focal or generalized periodic and quasi-periodic discharges typically elicited in stuporous or comatose patients upon stimulation—usually abating after the stimulus recedes.
   - Some may represent an arousal process while some represent definite seizures (eg, when associated with facial or limb jerking).
   - SIRPIDs are another pattern that may lie along an "ictal–interictal continuum."

7. **Triphasic Waves**
   - Bursts of moderate-to-high voltage (100–300 μV) complexes, often at 1 to 2 Hz, with an initial blunted, low-voltage negative spike-like phase; a second slowly rising high-voltage positive component; and a third phase of a lower voltage, broad negative slow wave.
   - Broadly distributed, with a frontal maximum.
   - May occur in clusters, or may be continuous at 0.5 to 2 Hz.
   - Often state-responsive, increasing with stimulation.
   - May be abolished with intravenous AEDs suggesting a diagnosis of NCSE, but benzodiazepines may also abolish typical TW that are due to an encephalopathy, but without clinical improvement.
   - TWs are often associated with diminished consciousness and occasionally myoclonus.
   - There is often an underlying toxic or metabolic state, including uremia, hepatic insufficiency, hypothyroidism, or medication toxicity.

8. **TWs versus epileptic discharges**
   - Are TWs epileptiform?
     ○ TWs may have "epileptiform" appearance on EEG but are generally not considered epileptic. Nevertheless, they may indicate seizures, especially with frequencies greater than 1 Hz.
     ○ TWs are usually broader and more blunted in appearance than epileptiform discharges, which usually have higher frequencies (mean 2.4 vs. 1.8 Hz),

more polyspikes (69% vs. 0%), sharper morphologies, and less background slowing than TWs.
- ○ TWs have a relative lack of phase reversal and longer duration.
- ○ An anterior to posterior "phase lag" occurs with many TWs, but not in NCSE.

B. EEG Monitoring in the ICU for Detection of NCSE
- Because seizures (including NCS) can be intermittent, prolonged cEEG can be necessary to detect them.
- Rapid detection of NCS requires frequent EEG review and interpretation by trained personnel, at least several times a day.
- Still, cEEG produces more data than is feasible for electroencephalographers to review, at least in raw form.
- Quantitative EEG (QEEG) can create graphic displays that allow rapid detection of EEG changes to identify paroxysmal rhythmic activity with increased voltage or frequency (compared to background activity).
- Automated detection programs can identify episodes of interest, such as epileptiform spikes or seizures that require more detailed review of the raw EEG.
- EEG in the ICU is susceptible to many types of artifacts that can mimic seizures
- Therefore, the original raw EEG data must be available in order to distinguish "true" seizures from other periodic patterns, changes in sleep–wake states, arousal, or artifacts.
- Computer analysis can aid in data compression but cannot replace expert electroencephalographers.

C. EEG Monitoring in the Management of NCSE
- Clinical signs of NCSE are nonspecific, subtle, or nonexistent, so even after NCSE is diagnosed in the ICU, cEEG monitoring is required to guide prolonged treatment and assess response to therapy.
- NCSE persists in 14–20% of patients after cessation of clinically evident seizures. cEEG must be reviewed to ensure that breakthrough or recurrent seizures do not occur.
- Relapse of NCSE is relatively common, especially in the first 24 hours—and when AEDs are tapered.
- Seizures can be missed if EEG monitoring is intermittent. An EEG may show a "postictal" encephalopathy, drug effect, isolated or periodic discharges, or a burst suppression tracing at one point, and nonconvulsive seizures or NCSE at another.
- cEEG may also provide important prognostic information.

D. Outcome of NCSE
- Morbidity of NCSE
  - ○ There is little evidence available on long-term morbidity due to NCSE itself, as opposed to that from the underlying illness that causes or precipitates NCSE.
  - ○ NCSE may exacerbate neuronal damage in patients with acute insults such as traumatic brain injury (TBI) or stroke, and some patients develop hippocampal edema during NCSE, with subsequent hippocampal atrophy.
  - ○ Pathologic studies are few after NCSE, as fatal SE is often associated with acute, severe brain injury that causes damage independently.

- ○ Cognitive deficits caused by NCSE, including memory and language dysfunction, can persist for months, but they are uncommon, occurring primarily in the most prolonged and severe cases.
- ○ GCSE is a major threat to health and warrants vigorous treatment, but evidence of lasting harm due to NCSE alone is modest.
- Longer-term outcome of NCSE.
  - ○ Depends mostly on the specific SE type (based on clinical and EEG findings), its cause and precipitants.
  - ○ Outcome may also be influenced by age, concomitant medical illness, duration of SE, and the effectiveness and complications of treatment.
  - ○ Simple partial SE and absence SE have minimal or no morbidity.
  - ○ Secondarily generalized NCSE in the setting of serious medical and neurologic illness, especially in the ICU, has major morbidity and a high risk of mortality.
  - ○ Etiology is the most important prognostic factor.
  - ○ Complications of treatment, particularly aggressive overtreatment, can also contribute to morbidity via hypotension or prolonged mechanical ventilation.
  - ○ Patients with anoxia or multiple medical problems, including sepsis, have a poor outcome.
  - ○ Patients with underlying strokes, tumors, trauma, infection, alcohol abuse, or other drugs have varied outcomes.
  - ○ The most favorable etiology is in patients with chronic epilepsy who have breakthrough seizures precipitated by a recent reduction in AEDs, or noncompliance.

REFERENCES

1. Drislane FW, Kaplan PW, Herman ST. Nonconvulsive status epilepticus, Chap 29. In: DL Schomer, F Lopes da Silva, eds. *Niedermeyer's Electroencephalography*, 6th ed. Philadelphia: Lippincott Williams & Wilkins;2010:595–643.
2. Granner MA, Lee SI. Nonconvulsive status epilepticus: EEG analysis in a large series. *Epilepsia.* 1994;35:42–47.
3. Towne AR, Waterhouse EJ, Boggs JG, et al.Prevalence of nonconvulsive status epilepticus in comatose patients. *Neurology.* 2000;54:340–345.
4. Young GB, Jordan KG, Doig GS . An assessment of nonconvulsive seizures in the intensive care unit using continuous EEG monitoring: An investigation of variables associated with mortality. *Neurology.* 1996;47:83–89.
5. Chong DJ, Hirsch LJ . Which EEG patterns warrant treatment in the critically ill? Reviewing the evidence for treatment of periodic epileptiform discharges and related patterns. *J Clin Neurophysiol.* 2005;22:79–91.
6. Jirsch J, Hirsch LJ . Nonconvulsive status epilepticus in critically ill and comatose patients in the intensive care unit, Chap 13. In: PW Kaplan, FW Drislane, eds. *Nonconvulsive Status Epilepticus.* New York: Demos Medical Publishing; 2009:175–186.

TWENTY-THREE

EEG Patterns in the Neonatal and Pediatric Population

Nicholas S. Abend, Courtney J. Wusthoff, Cecil D. Hahn, Tammy Tsuchida, and James J. Riviello

KEY POINTS

- Neonatal EEG interpretation requires knowledge of patient postmenstrual age and state.
- Neonatal EEG interpretation focuses on background continuity–discontinuity and seizure identification.
- Non-neonatal pediatric EEG interpretation is similar to adult EEG interpretation.

I. BACKGROUND

A. Neonatal EEG

- A limited array montage is often used in which anterior–posterior electrodes are double distance and the frontal electrodes are slightly more posterior than in standard adult montages.
- A standard montage is generally used after 46 to 48 weeks postmenstrual age.
- Neonatal EEG is often displayed at faster paper speed (15 to 20 seconds per screen) to enhance visualization of slow activity which predominates.
- Extracerebral channels including eye and respiratory channels are important in assessing patient state (awake, active sleep, or quiet sleep).
- Technologist notations are important in determining behavioral state (eyes open or closed) and identifying artifact.
- American Clinical Neurophysiology Guidelines describe that the first hour of EEG should be interpreted as soon as possible by the clinical neurophysiologist and subsequent review should occur at least twice per 24-hour epoch, unless clinical circumstances dictate more frequent review is needed. Written reports should be completed daily (1).

B. Pediatric EEG
- In non-neonatal critically ill children, EEG interpretation is similar to adults.

II. BASICS

A. Neonatal EEG
- EEG background activity
  - Normal Behavioral States:
    - Awake—eyes open, irregular respirations and spontaneous movements. EEG demonstrates mixed frequencies of 25 to 50 μV with a predominance of theta and delta activity. Continuity is dependent on postmenstrual age (see below).
    - Active sleep—eyes closed, rapid eye movements, irregular respirations. EEG similar to the awake state.
    - Quiet sleep—eyes closed, no rapid eye movements, and regular respirations. EEG demonstrates some discontinuity (ie, tracé alternant and tracé discontinu) with interburst interval dependent on postmenstrual age (see below).
    - NOTE: Encephalopathic neonates spend much time in indeterminate sleep.
  - In contrast to the older child or adult, a few weeks' age difference is associated with substantial differences in normal EEG features.
    - Dysmaturity refers to EEG background activity with features that are normal for an infant 2 weeks younger than the stated postmenstrual age.
  - Normal neonatal tracings may contain some discontinuity, and knowledge of the neonate's postmenstrual age is critical in determining whether discontinuity is normal or excessive for age.
    - Discontinuity refers to "on" periods, called bursts, and "off" periods, called interburst intervals.
    - Postmenstrual Age = Gestational Age + Legal Age.
    - A baby born at 30 weeks (gestational age = 30 weeks) who is 10 weeks old (legal age = 10 weeks) has a postmenstrual age of 40 weeks.
    - Discontinuity is measured by the interburst interval, often defined as the period with activity of less than 25 μV (Figure 23.1). Normal interburst intervals are provided in Table 23.1.
  - Tracé discontinu and tracé alternant refer to normal patterns.
    - Tracé discontinu is a normal discontinuous pattern in premature infants (about 30–34 weeks postmenstrual age) in which there is activity separated by an interburst interval that may be less than 25 μV.
    - Tracé alternant is a normal pattern seen in quiet sleep from about 36 to 37 weeks postmenstrual age in which bursts of high amplitude 50 to 100 μV activity are superimposed on 25 to 50 μV activity. Fragments of tracé alternant may persist until 44 weeks during quiet sleep.
  - Burst suppression refers to a pattern with interburst intervals of low amplitude (often defined as less than 5 μV) alternating with higher amplitude bursts. It is nonreactive and invariant. In contrast, an excessively discontinuous record will generally remain reactive with some variability.
  - Brief periods of attenuation, particularly when accompanied by muscle artifact, may be due to normal arousal (both spontaneous and provoked).

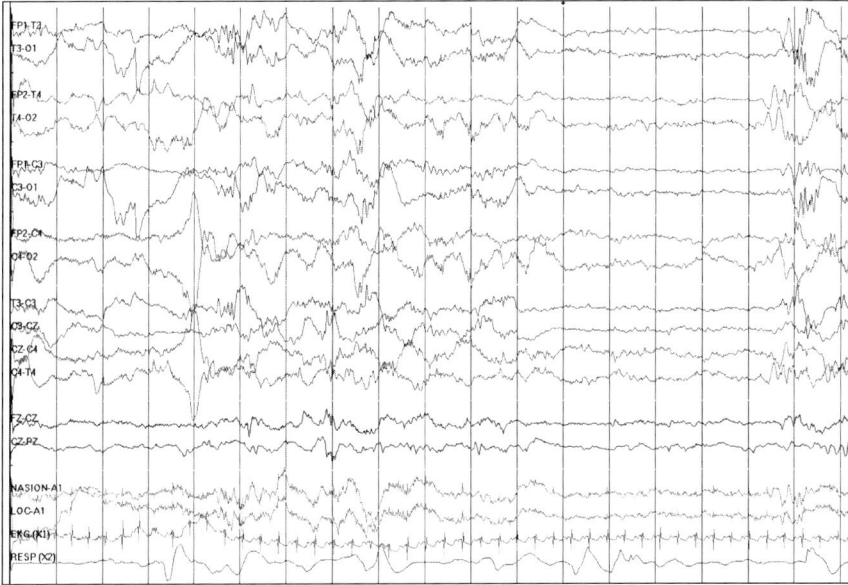

FIGURE 23.1   Neonate with discontinuous tracing. Determining whether the degree of discontinuity is normal or excessive requires knowledge of the postmenstrual age.

○ Synchrony is also age dependent. Background activity should be synchronous in premature (less than 29 weeks postmenstrual age) and term (greater than 37 weeks postmenstrual age) neonates. Asynchrony is normal between 29 and 36 weeks postmenstrual age.

TABLE 23.1   Neonatal EEG Characteristics

• Interburst (IBI): Upper Limit of Normal
○ less than 30 weeks PMA: 35 seconds (median 10 seconds)
○ 30–33 weeks PMA: 20 seconds
○ 34–36 weeks PMA: 10 seconds
○ 37–40 weeks PMA: 6 seconds (median 2–4 seconds)
• Normal Interburst Amplitude
○ less than 35 weeks PMA: < 25 uV
○ greater than 35 weeks PMA: > 25 uV

PMA, postmenstrual age

○ Reactivity refers to a clinical (EMG activity, respiratory pattern change) and/or EEG response (increased continuity, amplitude reduction, frequency change) to external stimulation.
○ Sharp waves may be physiologic (normal) or pathologic.
  • Physiologic sharp waves tend to be rare and often central–temporal predominant, while pathologic sharp waves are more frequent (greater than 11 per hour for preterm and greater than 13 per hour for term) or repetitive and unifocal.
  • Sharp waves may be more frequent in discontinuous periods (quiet or indeterminate sleep).
  • Sharp waves in neonates may be negative or positive in polarity, and may have a more limited field (ie, one channel) than seen in older children.
• Brief Rhythmic Discharges (BRDs), Seizures, and Status Epilepticus
  ○ Neonatal Seizure = a sudden rhythmic evolving and stereotyped event of abnormal electrographic activity with a duration of at least 10 seconds.
    • Evolving means EEG activity progresses in frequency, morphology, or distribution (Figure 23.2).
  ○ Most neonatal seizures last about 1 to 2 minutes (2).
  ○ Most neonatal seizures are electrographic-only (subclinical, nonconvulsive) (3).
  ○ Electro-mechanical uncoupling may occur following anticonvulsant administration, meaning clinical seizures cease but electrographic seizures persist (4).
  ○ Diagnosis of neonatal seizures by clinical observation is difficult (5).

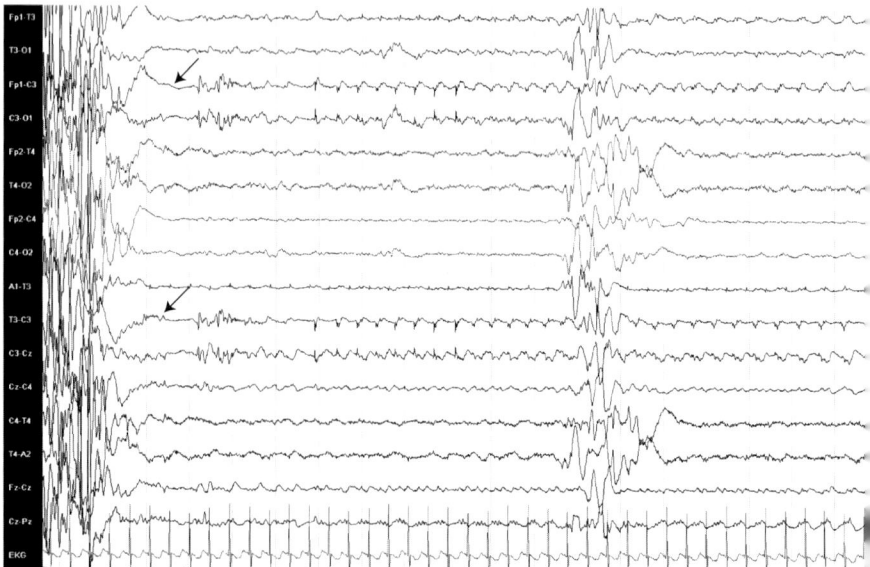

FIGURE 23.2   One-week-old term infant with hypoxic–ischemic encephalopathy. Suppression-burst background pattern with recurrent low-amplitude focal seizures arising from left central head region (sensitivity 3uV/mm).

- The most common clinically evident events with an electrographic correlate include focal clonic or tonic seizures (6).
- "Generalized tonic-clonic" seizures are extremely rare in neonates, and use of this term usually implies an inaccurate diagnosis.
  ○ Neonatal seizures are usually focal or multifocal, and may be restricted to only one electrode.
  ○ Brief Rhythmic Discharges (BRDs) refer to electroencephalographic events which are less than 10 seconds in duration, but otherwise appear as electrographic seizures.
  ○ There is no uniform system for calculating seizure burden and thus no standardized definition for status epilepticus in neonates.
  ○ One proposed definition of status epilepticus is when seizures comprise more than 50% of a 1 hour epoch.
- Amplitude integrated EEG (aEEG)
  ○ aEEG monitoring using one or two channels provides a bedside display of compressed EEG (Figure 23.3).

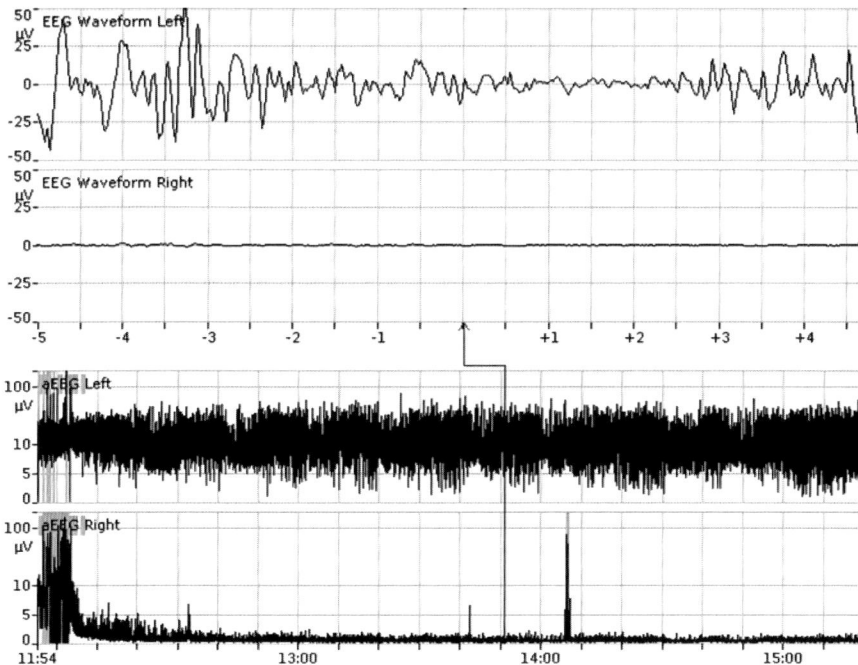

FIGURE 23.3 This two-channel (four electrode) aEEG tracing allows comparison of aEEG recording from the left and right hemispheres. The top two boxes show 10 seconds of the source EEG tracing at the point indicated by the cursor below. The two lower boxes show the processed aEEG signal, giving a trend over roughly 3 hours. In this example from a 40-week postmenstrual age newborn, there is initially activity in both the left and right hemispheres, but activity on the right hemisphere rapidly becomes markedly suppressed. In this case, the neonate had suffered a very large right subdural hemorrhage.

○ aEEG has fair-to-moderate agreement with conventional EEG in terms of background description.

○ Conventional full array EEG monitoring is superior to limited channel aEEG for seizure identification. However, when interpreted by a skilled user limited channel aEEG can identify seizures in many neonates.

○ Studies that have evaluated limited channel aEEG for seizure identification report that about half of seizures identified on conventional EEG are identified by aEEG, with the best identification when aEEG electrodes are placed at C3 to C4 (7).

○ Artifacts and nonseizure movements are common on aEEG, and must be distinguished from electrographic seizures.

B. Pediatric EEG
- Common Background Patterns
  ○ *Normal Predominant Frequencies*: With normal development, the predominant and posterior dominant frequencies increase.
    - Normal frequencies include 3 to 4 Hz at 4 months, 5 to 6 Hz at 1 year, 8 Hz at 3 years, and 9 to 10 Hz by 9 years.
  ○ *Mild Background Slowing*: Slowing of the background or posterior dominant rhythm compared to age-dependent norms (see above). This is a sensitive indicator of encephalopathy, but is nonspecific in etiology.
  ○ *Slow Activity*: Slowing can be focal or diffuse, intermittent or continuous, and polymorphic or rhythmic.
    - Diffuse continuous polymorphic slowing is common in encephalopathy but is nonspecific in etiology and can occur with metabolic encephalopathy, intoxication, or cerebral lesions.
    - Focal or multifocal slowing suggests a focal structural or functional abnormality, and neuroimaging is generally indicated.
  ○ *Low Voltage, Slow, Nonreactive*: Mostly delta and theta frequencies, amplitude of less than 20 μV, and lack of reactivity to auditory or tactile stimulation.
    - This is generally seen with diffuse cortical and subcortical damage due to anoxic encephalopathy, severe traumatic brain injury, encephalitis, or diffuse cerebral edema.
    - In these cases, the pattern is generally associated with an unfavorable prognosis. However, this pattern may also occur with high doses of sedating and anesthetic medications which may be associated with a more favorable prognosis.
  ○ *Burst Suppression*: Describes periods of activity with admixed periods of generalized background suppression (Figure 23.4). This is a nonspecific pattern that can occur with metabolic encephalopathy, diffuse structural or hypoxic–ischemic brain injury, intoxication or high-dose benzodiazepine, barbiturate, or other anesthetic therapy.
  ○ *Rhythmic Coma Patterns*: Rhythmic coma patterns are reported to occur in as many as 30% of comatose children (8).
    - The rhythmic coma patterns are etiologically nonspecific. Etiologies include toxic-metabolic encephalopathies which may have a favorable outcome and anoxic brain injury which often has an unfavorable outcome.

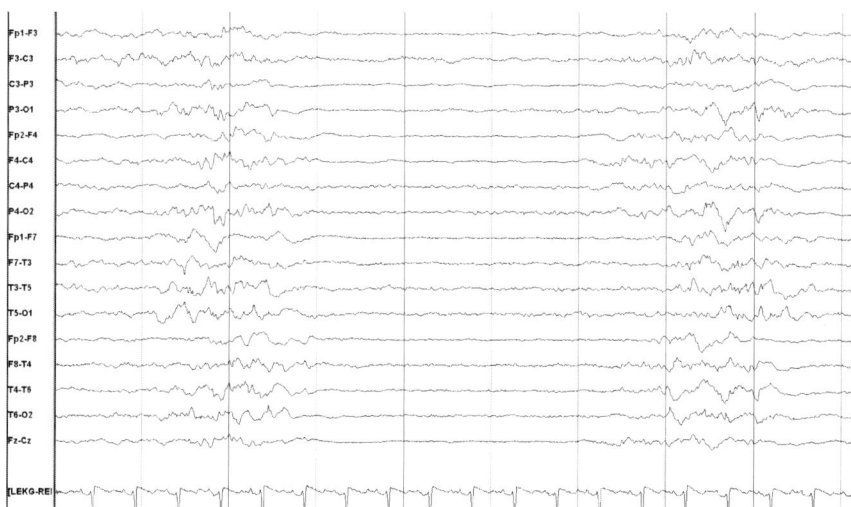

FIGURE 23.4 10-year-old with hypoxic ischemic encephalopathy after cardiac arrest with burst-suppression.

- Reactivity is associated with a more favorable prognosis.
- Alpha coma is the most common rhythmic coma pattern seen in children (8). It refers to diffuse monomorphic alpha activity (Figure 23.5). Alpha coma may alternate with other patterns and constitute a mixed alpha–theta or alpha-spindle coma pattern.
- Spindle coma may be associated with a better prognosis, especially after head trauma.
- Beta coma consists of generalized beta activity (12–16 Hz) that is often bi-frontally predominant. This beta activity may override slower frequencies including alpha, beta, or delta frequencies. Reactivity may be present or absent. Beta coma is most commonly caused by administration of high doses or overdoses of sedative medications including benzodiazepines and barbiturates. Medical support is required during the acute intoxication phase, but prognosis is generally favorable.
  ○ *Electrocerebral Inactivity*: No identifiable cerebral EEG activity recorded with scalp electrodes when the EEG is performed according to specific technical criteria (9).
    - When present in the appropriate clinical context, this is consistent with brain death.
    - Based on the recently updated guidelines, an ancillary study is required only if (1) any components of the examination or apnea testing cannot be completed; (2) there is uncertainty about the results of the neurologic examination; or (3) a medication effect may be present.
    - Intoxication with high doses of sedating and anesthetic medications agents or extreme hypothermia may all produce electrocerebral silence.

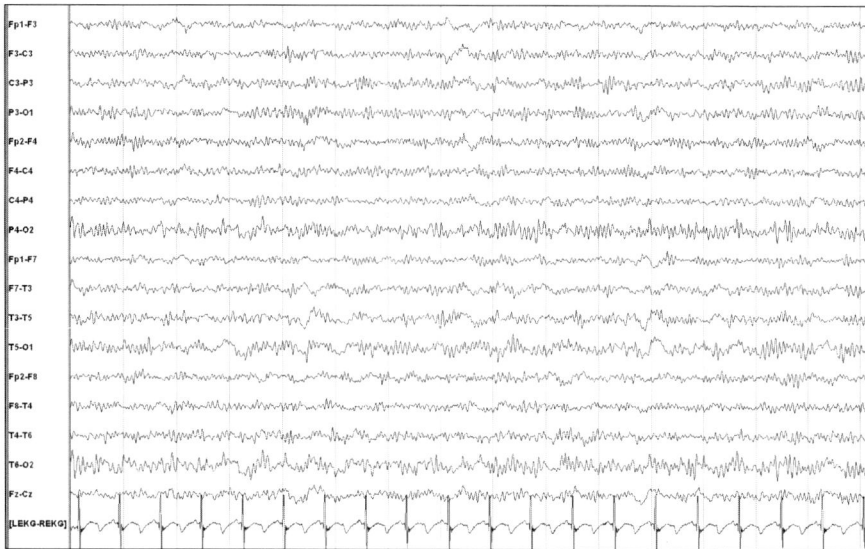

FIGURE 23.5   7-year-old with hypoxic ischemic encephalopathy after near-drowning with alpha coma.

- Seizures, status epilepticus, refractory status epilepticus, and nonconvulsive status epilepticus
  - ○ Clinical and electrographic seizures
    - Clinical and electrographic seizures have the same progressive sequence during status epilepticus in children as in adults: discrete seizures, merging seizures, continuous seizures, continuous ictal activity with admixed flat periods (electrodecrements), and periodic discharges (PDs) on a flat background (10).
  - ○ Refractory status epilepticus
    - EEG monitoring is used to guide treatment of electrographic status epilepticus.
      - It is unclear whether treating to any of the following EEG "endpoints" improves outcome: seizure suppression, burst suppression, or complete electroencephalographic suppression (electrocerebral inactivity).
      - The greater the degree of EEG suppression, the greater the chance of adverse events, especially hypotension.
      - It is also important to recognize that a pattern of PDs can be the end stage of status epilepticus and not just a post-ictal finding.
  - ○ Nonconvulsive seizures and nonconvulsive status epilepticus
    - Studies have reported that about 10% to 40% of children who undergo long-term EEG monitoring in pediatric intensive care unit or emergency departments experience nonconvulsive seizures (NCS) or NCSE (11–15).

- Clinical risk factors for NCS and NCSE in children include younger age (11), prior convulsive status epilepticus (14) or seizures (15), acute structural brain injury (15), traumatic brain injury (14), and cardiac arrest (16).
- Electrographic risk factors for NCS and NCSE include epileptiform discharges (14), periodic epileptiform discharges (12,15), and lack of background reactivity (12).
- The majority of patients with NCS and NCSE experience electrographic seizures without any clinical correlate which would not be identified without EEG monitoring.
- About 80% to 90% of patients with NCS or NCSE are identified with 1 to 2 days of EEG monitoring.
- NCSE may occur with specific epilepsy syndromes such as Dravet syndrome, myoclonic–atonic epilepsy, malignant migrating partial seizures of infancy, Lennox Gastaut syndrome, Panayiotopoulos syndrome (autonomic epilepsy), or nonprogressive encephalopathies (Angelman syndrome, Ring chromosome 20 epilepsy syndrome).
  ○ The ictal–interictal continuum:
    - The ictal–interictal continuum is also similar in children and adults.

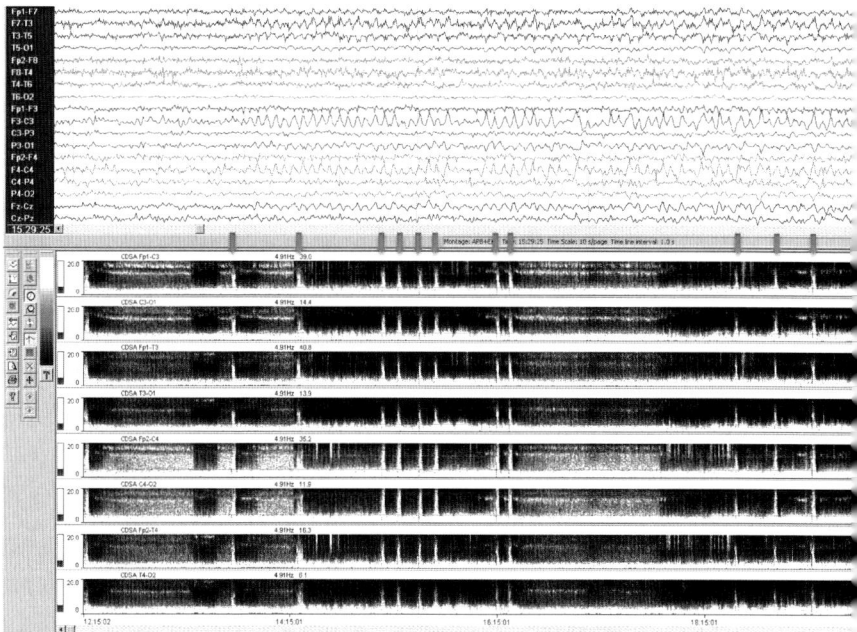

FIGURE 23.6 2-year-old girl with focal status epilepticus. Continuous EEG captured frequent electroclinical seizures consisting of right centrotemporal spike-wave discharges and rhythmic theta. Clinically, seizures consisted of facial twitching or elevation of the left arm. Top half of figure illustrates a typical seizure on raw EEG. Bottom half of figure depicts an 8-hour quantitative EEG (CDSA) display illustrating repetitive seizures (gray arrows).

- Lateralized periodic discharges (LPDs), generalized periodic discharges (GPDs) (17), and stimulus-induced rhythmic, periodic, or ictal discharges (SIRPIDs) (Figure 23.6) have all been reported in children.
  - Quantitative EEG
    - Quantitative EEG (QEEG) displays of EEG waveforms have long been used to monitor for seizures in the neonatal ICU, especially the amplitude integrated EEG (aEEG).
    - QEEG displays have also been shown to be useful in the interpretation of continuous EEG in the pediatric intensive care unit, including the compressed spectral array (18,19) (Figure 23.6).

III. FURTHER CONSIDERATIONS/REMAINING QUESTIONS

A. Further study is needed regarding the use of EEG for prognostication in neonates and children. EEG monitoring could be developed into a real-time marker of neurologic function that could be used to guide ongoing care.

B. Further study is needed to understand whether seizures in critically ill neonates and children worsen neurodevelopmental outcome, and if so, how to optimize seizure identification and management.

REFERENCES

1. Shellhaas RA, Chang T, Tsuchida T, et al. The American Clinical Neurophysiology Society's guideline on continuous electroencephalography monitoring in neonates. *J Clin Neurophysiol.* 2011;28:611–617.
2. Shellhaas RA, Clancy RR. Characterization of neonatal seizures by conventional EEG and single-channel EEG. *Clin Neurophysiol.* 2007;118:2156–2161.
3. Clancy RR, Legido A, Lewis D. Occult neonatal seizures. *Epilepsia* 1988;29:256–261.
4. Scher MS, Alvin J, Gaus L, et al. Uncoupling of EEG-clinical neonatal seizures after antiepileptic drug use. *Pediatr Neurol.* 2003;28:277–280.
5. Malone A, Anthony Ryan C, Fitzgerald A, et al. Interobserver agreement in neonatal seizure identification. *Epilepsia.* 2009.
6. Mizrahi EM, Kellaway P. Characterization and classification of neonatal seizures. *Neurology.* 1987;37:1837–1844.
7. Wusthoff CJ, Shellhaas RA, Clancy RR. Limitations of single-channel EEG on the forehead for neonatal seizure detection. *J Perinatol.* 2009;29:237–242.
8. Ramachandran Nair R, Sharma R, Weiss SK, et al. A reappraisal of rhythmic coma patterns in children. *Can J Neurol Sci.* 2005;32:518–523.
9. Guideline three: Minimum technical standards for EEG recording in suspected cerebral death. American Electroencephalographic Society. *J Clin Neurophysiol.* 1994;11:10–13.
10. Mikati MA, Werner S, Shebab L, et al. Stages of status epilepticus in the developing brain. *Epilepsy Res.* 2003;55:9–19.
11. Abend NS, Gutierrez-Colina AM, Topjian AA, et al. Non-convulsive seizures are common in critically ill children. *Neurology.* 2011;76:1071–1077.

12. Jette N, Claassen J, Emerson RG, et al. Frequency and predictors of nonconvulsive seizures during continuous electroencephalographic monitoring in critically ill children. *Arch Neurol.* 2006;63:1750–1755.
13. Shahwan A, Bailey C, Shekerdemian L, et al. The prevalence of seizures in comatose children in the pediatric intensive care unit: A prospective video-EEG study. *Epilepsia* 2010;51:1198–1204.
14. Williams K, Jarrar R, Buchhalter J. Continuous video-EEG monitoring in pediatric intensive care units. *Epilepsia.* 2011;52:1130–1136.
15. McCoy B, Sharma R, Ochi A, et al. Predictors of nonconvulsive seizures among critically ill children. *Epilepsia.* 2011;52:1973–1978.
16. Abend NS, Topjian A, Ichord R, et al. Electroencephalographic monitoring during hypothermia after pediatric cardiac arrest. *Neurology.* 2009;72:1931–1940.
17. Akman CI, Riviello JJ, Jr. Generalized periodic epileptiform discharges in critically ill children: A continuum of status epilepticus or an epiphenomenon? *J Clin Neurophysiol.* 2011;28:366–372.
18. Akman CI, Micic V, Thompson A, Riviello JJ, Jr. Seizure detection using digital trend analysis: Factors affecting utility. *Epilepsy Res.* 2011;93:66–72.
19. Stewart CP, Otsubo H, Ochi A, et al. Seizure identification in the ICU using quantitative EEG displays. *Neurology.* 2010;75:1501–1508.

TWENTY-FOUR

Postanoxic Encephalopathy

Elizabeth Waterhouse

KEY POINTS

- Postanoxic encephalopathy is most often seen following a cardiac or respiratory arrest. It may also be caused by severe anemia or hypotension.
- The EEG may show various patterns, including generalized slowing, alpha or theta coma, generalized suppression, generalized or bilateral periodic discharges, or a burst-suppression pattern.
- Patterns may wax and wane during the EEG and generalized, focal, or multifocal seizures or status epilepticus (SE) may also occur.
- EEG is performed on the postanoxic patient to evaluate cerebral activity, monitor for treatable conditions such as seizures, and assess prognosis. Prolonged continuous EEG monitoring is preferred, because EEG patterns may change over time.
- The most reliable EEG indicator of poor prognosis following anoxic injury is myoclonic SE. The EEG patterns of generalized suppression, generalized periodic discharges on a suppressed background, and burst suppression are strongly, but not invariably, associated with poor outcomes.
- In the intensive care unit, other factors such as therapeutic hypothermia and continuous infusions of sedative or anesthetic drugs, may complicate the interpretation of the EEG.

I. BACKGROUND

A. Neuronal Activity Is Coupled With Cerebral Blood Flow

- EEG changes occur within seconds of cerebral hypoperfusion.
  - Initial EEG changes include decreased fast activity and increased slowing.
  - When cerebral blood flow (CBF) less than 10 mL/100 g brain tissue per minute, all frequencies are suppressed.
- The development of cellular necrosis and infarction depends upon the duration of time that CBF remains below a certain level.

- Tissue that is functionally impaired but structurally intact is considered the "penumbra" and has the potential to improve or recover (1).

B. Survival Rates Following Cardiac Arrest (2)
- The overall rate of return of spontaneous circulation is 44%.
- Patients with arrests due to ventricular fibrillation or pulseless ventricular tachycardia have the highest rates of survival to hospital discharge (34%–35%).
- Only 10% of patients with asystole or pulseless electrical activity survive to hospital discharge.
- Fewer than 20% of in-hospital cardiac arrests survive until discharge.
- The survival rate for out-of-hospital cardiopulmonary resuscitation is less than 10%.
- Of patients who die, more than half are declared "Do Not Resuscitate," and about 40% have life support withdrawn, skewing the statistics toward poor outcomes.

II. BASICS

A. EEG Patterns After Anoxic Brain Injury
- Burst suppression (Figure 24.1)

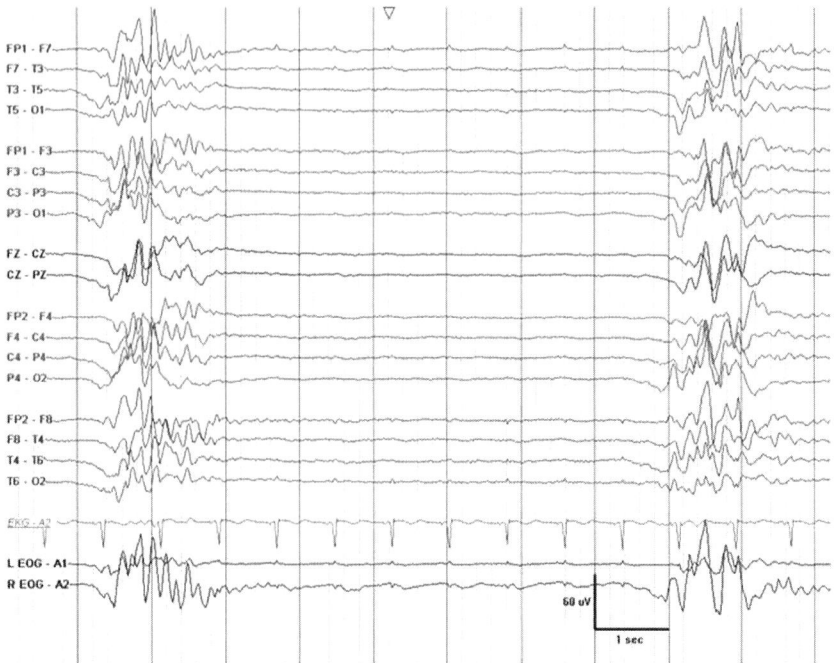

FIGURE 24.1   Burst-suppression pattern, with a 6-second interval between bursts. (Used with permission of VCUHS EEG Laboratory.)

- ○ Generalized very low voltage or flat background.
- ○ Intervals ("bursts") of higher-voltage activity lasting greater than 0.5 seconds and crossing the baseline at least 4 times.
- Generalized slowing (Figure 24.2)
  - ○ Often theta activity, but other frequencies may be intermixed.
- Generalized periodic discharges (Figure 24.3)
  - ○ Background is suppressed.
  - ○ Periodic discharges are waveforms with relatively uniform morphology, often sharp waves or spikes, lasting 0.5 seconds or less, and recurring at nearly regular intervals.
- Alpha coma (Figure 24.4)
  - ○ EEG shows diffuse invariant alpha activity, often anteriorly predominant.
  - ○ The pattern is not specific to postanoxic encephalopathy: may also occur with head trauma, brainstem stroke, or toxic/metabolic encephalopathy.
  - ○ The prognosis of patients with alpha coma is associated with the underlying etiology.

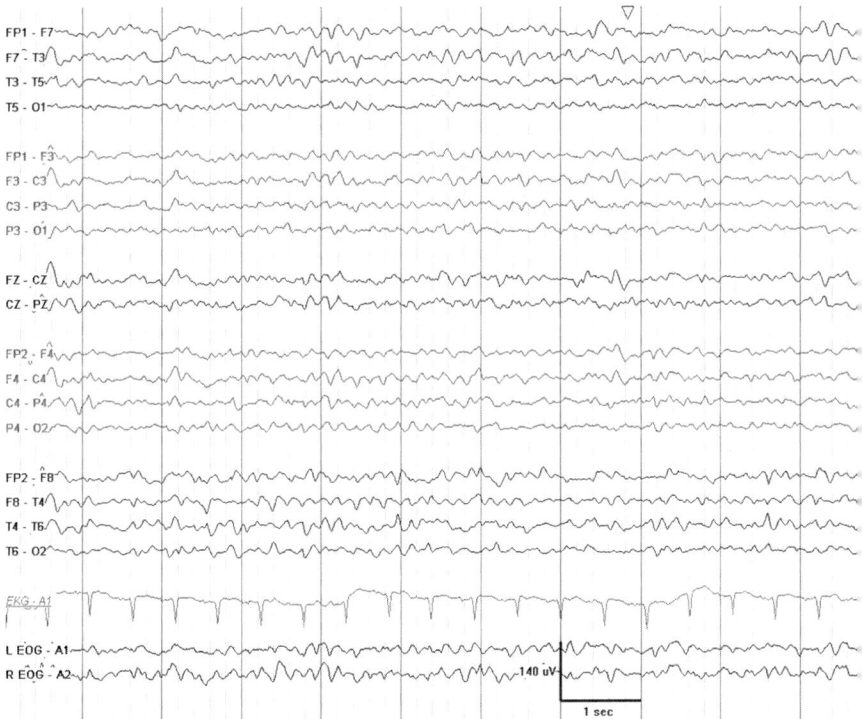

FIGURE 24.2 Generalized theta slowing. (Used with permission of VCUHS EEG Laboratory.)

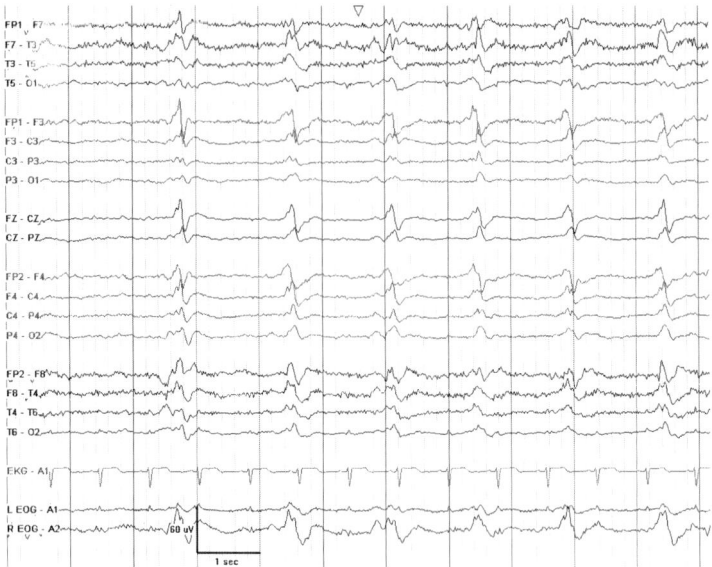

FIGURE 24.3 Generalized periodic discharges, occurring every 1 to 1.5 seconds (Used with permission of VCUHS EEG Laboratory.)

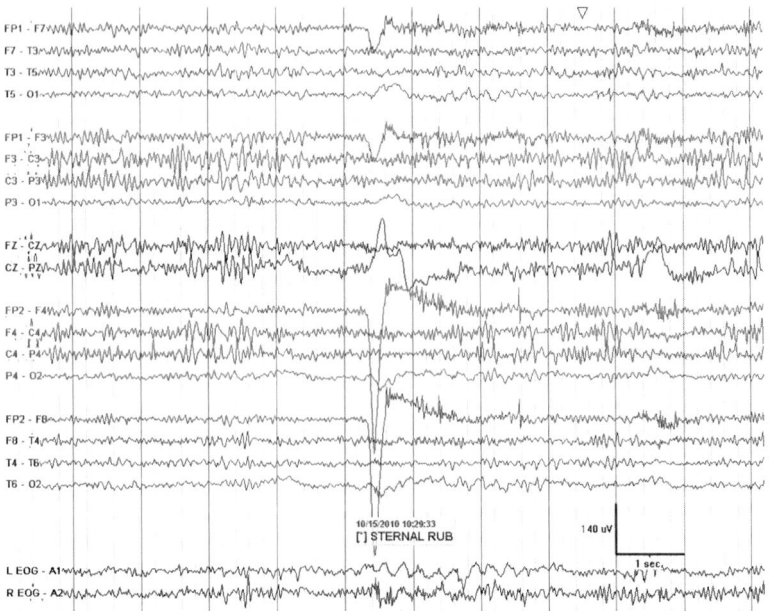

FIGURE 24.4 Alpha–beta coma, with generalized nonreactive fast activity. This patient was receiving fentanyl and midazolam following cardiac arrest. (Used with permission of VCUHS EEG Laboratory.)

- Kaplan et al. found the following mortality rates in patients with alpha coma: cardiopulmonary arrest, 88%; hypoxia without cardiac arrest, 61%; stroke, 90%; and drug-induced encephalopathy, 8% (3).
  - A reactive alpha coma pattern correlates with improved survival.
    - Eight of 15 patients with EEG reactivity regained consciousness, while only three of 19 patients without reactivity regained consciousness, one with persistent vegetative state (3).
  - The presence of brainstem reflexes in patients with alpha coma does not correlate with survival.
  - An alpha coma pattern does not invariably herald a poor prognosis (3).
    - When alpha coma patients (of various etiologies) were matched by age and coma etiology with non-alpha coma controls, a similar proportion of both groups (36%–39%) regained consciousness.
    - Among the subset of alpha coma patients who had suffered cardiopulmonary arrest, 19% regained consciousness.
    - An equal proportion of the control patients with cardiopulmonary arrest regained consciousness.

B. Ictal Patterns Associated With Postanoxic Encephalopathy

- Seizure activity occurs in up to 35% of postanoxic patients monitored with EEG (4,5).
- Since seizures and SE in this setting are frequently nonconvulsive, EEG is required to make the diagnosis.
- Seizures often contribute to decreased level of consciousness, and they have implications for prognosis.
- Electrographic seizures may be focal, multifocal, or generalized.
  - May arise from a continuous background, a suppressed background, or a burst suppression pattern (Figure 24.5).
  - May be of any frequency, and typically shows evolution of frequency, voltage, morphology, and/or field.
- One study by Rossetti et al found that postanoxic SE is associated with death independent of acute cardiac rhythm or hypothermia treatment (6)
  - SE occurred in 45% of those patients who died and in 8% of survivors.
- Myoclonic SE occurs when there is spontaneous, sustained, repetitive, generalized, or multifocal myoclonus in a comatose patient.
  - EEG typically shows a burst-suppression pattern, with myoclonic jerks synchronized with the bursts.
  - Generalized periodic discharges of 0.5 to 2 Hz may also be seen.
  - Myoclonic SE is associated with a poor prognosis.

C. Predicting Outcomes

- The American Academy of Neurology has published evidence-based guidelines concerning the prediction of outcome in comatose survivors of cardiopulmonary arrest (7). However, it should be noted that these guidelines are based on data prior to the era of therapeutic hypothermia (see "Potential Pitfalls" below).

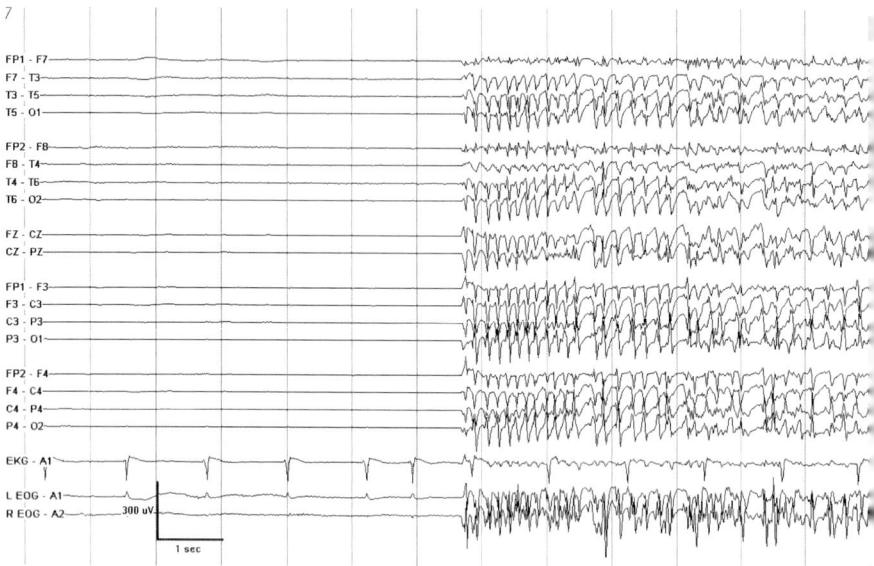

FIGURE 24.5 Sudden onset of generalized ictal activity, arising from generalized suppression. (Used with permission of VCUHS EEG Laboratory.)

- There is good evidence that patients with myoclonic SE within the first day after a primary circulatory arrest have a poor prognosis.
  - Not applicable, however, to patients with single seizures or sporadic focal myoclonus.
- Several EEG patterns are strongly, *but not invariably*, associated with a poor outcome following anoxic injury:
  - Burst suppression
  - Generalized suppression, with all activities less than or equal to 20 μV
  - Generalized periodic discharges on a flat background.
- Since the false-positive rate for poor outcome is 3%, the prognostic accuracy for these patterns is considered insufficient.
- EEG reactivity and variability have been suggested to favorably predict recovery of consciousness, but this has not been independently demonstrated.
- Strong evidence supports a poor prognosis for patients with absent pupillary or corneal reflexes, or absent or extensor motor responses 3 days after cardiac arrest.
- Strong evidence supports a poor prognosis for patients with bilaterally absent somatosensory cortical-evoked potentials (N20 wave) within 1 to 3 days of cardiac arrest.

D. Artifacts
- Sources for EEG artifacts abound in the intensive care unit.
- Artifacts are magnified by the high-sensitivity settings used for these often low-voltage EEG recordings.

- Rhythmic or regularly occurring EEG discharges are not always cerebral.
- EKG or pulse artifacts may be widespread on the EEG, and can be mistaken for periodic discharges by an inexperienced interpreter. Conversely, cerebral periodic discharges that occur at a rate approximating the heart rate may be attributed mistakenly to EKG artifact.
  - Artifactual discharges often show up in the EKG/chest lead. This is a clue that they are not of cerebral origin, assuming that the chest electrode is not paired with a cerebral reference.
  - Mechanical artifacts do not abate with increasing doses of anesthetic medications, whereas all cerebral activity eventually becomes suppressed with sufficient doses of anesthetic medications.
  - Temporary neuromuscular blockade abolishes artifacts due to shivering, twitching, eye blinking, and other muscular activity in a ventilated patient, allowing better visualization of cerebral activity.
- EEG activity that is extremely rhythmic, occurs at exact intervals, does not evolve in frequency or voltage, or lacks an appropriate electrographic field, should raise the suspicion of artifact.
- Video EEG is helpful for identifying human and mechanical sources of artifact, such as patting, sternal rub, ongoing dialysis, or automated chest therapy.

E. Potential Pitfalls

- Several important clinical variables can confound the prognostic value of the EEG and the clinical exam of patients following cardiopulmonary resuscitation.
- Since anoxic encephalopathy, anesthetic effects, and hypothermia may manifest similar EEG patterns, it is often difficult to determine whether EEG findings are due to one, or a combination, of these factors.
- Concurrent or prior use of sedatives is associated with EEG patterns similar to those caused by anoxic encephalopathy, and contributes to decreased level of consciousness.
- Neuromuscular blocking agents suppress myoclonus, masking the diagnosis of myoclonic SE. They also interfere with the clinician's ability to obtain useful findings on the neurological exam.
- Induced therapeutic hypothermia may cause suppression, generalized low-voltage slowing, alpha or theta coma, burst suppression, periodic discharges, or ictal activity on EEG. It also contributes to a decreased level of consciousness.
  - AAN guidelines for prognosis should be applied with caution in patients treated with therapeutic hypothermia following cardiac arrest, as there is higher false-positive rate for prediction of mortality (7).
- The presence of organ failure, which may be reversible, contributes to EEG changes, and to a decreased level of consciousness.
- Cardiogenic shock leads to ongoing hypoperfusion, but may be reversible.
- Studies in comatose patients after CPR have not systematically addressed the impact of the above factors on the reliability of clinical neurologic examination and tests (8).

- ○ Thus, it is essential to take the clinical context into account when interpreting the EEG.
- ○ The EEG interpreter must be aware of the patient's medications, body temperature, blood test results, and other pertinent clinical findings.
- Although serial or continuous EEGs are believed to be more accurate and valid than single EEGs, this has not been adequately tested.
- However, it is clear that postanoxic EEG patterns often change over time, and prognosis should not be assessed on the basis of a single EEG obtained in the hours immediately following cardiopulmonary resuscitation. Therefore, continuous EEG monitoring should be considered for a more accurate assessment of prognosis over time.

III. FURTHER CONSIDERATIONS/REMAINING QUESTIONS

A. Further research is needed to address these important questions regarding postanoxic encephalopathy.
- What factors predict good outcome following anoxic brain injury?
- Does treatment of electrographic seizures improve outcome?
- Does treatment of EEG patterns with periodic discharges improve outcome?

B. Although hypothermia treatment improves survival following cardiac arrest, many questions remain regarding the optimal parameters for this therapy.
- These include time to initiate hypothermia, time to reach target temperature, duration and degree of hypothermia, and re-warming rate.
- The optimal regimens of sedation, analgesia, and muscle relaxation are also yet to be determined.

REFERENCES

1. Astrup J, Siesjö BK, Symon L. Thresholds in cerebral ischemia—The ischemic penumbra. *Stroke.* Nov-Dec 1981;12(6):723–725.
2. Peberdy MA, Kaye W, Ornato JP, et al. Cardiopulmonary resuscitation of adults in the hospital: A report of 14720 cardiac arrests from the National Registry of Cardiopulmonary Resuscitation. *Resuscitation.* Sep 2003;58(3):297–308.
3. Kaplan PW, Genoud D, Ho TW, Jallon P. Etiology, neurologic correlations, prognosis in alpha coma. *Clin Neurophysiol.* Feb 1999;110(2):205–213.
4. Krumholz A, Stern BJ, Weiss HD. Outcome from coma after cardiopulmonary resuscitation: Relation to seizures and myoclonus. *Neurology.* Mar 1988;38(3):401–405.
5. Friedman D, Claassen J, Hirsch LJ. Continuous electroencephalogram monitoring in the intensive care unit. *Anesth Analg.* 2009;109:506–523.
6. Rossetti AO, Logroscino G, Liaudet L, Ruffieux C, Ribordy V, Schaller MD, Despland PA, Oddo M. Status epilepticus: An independent outcome predictor after cerebral anoxia. *Neurology.* 2007;69:255–260.

7. Wijdicks EF, Hijdra A, Young GB, et al. Quality standards subcommittee of the American Academy of neurology. Practice parameter: Prediction of outcome in comatose survivors after cardiopulmonary resuscitation (an evidence-based review): Report of the quality standards subcommittee of the American Academy of Neurology. *Neurology.* Jul 2006;67(2): 203–210.
8. Young GB. Neurologic prognosis after cardiac arrest. *NEJM.* 2009;36(6):605–611.

TWENTY-FIVE

EEG Correlates of Ischemia

William O. Tatum

KEY POINTS

- EEG abnormalities can indicate cerebral ischemia even when changes are not evident on neuroimaging or clinical exam.
- A sequence of progressive EEG changes is seen in association with ongoing ischemia as well as recovery from an ischemic event.
- Both nonepileptiform and epileptiform EEG features may help guide clinical assessment and treatment of patients with suspected cerebral ischemia.
- EEG patterns can aid in determination of prognosis following ischemic insults to the brain.

I. BACKGROUND

A. Cerebral Ischemia
- The brain is extremely sensitive to hypoxic injury.
- Ischemic destruction of brain neurons is irreversible and a frequent complication in critically ill patients with acute neurological injury.
- Sensitive diagnostic modalities are needed to detect the earliest phase of cerebral hypoxia and monitor response to therapy (1).

B. EEG Analysis
- The EEG is a dynamic indicator of brain function and a useful tool to detect focal and diffuse ischemic processes that disrupt the integrity of the central nervous system (2).
- There is a physiologic coupling of EEG morphology, frequency, and amplitude with changes in cerebral blood flow (Table 25.1).
- EEG is a practical and inexpensive adjunct to clinical assessment that is readily obtained by either serial or continuous recording during hospital evaluations.
- Focal abnormalities on EEG produced by ischemia may be more informative than initial neuroimaging.

TABLE 25.1 Blood Flow Thresholds Relative to Potential Brain Ischemic Injury and EEG Features

RCBF MG/100 G/MIN	BRAIN INJURY	EEG FREQUENCY
>35	None	Normal
25–35	Usually none	Decreased fast activity, less than 13 Hz Beta
18–25	Potential risk	Diffusely slow, 5–7 Hz Theta
12–18	Expected risk	Diffusely slow, less than 4 Hz Delta
<8–10	Neuronal death	Suppression

Adapted from Jordan KG. *JCN*. 2004;21:341–352.

rCBF, regional cerebral blood flow.

- Early detection of ischemia at a potentially reversible stage might facilitate treatment changes that improve outcome.

II. BASICS: EEG FEATURES OF ISCHEMIA

A. Nonepileptiform Activity: Focal Ischemia
- Focal ipsilateral polymorphic delta slowing corresponds to the ischemic brain region(s) following the distributions of the anterior, posterior, or middle cerebral artery.
- Acute occlusion of the carotid or middle cerebral artery can also result in generalized voltage attenuation (Figure 25.1).
- Other EEG features of focal ischemia may include ipsilateral background attenuation, slowing of alpha frequency, reduction in beta activity, or appearance of asymmetric frontally predominant intermittent rhythmic delta activity (FIRDA).
- As viable tissue recovers, focal abnormalities improve over time to become less continuous, with a corresponding increase in faster background frequencies.

B. Nonepileptiform Activity: Diffuse Ischemia
- Complete arrest of cerebral circulation leads to corresponding EEG changes within seconds.
- Lack of cerebral blood flow for 4 minutes or longer results in disruption of the brain's energy state and ion homeostasis which leads to irreversible neuronal death and electrocerebral inactivity (ECI).
- EEG changes from acute cerebral ischemia occur along a continuum (Figure 25.2) (3).
  - Intermixed theta slowing
  - Intermittent delta slowing (rhythmic or arrhythmic)
  - Diffuse background slowing
  - Low-amplitude unreactive diffuse slowing
  - Background attenuation

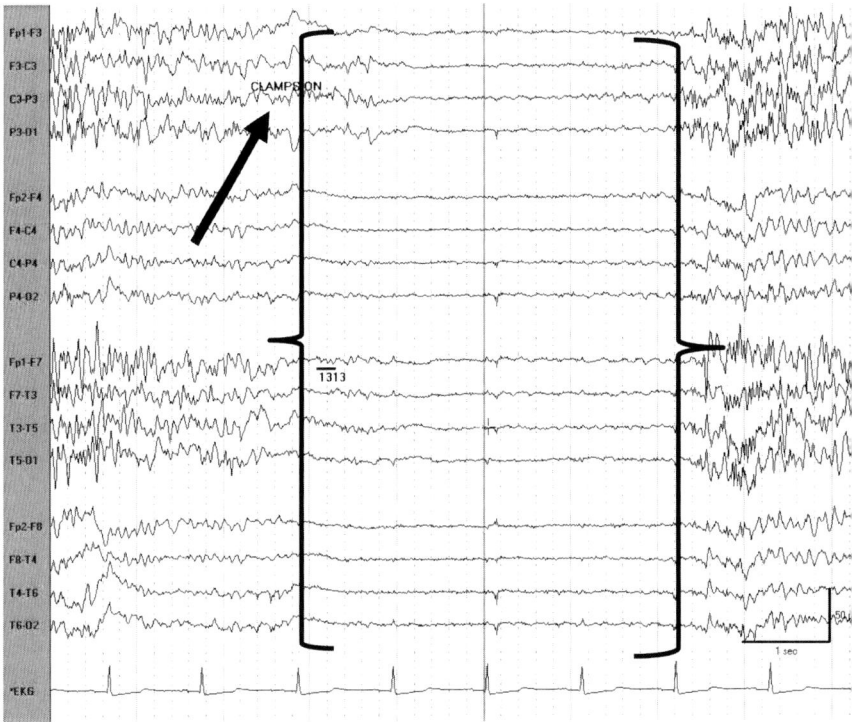

FIGURE 25.1 Bilateral attenuation (brackets) following right carotid clamping (arrow) during carotid endarterectomy. Following shunt placement, the EEG returned to baseline and the patient awoke without deficit. Recording parameters: 1to 70 μV/mm (60 Hz on) at 30 mm/sec.

- ○ Burst suppression (Figure 25.3)
- ○ Electrocerebral silence (ECI)
- • Brainstem and subcortical ischemia often do not result in changes in the scalp EEG.
- • Quantitative EEG and multimodal analyses may increase the sensitivity of EEG to detect ischemia compared with visual analysis of raw EEG.

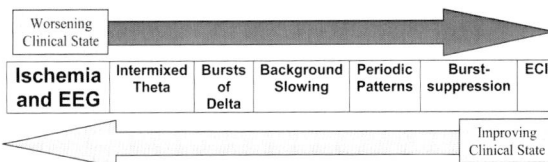

FIGURE 25.2 The progression of abnormalities following cerebral ischemic-induced hypoxia (top darker arrow) and following improvement (bottom arrow).

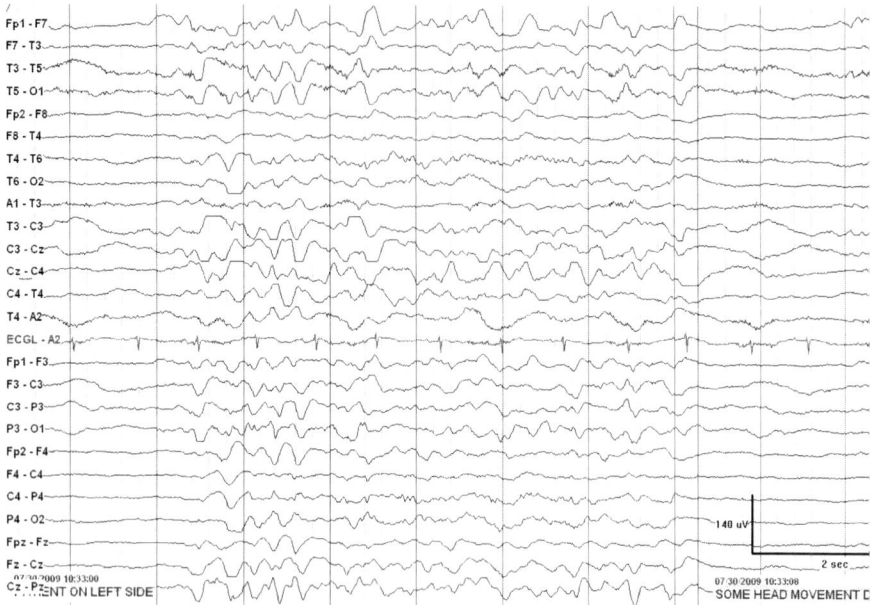

FIGURE 25.3 Burst-suppression pattern in a patient with global hypoxia due to traumatic cardiac tamponade.

C. Epileptiform Activity
- Epileptiform discharges and periodic patterns with bilateral involvement reflect a poor prognosis and high mortality when seen with (multi)focal or diffuse ischemic cerebral injury (2,4).
- Lateralized periodic discharges (LPDs) may be seen with acute *focal* ischemic injury (commonly hemorrhagic infarct).
- 80% to 90% of patients with LPDs following ischemic injury experience seizures which usually resolve in less than 1 month.
- LPDs with superimposed fast or rhythmic discharges (LPDs Plus) carry a greater risk of status epilepticus (Figure 25.4).
- Bilateral periodic discharges (BIPDs) and generalized periodic discharges (GPDs) usually reflect a severe *generalized* cerebral insult such as global anoxia and indicate a worse prognosis (Figure 25.5).

III. FURTHER CONSIDERATIONS/REMAINING QUESTIONS

A. Cerebrovascular Disease: Detection and Prognosis
- An evolving stroke may be identified on continuous EEG monitoring even prior to clinical deterioration.

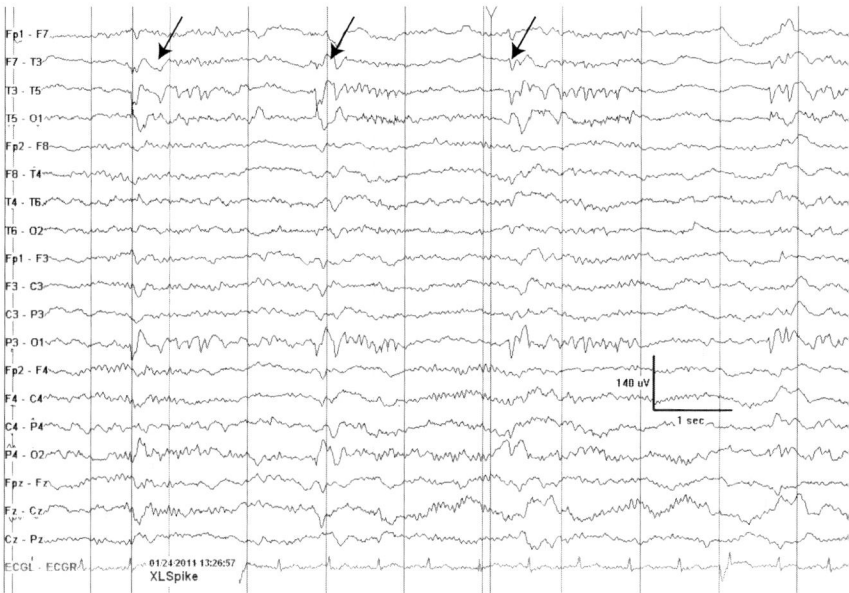

FIGURE 25.4   An ICU patient with basilar ischemia presented with blindness and confusion. The initial CT brain was normal although EEG revealed left posterior temporal-occipital LPDs Plus (above). The patient received antiepileptic drugs and later made a full recovery.

- Almost one-third of patients with subarachnoid hemorrhage suffer secondary injury from ischemia due to vasospasm that may be detected and treated much earlier with the use of EEG monitoring.
- Regional attenuation without delta activity (RAWOD) may identify massive infarcts that respond poorly to thrombolysis. However, the absence of delta slowing and the presence of beta frequencies within the focal ischemic area is a more favorable sign than diffuse slowing and focal delta activity (5).

B. Cerebral Ischemia and Mental Status Changes

- EEG is crucial to distinguish between a patient with locked-in syndrome secondary to brainstem ischemia (normal EEG) and patients with encephalopathy or coma secondary to widespread cortical ischemia (abnormal EEG).
- A greater degree of background slowing on EEG corresponds with a greater reduction in cerebral metabolism which may either precede or follow clinical deterioration associated with ischemic injury.
- Hypothermia may protect against ischemic injury by reducing cerebral metabolism. However, hypothermia may also introduce background slowing or attenuation of the EEG.
- In comatose patients with ischemia, EEG suppression, lack of EEG reactivity, and generalized periodic discharges are features that correlate with poor outcome and

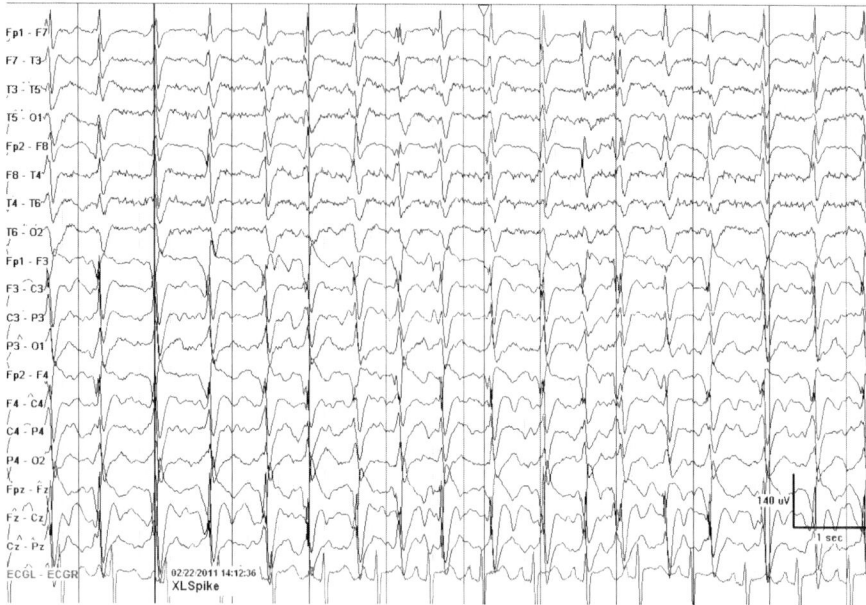

FIGURE 25.5 GPDs in a comatose patient after cardiac arrest. Treatment for nonconvulsive status epilepticus was unsuccessful and the patient died 3 days later.

high mortality. Focal epileptiform activity, regional delta slowing and reactivity are EEG features that favor survival.

C. Cerebral Ischemia and Seizures

- Mutism, face and limb twitching, eye deviation, myoclonus, and psychiatric features may occur with either an ischemic or epileptiform process requiring EEG for accurate diagnosis.
- The presence of epileptiform discharges may support the need for treatment with AEDs in patients with acute cerebral ischemia which otherwise may not have been evident without the use of EEG.
- Focal epileptiform discharges as well as LPDs in patients with acute focal ischemia are highly associated with seizures
- Focal seizures arising from an area of ischemia may have bilateral manifestations both clinically and electrographically.

REFERENCES

1. Hirsch LJ, Brenner RP, Drislane FW, et al. The ACNS subcommittee on research terminology for continuous EEG monitoring: Proposed standardized terminology for rhythmic and periodic EEG patterns encountered in critically ill patients. *J Clin Neurophysiol.* 2005;22:128–135.

2. Jordan KG. Emergency EEG and continuous EEG monitoring in acute ischemic stroke. *JCN.* 2004;21:241–252.
3. Hockaday JM, Potts F, Epstein E, et al. Electroencephalographic changes in acute cerebral anoxia from cardiac or respiratory arrests. *Electroencephalogr Clin Neurophysiol.* 1965;18:575–586.
4. Husain AM, Mebust KA, Radtke RA. Generalized periodic epileptiform discharges: Etiologies, relationship to status epilepticus, and prognosis. *J Clin Neurophysiol.* 1999;16:51–58.
5. Hilker BL, Dohmen C, Bosche B, et al. Early electroencephalography in acute ischemic stroke: Prediction of a malignant course? *Clin Neurol Neurosurg.* 2007;109:45–49.

ADDITIONAL READING

Friedman D, Claasen J, Hirsch LJ. Continuous electroencephalogram monitoring in the intensive care unit. *Anesth Analg.* 2009;109(2):506–523.
Blanco M, Lizasoain I, Sobrino T, et al. Ischemic preconditioning: A novel target for neuroprotective therapy. *Cerebrovasc Dis.* 2006:21(Suppl 2);38–47.

TWENTY-SIX

Artifacts

Sarah Schmitt

KEY POINTS

- Artifacts are particularly common in the ICU because of the presence of many electrical devices as well as frequent patient movements that can be either spontaneous or induced during the course of patient care.
- Artifacts are classified as physiologic or nonphysiologic depending on whether they originate in the patient's body or from the surrounding environment.
- The difficulty of distinguishing between artifacts and seizures can hinder optimal treatment.
- Although techniques exist for the digital removal of electromyography (EMG), eye movement, cardiac and blink artifacts, better ways are needed for the removal of other artifacts from EEG recordings in ICU patients.

I. BACKGROUND

A. Understanding Artifacts
- In EEG, an artifact is a recorded electrical potential that does not originate in the brain.
- Two primary concerns
  - Artifacts may resemble abnormal activity (eg, seizures, epileptiform discharges, etc).
  - Artifacts may obscure underlying EEG activity.
- Artifacts are especially common in the ICU.
  - Artifact-inducing electrical devices may be present in the room.
  - Patient movements are common.
  - Rooms are often "busy," with frequent movement of visitors and staff within the room.
- Understanding and identifying artifacts is critical to appropriate interpretation of EEG.

B. Two Basic Types of Artifacts
- Physiologic—artifacts originating within the patient's body, but not originating within the brain.
- Nonphysiologic—artifacts arising from the external environment.

II. BASICS

A. Physiologic Artifacts
- Eye-movement artifacts
  - The cornea is positively charged relative to the retina, with a 50 to 100 mV difference between the two structures.
    - These electrical potentials are most prominent in the frontal EEG leads (eg, Fp1, Fp2, F7, F8, and F3, F4).
    - Rotation of the eye toward an electrode creates a high-amplitude positive potential (downward deflection on EEG).
  - *Blink artifact*: during blinks, the positively charged cornea moves upward (toward the frontal electrodes, especially Fp1/Fp2), producing symmetric downward deflections on EEG.
  - *Eye flutter artifact*: repetitive blinks produce symmetric, rhythmic frontally predominant delta waveforms.
  - *Lateral rectus spike*: a brief, less than 50 msec spike caused by activation of the lateral rectus muscle during horizontal eye movements; most prominent in F7/F8.
- To address eye movement/blink artifacts:
  - Use electrodes at the lateral canthi (left upper canthus, right lower canthus) to differentiate eye movements.
  - Consider taping or holding eyes closed if elimination of blink/eye flutter artifact is important to distinguish seizures from artifact.
- EKG artifact
  - Caused by the electrical dipole generated by cardiac depolarization; most prominent in ear (A1, A2) electrodes but can also be seen in parasagittal/midline electrodes.
  - More prominent in patients with short, wide necks.
  - May vary with respiration.
  - Because of the high incidence of pacemakers and cardiac arrhythmias in the ICU population, EKG artifact may be more challenging to isolate and identify.
    - Ectopic QRS complexes, such as premature ventricular complexes, may be seen more prominently in temporal electrodes and less prominently in parasagittal electrodes.
    - Pacemakers result in variable-amplitude spike(s) immediately prior to the QRS complex; these spikes may occasionally be confused with epileptiform activity.
  - Any repetitive EEG abnormality should be compared to the EKG lead in order to determine whether or not it is artifactual.
- Pulse artifact
  - Seen when an electrode is placed over a pulsating artery or tissue.

- ○ A rhythmic, slow artifact seen 200 to 300 msec after the QRS complex.
- ○ Can be eliminated or reduced by moving the electrode away from pulsating arteries/tissues.
- Ballistocardiographic artifact
  - ○ Caused by subtle vibrations of the body in conjunction with systolic pulse waves.
  - ○ Produces low voltage, rhythmic delta activity.
- EMG artifact
  - ○ Occurs with muscle activation, particularly with muscles of the face, jaw, scalp, and neck (especially temporalis and frontalis).
  - ○ Typically a fast, spiky artifact that may be confused with beta activity (particularly when used with a high-frequency filter).
  - ○ Rhythmic EMG artifact can be seen with chewing or biting on endotracheal tubing.
    - If EMG artifact is severe and cannot be eliminated, consider transient neuromuscular paralysis with neuromuscular blocking agent (eg, vecuronium) in intubated, comatose patients.
- Movement artifacts
  - ○ Voluntary and involuntary movements can create a variety of artifacts.
  - ○ Rhythmic movements may create a rhythmic artifact on EEG that can resemble epileptiform or focal seizure activity (Figure 26.1). Rhythmic movement artifacts are often seen with:
    - Tremor
    - Clonus
    - Myoclonus
  - ○ However, rhythmic EEG activity can accompany rhythmic movements associated with clinical seizures.
  - ○ *Sternal rub artifact*: repetitive, diffuse, high amplitude, rhythmic, or semirhythmic artifact caused by physician or nurse evaluation of the patient using sternal rub.
  - ○ *Cardiopulmonary resuscitation (CPR) artifact*: Rhythmic, 1 to 2 Hz highamplitude artifact caused by CPR; waveforms are time-locked with chest compression (Figure 26.2).
- *Glossokinetic artifact*: artifact produced by tongue movements, caused by the negative polarity of the tip of the tongue with respect to the tongue base.
  - ○ May be unilateral or bilateral, positive or negative.
  - ○ Appears as a burst of frontally predominant slowing, most prominent at Fp1/Fp2.
  - ○ In alert patients, it can generally be reproduced by asking the patient to repeat a word or phrase that produces tongue movements, for example, "la la la."
  - ○ Can also be assessed by recording the same pattern from an electrode placed on submental muscle.
- Sweat artifact
  - ○ In the ICU, most commonly seen in patients with fever.
  - ○ Associated with slow (typically less than 1 Hz) delta activity.
  - ○ May be reduced by use of the low-frequency filter.
  - ○ May also be reduced by drying the scalp before electrode application, or cooling the patient (eg, using a fan, applying a cooling blanket).

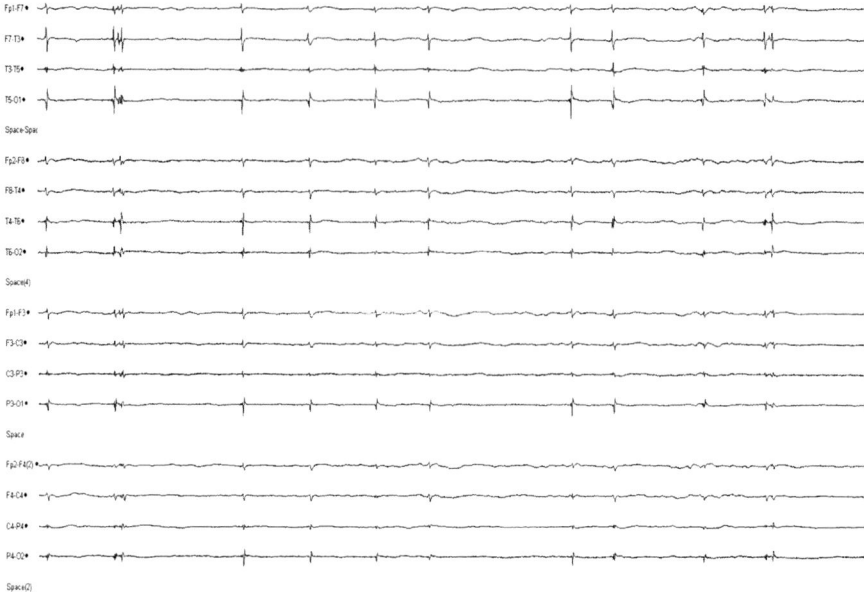

FIGURE 26.1 EMG artifact in a patient with semi-rhythmic myoclonic movements. These spiky appearing discharges can be confused for epileptiform activity. However, this activity disappeared after administration of paralytics confirming EMG artifact.

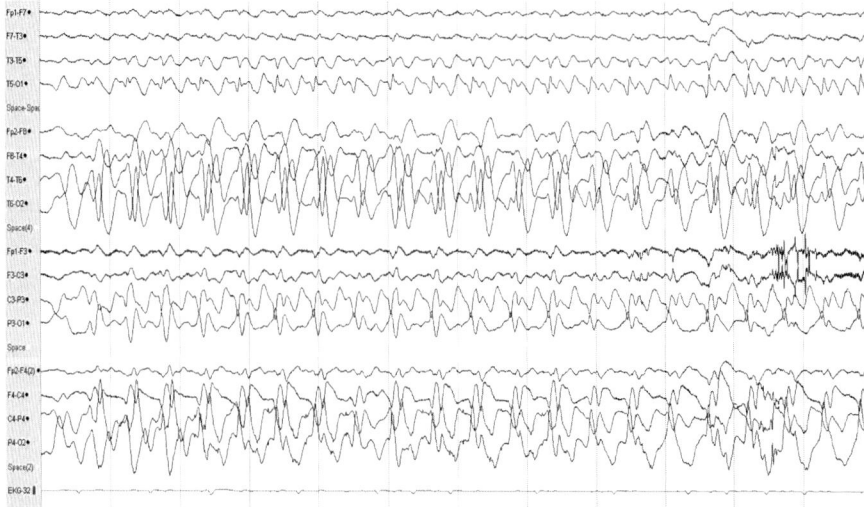

FIGURE 26.2 CPR artifact. Waveforms are time-locked to chest compressions.

B. Nonphysiologic Artifacts

- AC current (60 Hz) Hz artifact
  - Caused by 50 or 60 Hz (depending on location) alternating current that supplies power to electrical outlets
  - In the ICU, often caused by electrical devices located near the patient
    - Electrically powered bed
    - Mechanical ventilators
    - IV infusion devices
    - Dialysis machines
    - EKG machine
    - Extracorporeal membrane (ECMO) devices
    - Line isolation monitors
  - Creates a 60 Hz sinusoidal artifact
  - Most prominent in high-impedance electrodes
  - Can decrease this artifact by reapplying high-impedance electrodes, moving or (if appropriate) unplugging offending electrical devices, or using notch filter
- Electrode artifact
  - Typically caused by high-impedance electrode (although damaged wires and electrode movement may create similar artifacts)
  - May lead to sharp-appearing activity or slow waves of varying amplitude and appearance
  - "Electrode pop" is caused by a sudden change in electrode impedance, which may have a sharp appearance on EEG
  - Electrode artifact is usually restricted to one electrode
  - Correct the problem by fixing or replacing the electrode.
- Instrumental artifacts
  - *Capacitative artifact*: typically caused by moving the input cable
  - *Electrostatic artifact*: caused by discharge of static electricity
- Environmental artifacts
  - Ventilator artifact (Figure 26.3)
    - Varies widely in morphology, amplitude, polarity.
    - Can create either single or multiple waveforms.
    - Monitoring the respiratory rate in a separate channel can aid in artifact identification.
    - A related, faster frequency artifact can be caused by charged water molecules in the ventilator tubing; this artifact is typically improved by suctioning.
  - *Bed percussion artifact*: 5 to 6 Hz rhythmic activity seen with mechanical chest percussion devices which may be seen in multiple electrodes (Figure 26.4).
  - *Radiofrequency artifact*: High-frequency, diffuse artifact related to activation of radiofrequency devices including cell phones.
  - Continuous renal replacement therapy (CRRT) artifact: Rotation of motor within CRRT device produces rhythmic, 5 to 12 Hz activity in multiple electrodes; activity may have a sharp or sawtooth appearance.
  - Extracorporeal membrane oxygenation (ECMO) artifact: can create a rhythmic 1 to 3 Hz square wave artifact.

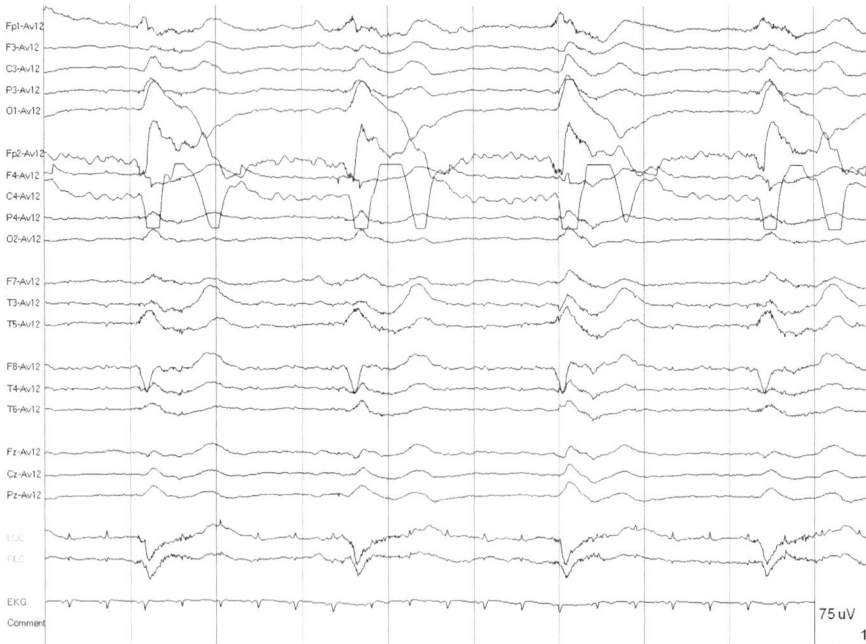

FIGURE 26.3 Mechanical ventilation artifact. This artifact has a highly variable appearance, but reoccurs with each respiration.

III. FURTHER CONSIDERATIONS/REMAINING QUESTIONS

A. Artifacts and EEG Misinterpretation
- The frequency with which artifacts are misinterpreted as ictal or epileptiform activity remains uncertain.
- Artifacts are one of the primary limiting factors in the development of digital seizure detectors as well as the use of quantitative EEG techniques for rapid record review.

B. Artifact Removal
- Many software packages have attempted to digitally remove certain types of artifact
  - Techniques have been developed for the digital removal of EMG, eye movement, cardiac, and blink artifacts but this technology is not widely available.
  - No reliable techniques have been developed for the elimination of most other artifacts, including movement, electrode, environmental, and instrumental artifacts.
- Artifact removal is not currently a part of routine clinical practice, but may be increasingly utilized as artifact removal techniques are improved and validated.

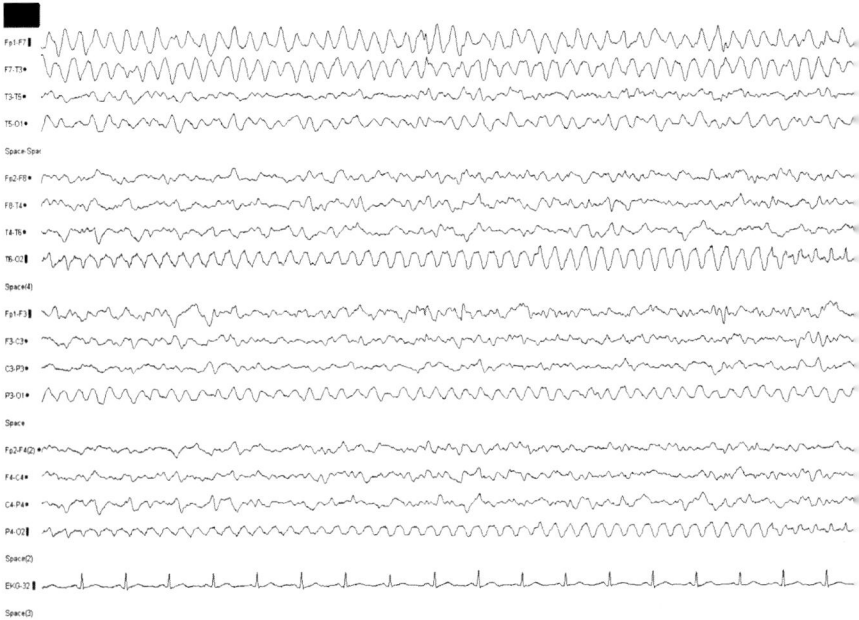

FIGURE 26.4　Chest percussion artifact. Mechanical chest percussion devices produce a rhythmic 5 to 6 Hz artifact in multiple electrodes.

ADDITIONAL READING

1. Blum DE. Computer-based electroencephalography: Technical basics, basis for new applications, and potential pitfalls. *Electroencephal Clin Neurophys.* 1997;106:118–126.
2. Ille N, Berg P, Scherg M. Artifact correction of the ongoing EEG using spatial filters based on artifact and brain signal topographies. *J Clin Neurophysiol.* 2002;19(2):113–124.
3. Lesser RP, Luders H, Dinner DS, et al. An introduction to the basic concepts of polarity and localization. *J Clin Neurophysiol.* 1985;2:45–61.
4. Shackman AJ, McMenamin BW, Slagter HA, et al. Electromyogenic artifacts and electroencephalographic inferences. *Brain Topogr.* 2009;22:7–12.

TWENTY-SEVEN

Quantitative EEG Basic Principles

Saurabh R. Sinha

KEY POINTS

- Immediate interpretation of ICU EEG recordings is desirable for providing feedback to the clinical team, but these recordings contain a large volume of data whose interpretation is labor-intensive.
- Quantitative EEG provides a potential tool for overcoming some of these challenges because it allows for post hoc analyses, the immediate detection of events such as ischemia or seizures, and can give nonneurophysiologists a simplified overview of the EEG data.
- Commercial EEG software increasingly includes quantitative EEG tools to aid in the analysis of EEG monitoring in the ICU as well as other EEG applications.

I. BACKGROUND

A. Analysis of Raw ICU EEG
- Routine evaluation of EEG consists of visual inspection of the data page-by-page.
  - Thus, reviewing 15 seconds of EEG data per page at a review speed of 5 pages per second, a 24-hour study would require a minimum of 20 minutes to screen.
  - A more in-depth analysis of the data would likely take much longer.
  - Furthermore, such detailed analyses require the expertise of a specialty trained neurophysiologist and are usually performed in a post-hoc manner and not in real time.
- The challenge: immediate interpretation and feedback of prolonged EEG recordings.

B. Quantitative EEG (QEEG)
- Defined as the application of mathematical and analytical techniques to characterize EEG signals.
- Many potential applications:
  - Characterization of normal activity.

○ Detection of abnormal activity for diagnostic purposes (including individual epileptiform discharges, seizures, and ischemia).

○ Detection of abnormal activity for treatment purposes (eg, responsive neural stimulators).

• Can also be used to summarize trends in the EEG data over longer periods of time and to look for subtle changes in the EEG, hence QEEG parameters are often referred to as "trends."

II. BASICS

A. Many Different QEEG Tools Are Available

• Historically, availability of QEEG tools depended upon development of technology, starting with hardware instruments with the ability to analyze analog EEG signals.

• Today, almost all QEEG analysis consists of software algorithms operating on digital EEG signals.

B. Commonly Used Nonfrequency-Based QEEG Tools

• Time-domain analysis

○ The analysis of how the EEG signal amplitude varies over time.

• Amplitude integrated EEG (aEEG)

○ Raw EEG is filtered, rectified, smoothed, and then displayed on a compressed time scale (Figure 27.1).

○ For each epoch, both the maximum and minimum amplitude of the smoothed signal are plotted, connected by a vertical line.

○ aEEG has been applied extensively to the analysis of EEG in neonates (1).

• Envelope trend analysis

○ Raw EEG is first filtered within a specified frequency range (eg, 2–6 Hz), then the median amplitude of the waveforms within this frequency range is plotted for each epoch (eg, 10–20 seconds) (2).

• Burst suppression measures

○ EEG suppression is usually defined as background amplitude less than 5 μV for greater than 0.5 seconds.

○ Traditionally, the most clinically relevant parameter is the duration of the periods of suppression, known as the interburst interval (IBI).

○ However, most QEEG programs calculate the burst-suppression ratio (BSR) instead, defined as % of time during each epoch that the EEG is suppressed.

C. Frequency Domain Analysis: Analysis of the Contribution of Different Frequencies to the EEG Signal

• Filtering can be applied to most QEEG parameters.

○ The EEG signal can be passed through analog or digital filters to remove the contribution from certain frequencies.

○ This allows for the removal of noise (60 Hz noise from electronic equipment, high-frequency artifact from muscle activity, low-frequency artifact from sweat).

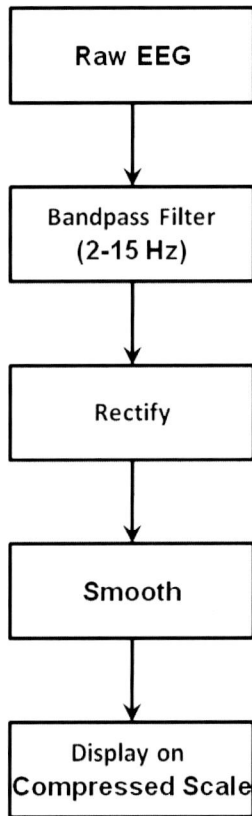

FIGURE 27.1 Algorithm for calculation of amplitude integrated EEG. The EEG is filtered, often to a range of 2 to 15 Hz, rectified (all values made positive), smoothed and then displayed on a highly compressed time scale.

- ○ This also allows for analysis of specific frequency bands.
  - ○ For example, by putting the EEG through an 8 to 13 Hz bandpass filter, the contribution of alpha frequencies can be isolated.
- Fourier spectrum
  - ○ The EEG signal is represented as the weighted sum of sine waves of different frequencies.
  - ○ For each frequency, there is an amplitude (the magnitude of the contribution made by the sine wave at that frequency) and a phase (the starting point of the sine wave of a given frequency).
  - ○ A plot of the amplitude versus frequency is the Fourier spectrum (Figure 27.2).
    - Fourier spectrum describes the contributions made by different frequencies to the EEG for a given epoch of time.

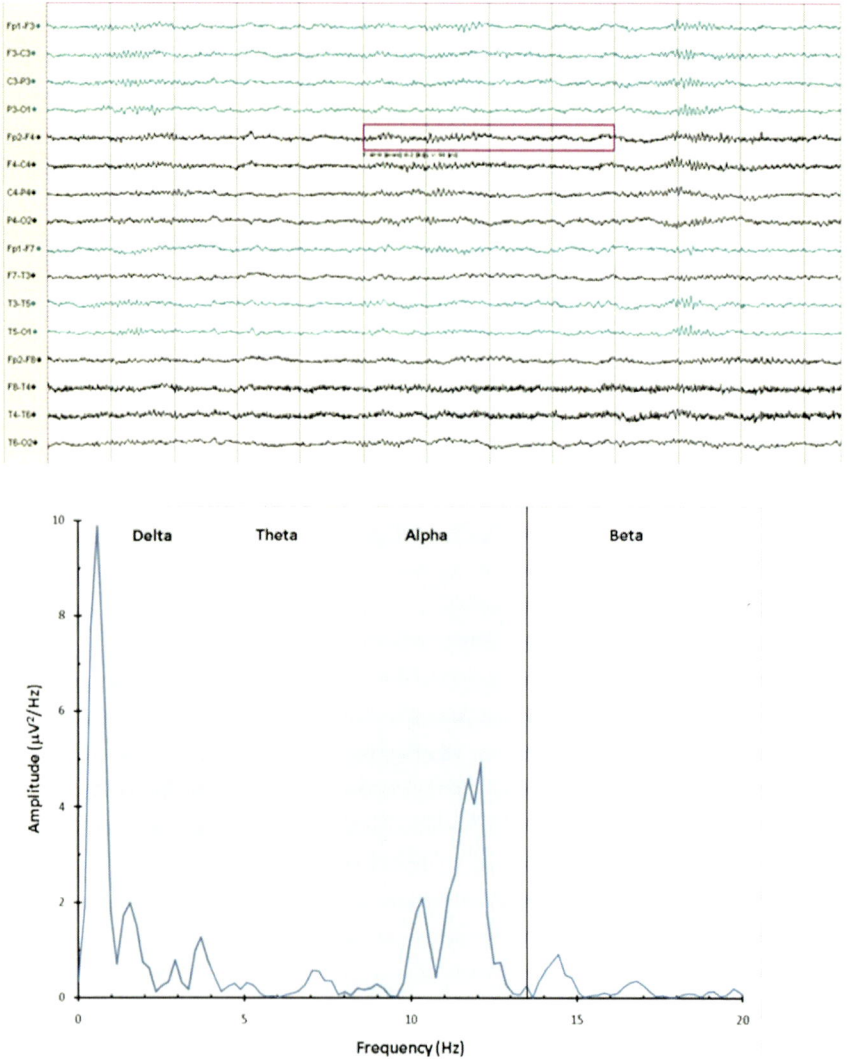

FIGURE 27.2 Fourier spectrum of EEG. A sample of EEG from an adult patient in stage 2 sleep is shown at the top. The Fourier spectrum for 4 seconds of EEG from the channel Fp2-F4 (purple box) is shown at the bottom. The amplitude is plotted versus frequency (stopped at 20 Hz). EEG frequency bands (delta, theta, alpha, beta) are indicated. The power in a frequency band is the area under the portion of this curve in that frequency band.

- Phase information is ignored in most types of QEEG analysis, although it can be used for some more complex types of analysis.
- Fourier spectrum analyses
  - Power
    - The area under the Fourier spectrum amplitude curve within a given frequency range.
    - For example, the alpha power would be the area under the curve from 8 to 13 Hz.
    - May be expressed as absolute power (the actual value) or relative power (ratio of power in a given frequency range to the total power over all frequency ranges).
  - Power ratio
    - Ratio of power in two frequency bands.
    - For example, alpha to delta ratio (ADR) is the ratio of power in the alpha frequency band (8–13 Hz) to that in the delta frequency band (1–3 Hz).
    - A potentially useful tool for monitoring for ischemia in the ICU setting (3).
  - Spectral edge frequency (SEF)
    - Represents the frequency below which a certain percentage of the total power resides.
    - For example, SEF95 = frequency below which 95% of the total power resides.
    - SEF is a potential parameter for monitoring for cerebral ischemia (4) or level of sedation (5).
- The Fourier spectrum of the EEG is not constant with time.
  - This includes both expected changes with activity and behavioral state (eg, sleep versus awake) and pathological changes (eg, during seizures or ischemia) (Figure 27.3).

D. Time–Frequency Analysis: How the Contribution of Different Frequencies Varies Over Time

- Because the EEG signal is a nonstationary signal (one whose frequency makeup is not constant over time), its power spectrum varies with time.
  - Time–frequency tools are used to describe this variation.
- Compressed spectral array (CSA) and density spectral array (DSA) are tools for displaying the power spectrum of the EEG versus time.
  - For CSA, the power spectrum at each time point is displayed as a line graph. CSA are rarely used now.
  - For DSA, the amplitude of the power spectrum is encoded in different colors and displayed versus time.
- Rhythmicity spectrogram is a proprietary QEEG tool that is included with the Persyst software package.
  - It highlights the frequency components of the DSA that have the highest amplitude and rhythmicity at a given time.
  - This can help highlight the rhythmic activity associated with seizures, especially if the most prominent frequency appears to change with time (evolution of frequency).

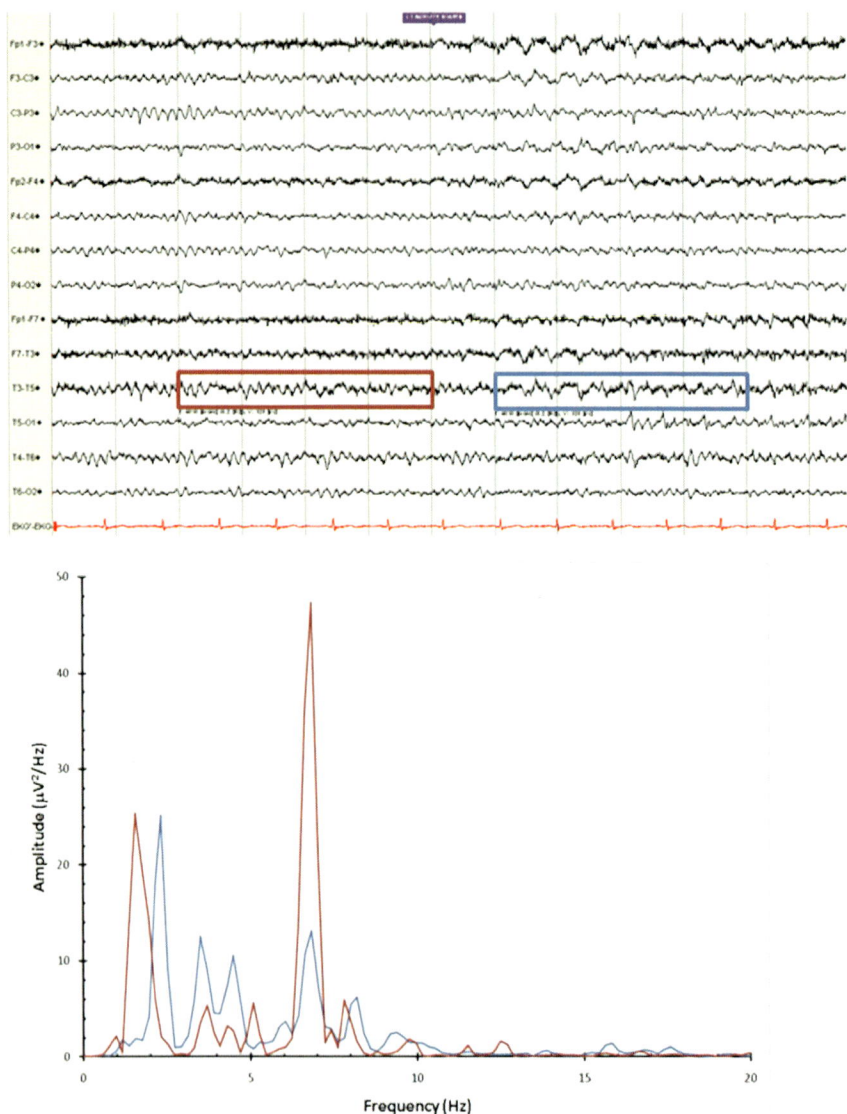

FIGURE 27.3 Fourier spectrum of EEG immediately before and during a seizure. A sample of EEG from an adult patient with left temporal-lobe epilepsy is shown at the top. The Fourier spectrum of 4 seconds epochs of EEG from channel T3 to T5 is show immediately before (red box in top, red trace on bottom) and at electrographic seizure onset (blue box in top, blue trace in bottom). At baseline, the predominant activity is at 6.8 Hz; at seizure onset the predominant frequency becomes 2.3 Hz.

E. Quantitative EEG tools offer the potential for automated detection of events of interest, such as seizures and ischemia

- This is of particular interest in prolonged recordings as an option for providing rapid feedback when continuous raw EEG review may not be possible.
  - ○ Seizure detectors rely on comparing morphological parameters of the EEG during a given epoch to preceding or following epochs.
  - ○ Owing to the highly variable nature of ictal patterns, this task is significantly more difficult than spike detection.
  - ○ Many seizure detector algorithms produce a value indicating the probability that a given epoch contains an electrographic seizure based on a combination of parameters.
  - ○ Most detectors are not generalizable and tend to have significant false-detection rates (6).
- For certain applications, such as detection of ischemia, monitoring of sedation or monitoring of pharmacological burst suppression during treatment of status epilepticus, it may be fairly straightforward to set thresholds for QEEG parameters to alarm the clinical team for a likely event.
  - ○ However, the sensitivity and specificity of such techniques remain unknown.

III. FURTHER CONSIDERATIONS/REMAINING QUESTIONS

A. The sensitivity and specificity of specific QEEG tools for detecting seizures and other abnormalities in prolonged ICU EEG remain largely unknown.

B. Limited data exist on the utility of bedside QEEG with automated detection algorithms for identification of seizures and other abnormalities by nonneurophysiologists.

- However, such applications have the potential for improving the availability and utilization of continuous EEG for monitoring and management of critically ill patients.

REFERENCES

1. Tao JD, Mathur AM. Using amplitude-integrated EEG in neonatal intensive care. *J Perinatol.* 2010;30:S73–S81.
2. Abend NS, Dlugos D, Herman S. Neonatal seizure detection using multichannel display of envelope trend. *Epilepsia.* 2008;49:349–352.
3. Claasen J, Hirsch LJ, Kreiter KT, et al. Quantitative continuous EEG for detecting delayed cerebral ischemia in patients with poor-grade subarachnoid hemorrhage. *Clin Neurophysiol.* 2004;115:2699–2710.
4. Diedler J, Sykora M, Bast T, et al. Quantitative EEG correlates of low cerebral perfusion in severe stroke. *Neurocrit Care.* 2009;11:210–216.
5. Roustan J-P, Valette S, Aubas P, et al. Can electroencephalographic analysis be used to determine sedation levels in critically ill patients. *Anesth Analg,* 2005;101:1141–1151.
6. Kuhlman L, Burkitt AN, Cook MJ, et al. Seizure detection using seizure probability estimation: Comparison of features used to detect seizures. *Ann Biomed Engr.* 2009;37: 2129–2145.

TWENTY-EIGHT

Quantitative EEG for Seizure Detection

Suzette M. LaRoche

KEY POINTS

- Quantitative EEG (QEEG) allows for visualization of up to several hours of EEG data in a single screen display.
- QEEG trends most useful for seizure detection are based on the following properties: amplitude, frequency, rhythmicity, and degree of asymmetry.
- A combination of QEEG trends utilizing each of these properties is likely to offer the best recognition of a variety of seizure types.
- Pitfalls in QEEG analysis include the high degree of false-positive detections due to common ICU artifacts in addition to false negatives from very brief, low-amplitude or slowly evolving seizures.
- QEEG should never replace raw EEG review, but can expedite seizure detection and treatment as well as allow for initial EEG screening by non-EEG-trained personnel.
- More research is needed to determine the best combination of QEEG trends, electrode "montages," and time, frequency, and amplitude scales for detection of the widest range of seizure presentations.

I. BACKGROUND

A. History of QEEG
- By definition, QEEG is the visual representation of mathematically or statistically compressed raw EEG waveforms.
- When used in ICU EEG monitoring, QEEG is commonly referred to as "trend analysis" or "trends."
- Quantitative analysis of brain potentials is not new; early physiological studies of electrical activity in animal brains used fast Fourier transformation with simple yet cumbersome equipment.
- QEEG emerged as a potentially useful clinical tool with the advent of digital EEG technology in the 1960s.

○ Compressed spectral array (CSA), a condensed display of EEG based on amplitude and frequency, was the first QEEG trend to be developed and is still utilized today.
○ In 1978, Dr. Bricolo from Verona, Italy commented on the use of CSA in EEG monitoring of comatose patients: "The advantages of such a technique are mainly due to its capacity of synthesizing EEG signals and to its clarity of presentation, which is easily grasped even by people not specifically trained in electroencephalography" (1).
  • This display of "clarity" is one of the major reasons for the use of QEEG in ICU EEG monitoring still today.
○ 1980s: Jean Gotman developed commercially available spike and seizure detection software (Stellate®), the first EEG software program routinely used to assist in the interpretation of raw EEG.
○ 1990s to today: QEEG finds increasing use in the clinical practice of ICU EEG monitoring.

B. Advantages of QEEG for Seizure Detection
• "Finding the needle in the haystack"
  ○ Allows rapid identification of rare or occasional seizures in a prolonged recording without the time required for visual screening of each 10 second display of raw EEG.
• "Seeing the forest for the trees"
  ○ Can provide a quick overview of seizure location, frequency, and duration as well as response to treatment.
  ○ Also reveals subtle background asymmetry, changes in state, reactivity, and rhythmic or periodic patterns that may fluctuate over the course of several hours.
• Typically consists of 1 to 4 hours of QEEG on a single screen as opposed to 10 seconds of raw EEG per screen with conventional EEG review.
• Cannot replace expert review of raw EEG, but rather focuses detailed analysis on specific points of interest and can expedite clinical decision making, particularly in the treatment of recurrent seizures and status epilepticus.

C. QEEG Versus Seizure Detection Algorithms in ICU Patients
• Current seizure detection algorithms are designed for identification of classic seizure patterns seen in the setting of the epilepsy monitoring unit.
• Typically, electrographic seizures in ICU patients have a very different morphology (often more slowly evolving at lower frequencies and amplitudes) and therefore, not detected as reliably with standard seizure detection algorithms (Figure 28.1).
• Seizure detection algorithms provide a binary output (seizure: yes/no) as opposed to a QEEG visual display which provides additional qualitative and quantitative information including frequency, location, and propagation patterns.

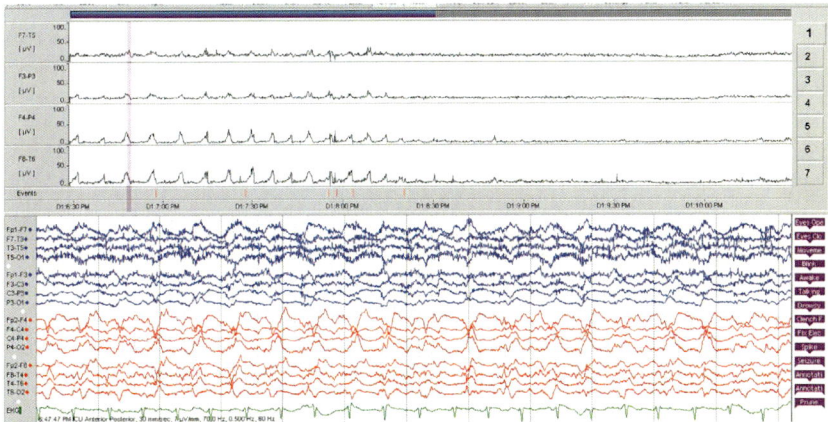

FIGURE 28.1   Seizure detection algorithm recognized 5/16 (31%) of right hemisphere electrographic seizures (red lines above time stamp) that were better detected by envelope trend, an amplitude-based QEEG measure (F4–P4 and F8–T6 channels).

II. BASICS

A. Amplitude-Based QEEG Trends

- Amplitude integrated EEG (aEEG)
  - Displays **minimum and maximum** amplitude of all background activities over a preset time interval (generally 1–2 seconds).
  - Seizures are represented by an increase in baseline amplitude.
  - Sensitivity for seizure detection can be variable, particularly with limited-channel aEEG in which case only about half of the seizures seen on conventional EEG are recognized on aEEG trends. (2)
  - Owing to the small sampling time interval and the fact that both minimum and maximum amplitude is represented, brief increases in amplitude seen on aEEG can be nonspecific and often represent artifact.
  - Provides a good measure of background activity, hence it is also known as Cerebral Function Monitor (CFM).
  - Very sensitive for recognition of burst-suppression pattern.
  - Has been utilized for many years for seizure detection and evaluation of background in neonates.
- Envelope
  - Displays **median** amplitude of all background activities over a preset time interval (generally 10–20 seconds).
  - Seizures are represented by an increase in median amplitude.
  - Filters short-duration artifacts and offers better visual resolution than aEEG.
  - More specific than aEEG, but could miss seizures that are shorter than the selected time interval.

B. Frequency-Based QEEG Trends

- Frequency-based trends use fast Fourier transform (FFT) to display a three-dimensional picture of EEG power over time at various frequencies.
- Power is a calculation based on amplitude.
  - Total power = sum of the area under the curve (uV^2) for a defined time period.
  - Band power = area under the curve at selected frequencies (uV^2/Hz) (Figure 28.2) (3).
- Visual display
  - Time is represented along the x-axis, frequency along the y-axis and power represented by a color scale along the z-axis.
  - Color scale varies depending on software vendor. Typically low power = dark or blue, high power = bright or dark red.
- Seizures are typically represented by increasing power (brighter color scale) that typically evolves from lower to higher frequencies along the y axis (or vice versa, by increasing power that evolves from higher to lower frequencies).
- By comparison, many artifacts such as muscle activity or electrode artifact will be represented by a prolonged or sudden increase in power at higher frequencies along the y-axis, with no evolution.
- Known by several different names:
  - Compressed spectral array (CSA)
  - Density spectral array (DSA)
  - Color density spectral array (CSDA)
  - FFT spectrogram or "spectrogram"

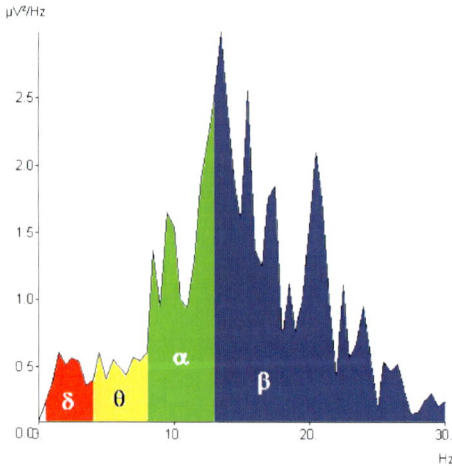

FIGURE 28.2   Band power is represented by the area under the curve at specific frequency intervals. In this example, the majority of the EEG power is in the beta frequency range (blue) with less alpha frequency power (green) and a small but nearly equal amount of theta (yellow) and delta (red) power (3).

C. QEEG Trends Based on Rhythmicity (Persyst Corp.): Rhythmicity Spectrogram

- A three-dimensional representation of the power of **rhythmic** EEG component at various frequencies.
  - ○ Time is represented along the x-axis, frequency along the y-axis, and the power of rhythmic EEG components is represented by a color scale along the z-axis.
  - ○ The y-axis utilizes a square root scale (logarithmic) in order to accentuate rhythmicity at lower frequencies which is prevalent in many seizure presentations in the ICU population.
  - ○ Color scale: less rhythmic activity = white to light blue, more rhythmic activity = darker blue to black (measured in uV/Hz).
- Seizures are often represented by a characteristic pattern (Figure 28.3).
  - ○ At initial seizure onset, rhythmic components appear at faster frequencies along the y-axis.
  - ○ As the seizure progresses, rhythmic components gradually decline in frequency (or vice versa, rhythmic components evolving to higher frequencies as the seizure progresses).

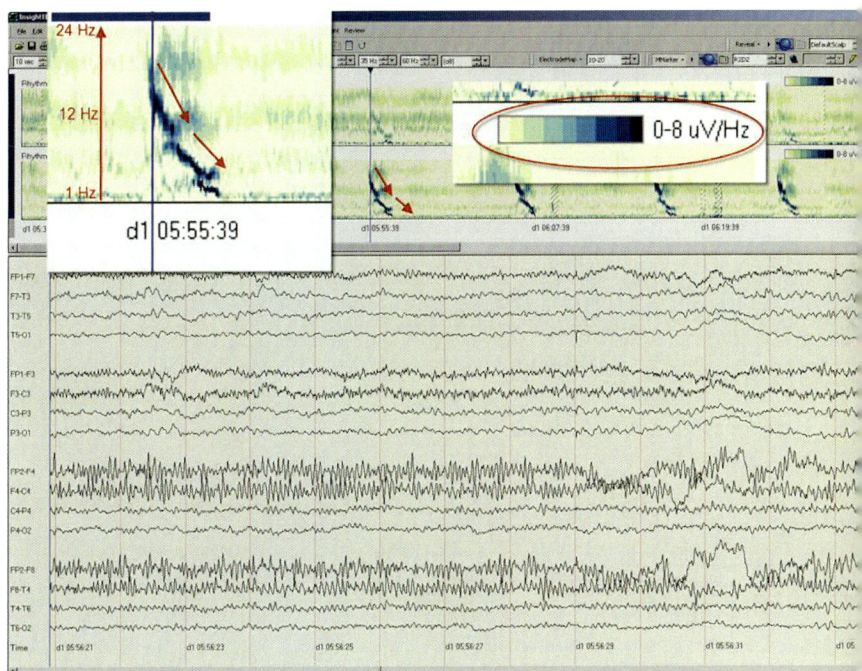

FIGURE 28.3 Characteristic seizure pattern on rhythmicity spectrogram of a right hemisphere electrographic seizure. Seizure begins with increased power of rhythmic 12–15 Hz activity; dark blue in bottom tracing. As the seizure progresses, the power is higher at lower frequencies representing seizure evolution to low frequency activity. Notice there is some propagation of the seizure to the left hemisphere evidenced by a similar pattern in the top tracing but of lower power (lighter blue). Courtesy of Mark Scheuer, Persyst Corporation.

○ Best viewed at shorter time displays (30–60 minutes).
○ Very specific, but less sensitive for some seizure types.

D. Asymmetry-Based QEEG Trends (Persyst Corp.)

- Compares differences in power between homologous electrodes (T3 vs. T4; C3 vs. C4, etc.); thus, measures power asymmetry between hemispheres.
- Most useful for lateralized or focal seizures.
- Relative asymmetry index
  ○ Upward deflection means higher power in the right hemisphere.
  ○ Downward deflection means higher power in the left hemisphere.
- Relative asymmetry spectrogram
  ○ Red indicates higher power over right hemisphere.
  ○ Blue indicates higher power over left hemisphere.
  ○ Deeper colors = more asymmetry
- Focal seizures over the left hemisphere will be represented by an increase in blue color while focal seizures over the right hemisphere are represented by an increase in red color (Figure 28.4).

E. Studies Evaluating the Utility of QEEG for Seizure Detection

- Hahn and colleagues compared the accuracy of CSA and aEEG in 27 ICU recordings in children, each with 8-channel trend display (4).
  ○ Trend displays were reviewed by three neurophysiologists with 2 hours of training each.
  ○ Sensitivity for seizure detection was similar between the two trends (CSA 83% vs. aEEG 81%).

(A)

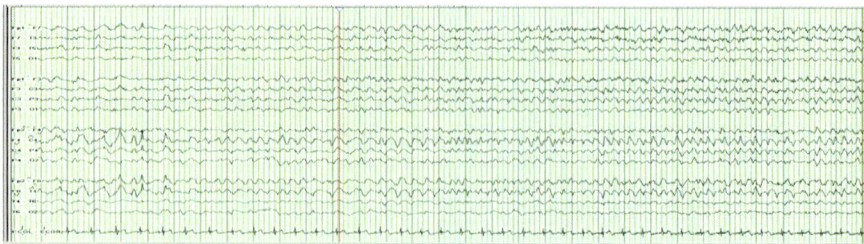

(B)

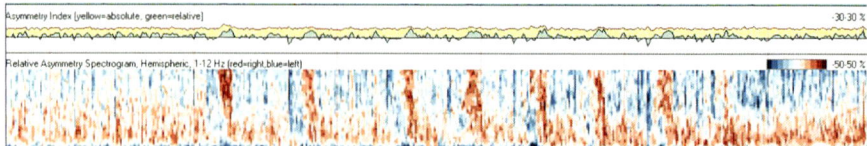

FIGURE 28.4 Raw EEG of recurrent right hemisphere seizures in a 55-year-female patient presenting with status epilepticus of unknown etiology. **(A)** A total of eight seizures are best seen on this 1 hour time display of relative asymmetry spectrogram where each seizure is represented by an increase in right hemisphere power (red), **(B)** bottom. Seizures appear more subtle on relative asymmetry index with a slight upward deflection (green), **(B)** top.

○ 10.5% of seizures identified on conventional EEG were missed by all three reviewers when viewing QEEG only.
○ Seizures that were missed were low amplitude, short duration, and focal.
- Akman et al. (5) identified factors that contribute to accurate seizure detection by comparing CSA and envelope trend.
  ○ Experienced QEEG readers were more accurate than inexperienced readers, particularly when using envelope trend (sensitivity of 87% vs. 52%).
  ○ Both experienced and inexperienced readers were more accurate in identifying seizures when CSA and envelope trends were viewed together as a panel.
  ○ CSA was more accurate when trends were viewed in a shorter time window (2-hour window = 78% vs. 4-hour window = 48%).
  ○ Seizure amplitude, duration, and frequency were other important determinants of QEEG accuracy.

F. Increasing the Sensitivity of QEEG for Seizure Detection

- A combination of QEEG trends based upon the four most important EEG properties for seizure detection (amplitude, frequency, rhythmicity, and asymmetry) is most likely to provide the best combination of sensitivity and specificity for a variety of seizure types.
  ○ High-amplitude, high-frequency seizures localized to one hemisphere are typically recognized on all QEEG trends (Figure 28.5).
  ○ Low-frequency seizures that predominantly evolve in amplitude might be best recognized on aEEG or envelope trend but not apparent at all on other trends.
  ○ Asymmetry index/spectrogram may detect very subtle focal seizures not seen on other trends while generalized seizures will not be visualized at all on asymmetry trends.
- Customization of QEEG measures
  ○ Similar to raw EEG, optimal QEEG display often involves adjustment of amplitude and frequency scales based upon an individual patient's baseline background activity.
  ○ After detection of an initial seizure, further adjustment of amplitude, frequency, and time scales as well as recognition of the visual features of the initial seizure can increase the sensitivity of QEEG for detection of subsequent seizures.

G. Pitfalls of QEEG

- False positive detections are common due to the high-amplitude, high-frequency, often rhythmic artifacts common in the ICU setting: ventilator, suctioning/oral care, bed percussion, and CPR (Figure 28.6).
- False negatives are typically encountered with brief, focal, low-frequency, low-amplitude seizures.

III. FURTHER CONSIDERATIONS/REMAINING QUESTIONS

A. How does QEEG change our approach to reviewing cEEG?

- QEEG can never replace raw EEG review but can focus and expedite EEG interpretation.
- QEEG allows for initial EEG screening by non-EEG trained personnel.

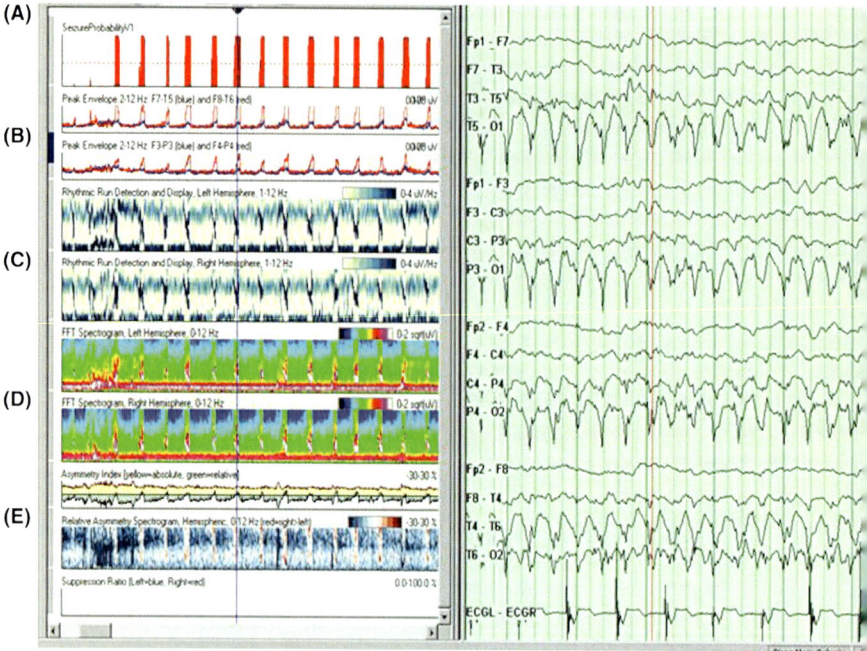

FIGURE 28.5 A combination of QEEG trends (trend panel) provides easy recognition of recurrent focal onset seizures, most prominent over the right posterior region. (A) *Seizure probability* (Persyst): proprietary seizure detection algorithm. (B) *Envelope trend*: each upward deflection of the red tracing represents increase in median amplitude over the right hemisphere (F8–T6 and F4–P4) which corresponds to each seizure. (C) *Rhythmicity spectrogram* (Persyst): dark blue vertical bands over both hemispheres represent an increase in power of rhythmic activity at higher frequencies. (D) *FFT spectrogram*: increase in bright color over both hemispheres represents an increase in power at higher frequencies. (E) *Asymmetry index and spectrogram* (Persyst): upward deflection of asymmetry index and increase in red of asymmetry spectrogram reflects increase in power over the right hemisphere. Note, in between seizures, power is relatively lower over the right hemisphere compared to the left (downward deflection on asymmetry index and increase in blue on asymmetry spectrogram) which signifies interictal right hemisphere dysfunction.

○ Bedside use of QEEG by nurses or EEG technologist with alarms set for specific thresholds is feasible but not yet optimized.

B. Further evaluation of the sensitivity and specificity of QEEG in patient populations with various seizure types is warranted.
- Which QEEG measures (or combinations) are best for recognition of specific seizure types needs to be defined.
- Optimum time, frequency, and amplitude scales should be established.
- Improved software programs with better recognition and rejection of artifacts would be useful.

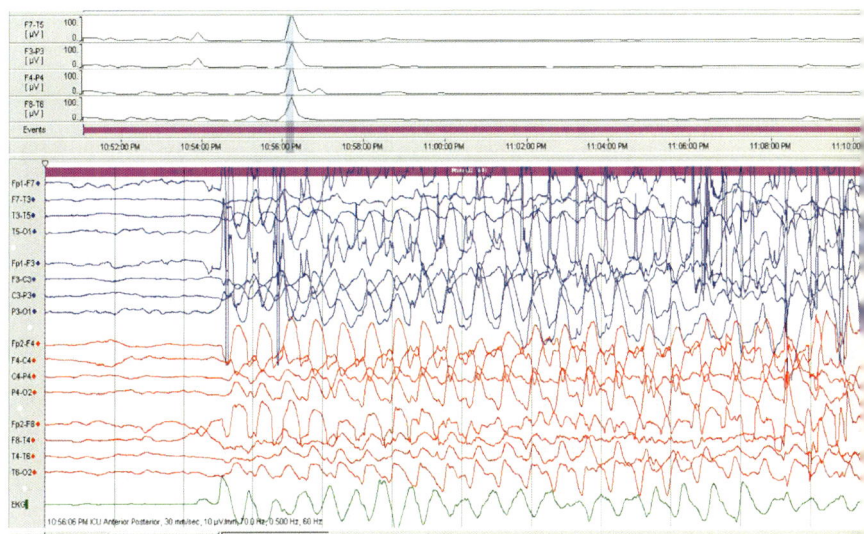

FIGURE 28.6 Increase in amplitude is seen in all channels at the 10:58:00 time stamp of this 20-minute envelope trend display (top). Raw EEG review including single-channel EKG lead reveals obvious rhythmic artifact that corresponded to CPR (false positive detection).

C. There are many challenges to performing clinical trials evaluating the utility of QEEG.

- Studies are labor intensive requiring expert review of raw EEG to score prolonged recordings to use as a "gold standard" for QEEG comparison.
- There is no clear consensus as to what EEG criteria constitute an electrographic seizure and studies on interrater agreement of the diagnosis of electrographic seizures is lacking.
- Large study populations are needed with a variety of acute and chronic neurological insults, varying seizure frequencies, and representation of all age groups from neonates to adults.
- Clinical outcomes of critically ill patients remain tightly linked to the primary neurological injury making it difficult to establish that detecting and treating forms of secondary injury such as seizures shortens length of stay or improves long-term function.

REFERENCES

1. Bricolo A, Turazzi S, Facciioli F, et al. Clinical application of compressed spectral array in long-term EEG monitoring of comatose patients. *Electroencephalogr Clin Neurophysiol.* 1978;45:211–225.
2. Wusthoff C, Shellhaas R, Clancy R. Limitations of single-channel EEG on the forehead for neonatal seizure detection. *J Perinatol.* 2009;29:237–242.

3. Moreno M, Anderson N. Introduction to the trending of EEG data for clinical monitoring In: ASET ed. *Pattern Recognition for the Bedside Caregiver: Continuous EEG in Adult Patients.* ASET: The Neurodiagnostic Society, Kansas City, MO, 2012.
4. Stewart CP, Otsubo H, Ochi A, et al. Seizure identification in the ICU using quantitative EEG displays. *Neurology.* 2010;75(17):1501–1508.
5. Akman CI, Micic V, Thompson A, et al. Seizure detection using digital trend analysis: Factors affecting utility. *Epilepsy Res.* 2011;93(1):66–72.

ADDITIONAL READING

Hirsch LJ, Brenner RP. Prolonged EEG monitoring and quantitative EEG techniques for detecting seizures and ischemia. In: *Atlas of EEG in Critical Care.* West Sussex: Wiley-Blackwell; 2010:217–261.

TWENTY-NINE

Quantitative EEG for Ischemia Detection

Susan T. Herman

KEY POINTS

- Quantitative EEG measures for detecting ischemia highlight the characteristic EEG changes that occur with decreased cerebral blood flow (CBF): loss of fast activity (beta and alpha frequencies) and increase in slow activity (polymorphic theta and delta activity).
- Quantitative EEG is most commonly used for the detection of delayed cerebral ischemia (DCI) after subarachnoid hemorrhage (SAH), but may also help with the diagnosis, monitoring, and prognosis of acute ischemic stroke and the detection of acute ischemia during and after neurosurgical or interventional radiology procedures.
- The most useful QEEG measures are alpha variability, alpha delta ratios (ADR), and asymmetry indices.
- For monitoring ischemia, quantitative EEG trends should include electrodes corresponding to the major supratentorial cerebral vascular territories: frontocentral-parasagittal for anterior cerebral artery (ACA) territories, centrotemporal or temporal for middle cerebral artery (MCA) territories, and parietal-occipital for posterior cerebral artery (PCA) territories.
- Since quantitative EEG trends are susceptible to artifacts commonly seen in the intensive care unit, artifact-rejection algorithms may reduce artifact; however, review of raw EEG tracings is imperative to confirm QEEG changes.

I. BACKGROUND

A. EEG Changes During Ischemia
- Within seconds, a decline in CBF results in predictable changes in EEG (1).
- Initial EEG changes (CBF 25–30 mL/100 g/min) consist of loss of fast activity: loss of beta activity, slowing or loss of alpha rhythm, and absence of sleep spindles.
- With more severe ischemia, polymorphic theta and delta activity is seen over the region of ischemia.

- With irreversible ischemia (CBF $<8-10$ mL/100 g/min), there is focal attenuation of all EEG activity.

B. Carotid Endarterectomy Monitoring
- The first use of EEG monitoring for reversible ischemia was to detect decreased CBF during carotid endarterectomy (CEA).
- Today, quantitative EEG (QEEG) is often used as an adjunct to visual review of the raw EEG during CEA.
  - Decreases in beta power, increases in delta power, changes in color spectrogram (decreased beta, increased delta), decreases in ADR, and changes in Brain Symmetry Index (BSI) may aid in detecting ischemia during carotid artery clamping (2).

C. Subarachnoid Hemorrhage
- DCI refers to clinical deterioration and/or cerebral infarction due to vasospasm after SAH.
- Typically a long-time window (hours to days) ensues between onset of vasospasm and irreversible infarct.
- Treatments such as volume expansion, hypertensive therapy, intra-arterial vasodilators, and angioplasty may prevent infarct, if initiated before irreversible ischemia occurs.
- Continuous EEG monitoring, particularly with utilization of QEEG trends, may detect ischemia at a reversible stage, allowing initiation of therapy to prevent infarct.
- In retrospective analyses, relative alpha variability (RAV) and ADR show excellent sensitivity and fair-to-good specificity for DCI (3–5).
- DCI generally causes widespread EEG changes that are not limited to the vascular territory of the vessels in vasospasm (5).
  - However, changes are usually maximal in the region of vasospasm.

D. Acute Ischemic Stroke
- Many QEEG techniques can be used to diagnose and monitor neurologic deterioration in acute ischemic stroke.
- BSI and paired BSI (pdBSI) values correlate with NIH stroke scale (NIHSS) and lesion volume on diffusion weighted MRI (DWI), thereby providing a quantitative measure of stroke severity (6,7).
- pdBSI has been shown to detect stroke even in patients with low (0–1) NIHSS scores, with a value less than 0.12 excluding stroke and greater than 0.19 being 90% specific for stroke.
  - pdBSI is also an independent predictor of neurologic deterioration: values greater than 0.22 have shown a sensitivity of 100% and specificity of 78% for acute decline (7).
- During continuous EEG monitoring, changes in BSI values suggest a change in the clinical status of the patient, either deterioration or improvement.
  - For example, changes in BSI during intravenous thrombolysis correlate significantly with changes in NIHSS (8).
- QEEG monitoring can also be considered for monitoring patients with recurrent or crescendo transient ischemic attack (TIAs), after interventional neuroradiology or vascular neurosurgical procedures, and for those at risk for secondary stroke extension.

- BSI changes are not specific for ischemia: hemorrhage, seizures, and artifact can all result in focal EEG abnormalities that affect BSI.

II. BASICS

A. Overview of Quantitative EEG Trends for Ischemia
- QEEG parameters for ischemia monitoring are designed to optimally represent the raw EEG changes seen during ischemia: loss of fast activity and increase in slow activity.
- These parameters include color spectrograms, trend analysis of total power, ratios of fast-to-slow frequency bands (eg, RAV, ADR), and asymmetry (or symmetry) indices.

B. Color Density Spectral Array (CDSA) or Spectrogram
- CDSA trends can be calculated for individual channels, brain regions, or hemispheres.
- The channels corresponding to the ischemic hemisphere will show increased power in the theta and delta frequency range and decreased power in the alpha and beta frequency range compared to the opposite hemisphere.

C. Trend Analysis of Total Power 1 to 30 Hz
- Labar et al studied two-channel QEEG (Cz–T3 and Cz–T4) in 11 patients with aneurysmal SAH (4).
- The total power from 1 to 30 Hz (2 seconds epochs averaged over 2 minutes) showed sensitivity of 100% for ischemia associated with focal lesions on CT, and 91% for all ischemic events.
- Other parameters showed lower sensitivity: alpha power ratio (7.5–15 Hz/1–7 Hz) sensitivity was 64% and percent delta power (1–3.5 Hz/1–30 Hz) sensitivity was 45%. Compressed spectral array showed sensitivity of 44%.
- QEEG changes preceded clinical changes in four cases. In five cases, QEEG changes accompanied asymptomatic radiologic findings.

D. Relative Alpha Variability (RAV): The Ratio of Theta–Alpha Power (6–14 Hz) to Total Power (1–20 Hz)
- Vespa et al studied 32 patients with aneurysmal SAH using RAV (5). EEG channels F4–T4, T4–P4, P4–O2, F3–T3, T3–P3, and P3–O1; 2 seconds epochs averaged over 2 minutes.
  - Qualitative analysis: RAV was classified every 8 to 12 hours into four grades based on visual appearance: excellent, good, fair, and poor (Figure 29.1).
  - A change of one grade was considered a significant decrease (5).
  - Quantitative analysis: RAV was calculated as (peak value–trough value)/(peak value + trough value) for each 8 to 12 hours trend.
  - 19/19 patients with angiographically verified vasospasm had a qualitative RAV decrease of two grades at the time of vasospasm.
  - Quantitative measures showed a similar decrease in RAV (Figure 29.2).
  - In half of the patients, RAV changes occurred at a mean of 2.9 days before clinical changes.

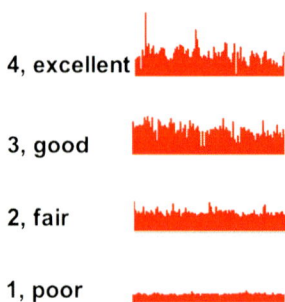

FIGURE 29.1   Visual scale for grading of RAV (5).

(A)

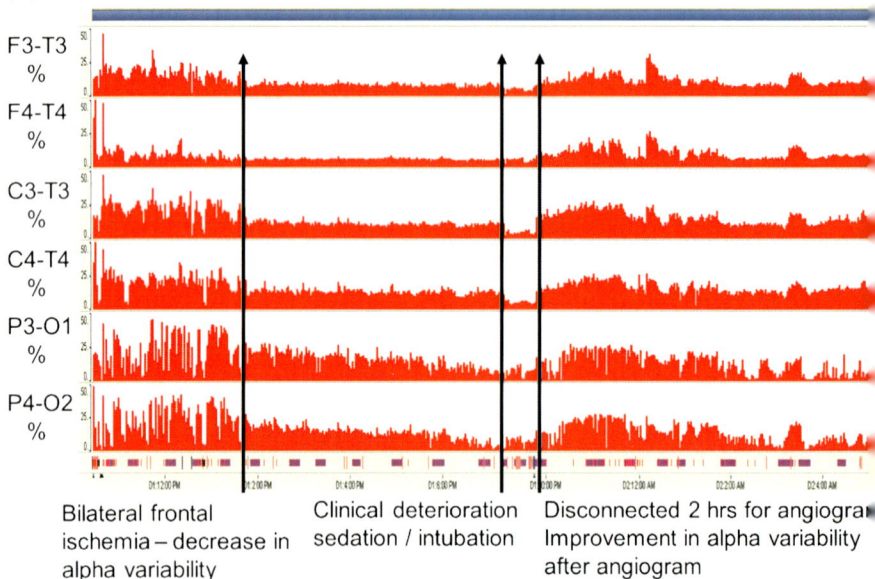

Bilateral frontal
ischemia – decrease in
alpha variability

Clinical deterioration
sedation / intubation

Disconnected 2 hrs for angiogram
Improvement in alpha variability
after angiogram

FIGURE 29.2   (**A**) Relative alpha variability (RAV) trends in a 57-year-old woman with SAH from right ACA aneurysm. At baseline, there is a mild decrease RAV in the right frontal region, likely from mild ischemia. At the first time point, a diffuse decrease in RAV is seen, maximal in the frontal regions, particularly on the right. The patient had no clinical deterioration at this time. Five hours after the RAV change, the patient had an acute clinical deterioration, becoming confused with bilateral leg weakness. She was intubated (second arrow) and taken to angiogram. After intra-arterial nicardipine, RAV trends show excellent RAV in all channels. The patient had no permanent neurologic deficits. (**B**) a, b, and c (*opposite*) show the raw EEG tracings. Initial diffuse theta activity in A is replaced by high voltage frontally maximal delta activity in B with onset of delayed cerebral ischemia. Diffuse severe slowing at C corresponds to clinical deterioration.

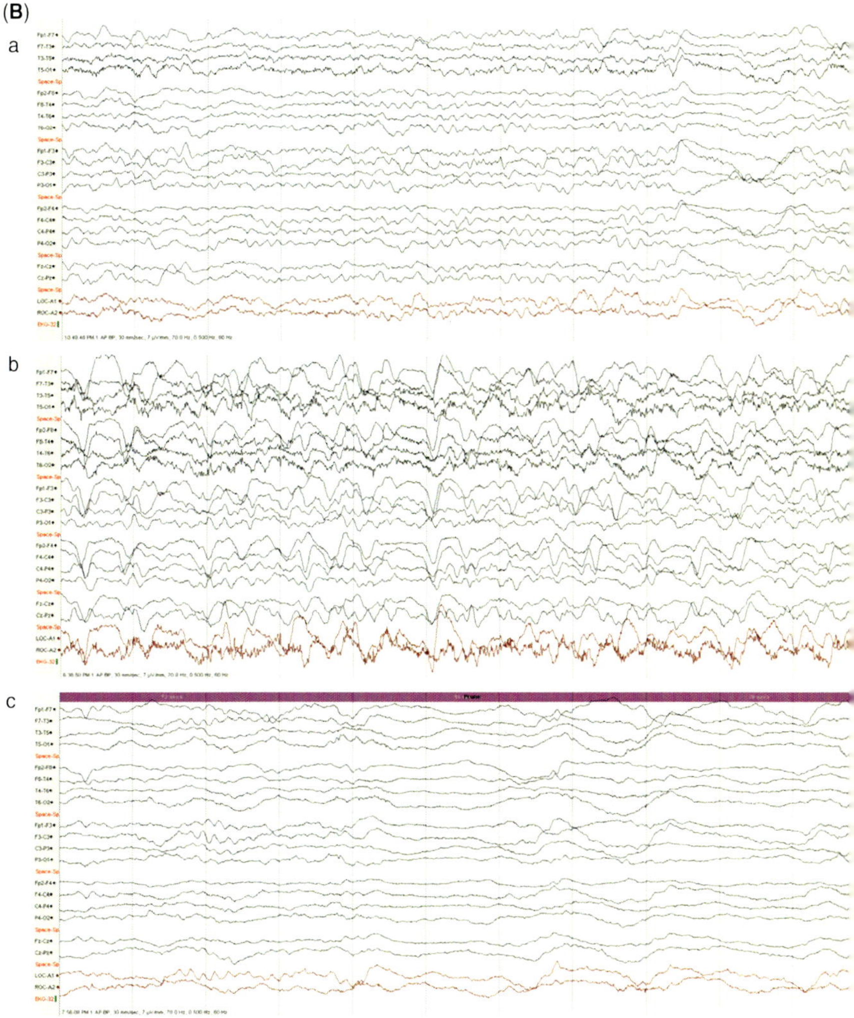

(B)

FIGURE 29.2 *Continued.*

E. Post-Stimulation Alpha–Delta Ratio (PSADR): Ratio of Alpha Power (8–13 Hz) to Delta Power (1–4 Hz) (Figure 29.3)

- Claassen et al. retrospectively studied 34 of 78 consecutive patients with poor-grade SAH (Hunt–Hess grade 4–5)(3).
  - EEG analysis was done on 20 artifact-free, 1-minute EEG clips after an alerting stimulus. Ten clips were done on monitoring day 1 (baseline) and 10 on days 4 to 6 (after clinical deterioration).

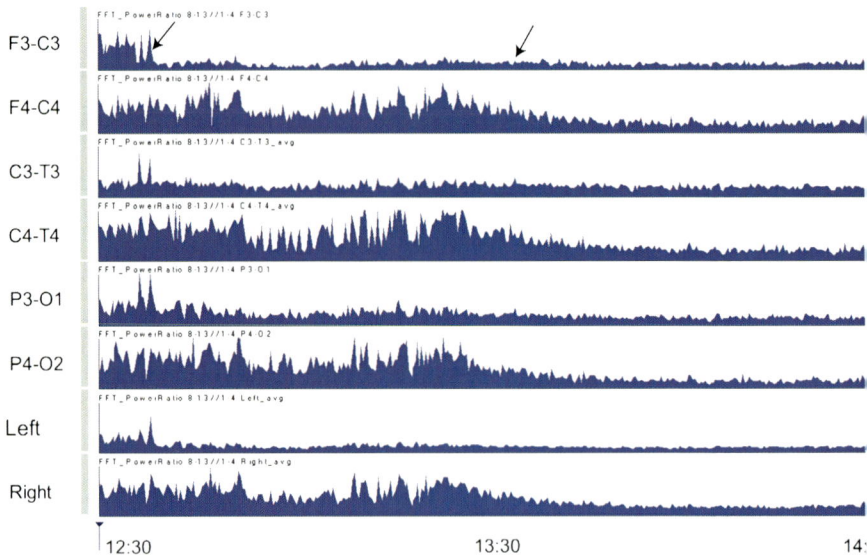

FIGURE 29.3 ADR trends in a 72-year-old man with a large left ACA aneurysm and SAH. On day 4 after SAH, ADR trends show a sudden severe decrease over the left hemisphere (first arrow), followed 1 hour later by similar decrease on the right (second arrow). Angiogram showed severe diffuse vasospasm, which was refractory to intra-arterial vasodilators.

- ○ Nine of 34 patients (26%) developed DCI. The ADR ratio was strongly associated with DCI, with median decrease of 24% in those with DCI, compared to increase of 3% without DCI.
- ○ The authors described two clinically useful cutoffs: (1) six consecutive epochs with greater than 10% decrease in PSADR compared to baseline (sensitivity 100%, specificity 76%) and (2) any single measurement with greater than 50% decrease in PSADR (sensitivity 89%, specificity 84%).

F. Asymmetry Indices
- The absolute asymmetry index compares the difference in power at each pair of homologous electrodes, sums the absolute values, and displays a total asymmetry score.
  - ○ This score is always positive, and goes up with increasing asymmetry in any frequency or direction.
- The relative asymmetry index calculates asymmetry at each pair of homologous electrodes, but shows laterality.
  - ○ If the trend is downgoing, there is more power on the left hemisphere, and if upgoing, there is more power on the right.
  - ○ Therefore, a loss of power over one hemisphere secondary to ischemia (eg, the right hemisphere) would result in relatively higher power over the contralateral

hemisphere (the left hemisphere) and therefore, a downward deflection of the relative asymmetry index (Figure 29.4, top).

- BSI is comparable to absolute asymmetry index. BSI is the mean of the absolute value of the difference in mean hemispheric power for frequencies between 1 and 25 Hz for channels F4–C4, F3–C3, C4–P4, C3–P3, P4–O2, P3–O1, F4–T4, and F3–T3 (6).
  - pdBSI is a revised measure evaluating asymmetry along homologous channel pairs (7).
- BSI is displayed as a trend of a single value over time.
  - Values range from 0 (perfect symmetry) to 1 (maximal asymmetry).

G. Relative Asymmetry Spectrogram (Persyst Corp.)

- The asymmetry spectrogram is similar to a color spectrogram, but shows the difference in power at each frequency from 1 to 18 Hz averaged over the entire hemisphere.
  - Perfect symmetry would show no color on this trend.
  - If there is more power on the right at a particular frequency, the spectrogram will show more red signal; if more power on the left, the spectrogram will show more blue.
  - Therefore, a loss of power over one hemisphere secondary to ischemia (eg, the right hemisphere) would result in relatively higher power over the contralateral hemisphere (the left hemisphere) and therefore, a predominantly blue signal (Figure 29.4, bottom).

H. Clinical Use of QEEG Trends for Ischemia

- Similar QEEG trends are used to detect ischemia regardless of the etiology of the ischemia.
- Monitoring for DCI after SAH:
  - CEEG recording should be started before the window for vasospasm (days 3–14), which is typically on day 1 or 2 after coiling or clipping of the aneurysm.
  - This allows for assessment of baseline EEG and any asymmetries that may be present from neurosurgical procedures (breach artifact), scalp edema, or intraparenchymal hemorrhage.

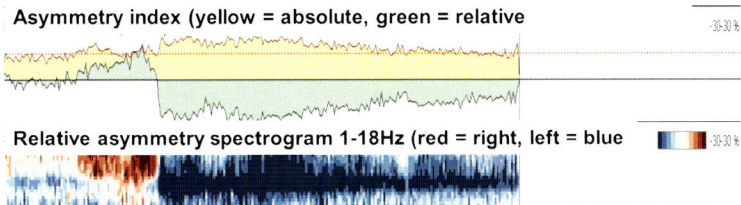

FIGURE 29.4 Relative and absolute asymmetry indices and relative asymmetry spectrogram. Loss of power over the right hemisphere secondary to ischemia results in relatively increased power over the left hemisphere seen as a downward trend on relative asymmetry index (top, green band) and a predominantly blue signal on relative asymmetry spectrogram (bottom).

TABLE 29.1   Suggested QEEG Trends for Ischemia

TRENDS	REGIONS OR CHANNELS
Spectrogram 0–30 Hz	L/R hemisphere
Alpha variability (6–14 Hz/1–20 Hz)	L/R hemisphere Single channel: F3–C3, F4–C4, C3–T3, C4–T4, P3–O1, P4–O2
Alpha-delta ratio (6–14 Hz/1–4 Hz)	L/R hemisphere Single channel: F3–C3, F4–C4, C3–T3, C4–T4, P3–O1, P4–O2
Amplitude integrated EEG	Single channel: F3–C3, F4–C4
Asymmetry indices (absolute and relative)	L/R hemisphere
Asymmetry spectrogram	L/R hemisphere

- ○ Optimally, CEEG should be continued throughout the vasospasm window, usually 10 to 14 days after SAH.
- QEEG trends for monitoring ischemia (Table 29.1)
  - ○ Trends should include electrodes corresponding to the major supratentorial cerebral vascular territories: frontocentral parasagittal for ACA territories, centrotemporal or temporal for MCA territories, and parietal–occipital for PCA territories.
  - ○ The ability to detect ischemia can be improved by combining multiple trends (Figure 29.5).
  - ○ No studies have examined the sensitivity and specificity of combined trend panels for detection of ischemia.
  - ○ Several analysis and display factors, such as number of channels in each trend, duration of EEG epochs, number of trends per screen, number of hours per screen, and color scales, can significantly affect the appearance of QEEG trends and the ability to detect ischemia. These factors have not been systematically evaluated.
- Quantitative EEG trends are susceptible to artifacts commonly seen in the intensive care unit, including muscle and electrode artifacts.
  - ○ Artifact rejection algorithms may reduce artifact, but review of raw EEG tracings is imperative to confirm QEEG changes.
- Because of the short time window for intervention in acute ischemic stroke, QEEG monitoring for this indication is not currently feasible in most intensive care units.

III. FURTHER CONSIDERATIONS/REMAINING QUESTIONS

A. Systematic studies are needed to determine the sensitivity and specificity of various QEEG trends and display panels for ischemia.
- In particular, there is little information about the effects of combining QEEG trends.

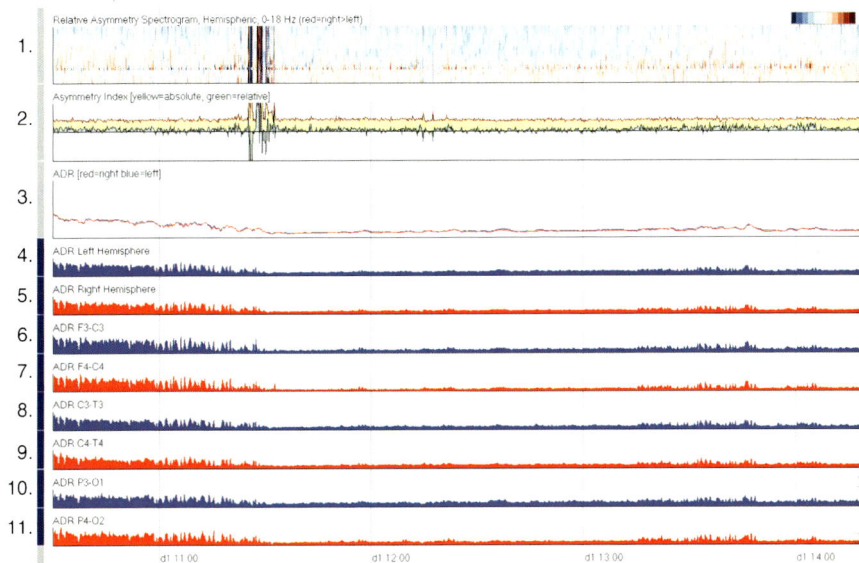

FIGURE 29.5 Example of a QEEG trend panel for ischemia monitoring. Trends include (top to bottom): 1. Hemispheric relative asymmetry spectrogram, 1 to 18 Hz. This shows slightly more slow activity over the right hemisphere (red color predominates at low frequencies) and loss of fast frequencies on the right (blue color predominates at higher frequencies). 2. Asymmetry index: No significant asymmetries. 3. ADR, hemispheric, left hemisphere: blue, right hemisphere: red. 4. ADR left hemisphere. 5. ADR right hemisphere. 6 through 11: ADR of single channels over homologous brain regions, left = blue, right = red. At approximately 11:30, there is a sudden decrease in all alpha-delta ratio trends, indicating diffuse ischemia. Since the change is relatively symmetric, the asymmetry trends do not detect this change. Shortly after 1300, ADR trends improve minimally after increase in systolic blood pressure with pressors, but this effect is not sustained.

B. **True real-time ischemia monitoring will likely become the standard of care in neurologic intensive care units as more reliable QEEG trends and reliable automated alerts are developed.**

C. **Prospective studies are essential to evaluate if interventions based on EEG findings lead to improved neurologic outcome after SAH and acute ischemia, or merely necessitate costly, potentially harmful diagnostic testing (eg, angiography).**

REFERENCES

1. Astrup J, Siesjo BK, Symon L. Thresholds in cerebral ischemia—The ischemic penumbra. *Stroke.* 1981;12:723–725.

2. van Putten MJ. Extended BSI for continuous EEG monitoring in carotid endarterectomy. *Clin Neurophysiol.* 2006;117:2661–2666.
3. Claassen J, Hirsch LJ, Kreiter KT, et al. Quantitative continuous EEG for detecting delayed cerebral ischemia in patients with poor-grade subarachnoid hemorrhage. *Clin Neurophysiol.* 2004;115:2699–2710.
4. Labar DR, Fisch BJ, Pedley TA, et al. Quantitative EEG monitoring for patients with subarachnoid hemorrhage. *Electroencephalogr Clin Neurophysiol.* 1991;78:325–332.
5. Vespa PM, Nuwer MR, Juhasz C, et al. Early detection of vasospasm after acute subarachnoid hemorrhage using continuous EEG ICU monitoring. *Electroencephalogr Clin Neurophysiol.* 1997;103:607–615.
6. van Putten MJ, Tavy DL3. Continuous quantitative EEG monitoring in hemispheric stroke patients using the brain symmetry index. *Stroke.* 2004;35:2489–2492.
7. Sheorajpanday RV, Nagels G, Weeren AJ, et al. Additional value of quantitative EEG in acute anterior circulation syndrome of presumed ischemic origin. *Clin Neurophysiol.* 2010;121:1719–1725.
8. de Vos CC, van Maarseveen SM, Brouwers PJ, van Putten MJ. Continuous EEG monitoring during thrombolysis in acute hemispheric stroke patients using the brain symmetry index. *J Clin Neurophysiol.* 2008;25:77–82.

ADDITIONAL READING

Claassen J, Mayer SA, Hirsch LJ. Continuous EEG monitoring in patients with subarachnoid hemorrhage. *J Clin Neurophysiol.* 2005;22:92–98.
Scheuer ML, Wilson SB. Data analysis for continuous EEG monitoring in the ICU: Seeing the forest and the trees. *J Clin Neurophysiol.* 2004;21:353–378.

Generalized Convulsive Status Epilepticus

Christa Swisher and Aatif M. Husain

KEY POINTS

- Generalized convulsive status epilepticus (GCSE) is the most common type of status epilepticus (SE).
- The morbidity and mortality of GCSE depend upon its etiology, with acute CNS injury, older age, and longer duration of GCSE at highest risk.
- GCSE is an emergency and must be aggressively treated: the longer an episode lasts, the more refractory the patient becomes to treatment.
- Lorazepam and diazepam are the preferred initial therapies for GCSE. Phenytoin, fosphenytoin or valproic acid should be used after benzodiazepines terminate the seizures or for treatment of ongoing seizures after benzodiazepines have failed.
- Approximately 30% of patients with GCSE will progress to nonconvulsive SE (NCSE) on EEG after clinical events cease.

I. BACKGROUND

A. Epidemiology
- GCSE is thought to be the most common type of SE.
- Estimated incidence in the United States is 65,000 to 150,000 patients each year (1).
  - There is a bimodal distribution of the incidence of SE.
  - Most common in ages less than 1 year and greater than 60 years of age.
- SE costs approximately $4 billion per annum in the United States.
- Relationship to epilepsy (2)
  - 12% to 30% of adults with epilepsy have SE as the initial presentation.
  - 40% of adult patients with SE have a history of epilepsy.
  - 15% of patients with epilepsy will experience SE in their lifetime.
- Patients with GCSE are at risk of developing GCSE again, and also at risk for developing epilepsy.

B. Morbidity and Mortality
- Determined primarily by the etiology of GCSE

- Mortality estimates range from 5% to 50% (3).
- In the VA Cooperative trial, the mortality rate was 26.8% for overt GCSE and 64.9% for subtle GCSE (4).
- Predictors of poor outcome are etiology, age, and duration of SE.
  ○ Patients with acute CNS insults including stroke, hypoxia, head trauma, CNS infection and sepsis, have the highest association with poor outcome.
  ○ Myoclonic SE after a hypoxic injury such as cardiac arrest is associated with an extremely poor prognosis.
  ○ Better prognosis is seen in patients with epilepsy who have breakthrough seizures from medication noncompliance, seizures in the setting of alcohol abuse, or seizures as a result of a preexisting stroke.
  ○ Mortality rate for patients greater than 80 years old is 50%.
  ○ When GCSE lasts longer than 1 hour, mortality begins to rise steeply, indicating the importance of early and aggressive treatment.

C. Clinical Features of GCSE
- Clinical research definition of GCSE: continuous, generalized seizure activity lasting longer than 30 minutes or *greater than or equal to* 2 generalized seizures within a 30-minute period without return to baseline between seizures.
- Because 90% of all seizures stop spontaneously within 2 minutes, a more practical definition of SE has been proposed: a single seizure lasting longer than 5 minutes or recurrent, discrete seizures without recovery in between.
  ○ These revised criteria will lead to more aggressive initial treatment and prevent recurrent SE.
  ○ This definition of SE encourages providers to aggressively treat any seizure lasting more than 5 minutes.
- Types of GCSE include generalized tonic–clonic, myoclonic, tonic, and clonic
  ○ Clinical seizure activity can be symmetric or asymmetric.
  ○ Always associated with marked impairment in consciousness and bilateral epileptiform activity on EEG.
- As GCSE continues, motor activity can diminish resulting in subtle GCSE. Motor activity in subtle GCSE can be as simple as eye twitching, finger twitching, and nystagmus.
- Eventually, all clinical seizure activity may cease, while the EEG still shows generalized electrical discharges. This is nonconvulsive status epilepticus (NCSE).
- Systemic features of GSCE
  ○ Pulmonary edema, respiratory failure and acidosis are common.
    ▪ Acidosis is a result of respiratory failure and lactate release and is often severe (pH < 7.0).
  ○ Hyperpyrexia can occur and has been found to correlate with poor outcomes in GCSE.
  ○ White blood cell count can be elevated.
  ○ A low-grade CSF pleocytosis may be seen (less than $30/mm^3$). However, CSF WBC count above $30/mm^3$ is concerning for infection.
  ○ Hypotension can be seen as early as 30 minutes after the start of GCSE.
  ○ Other cardiovascular complications include arrhythmias and tachycardia.

○ Renal failure may occur secondary to rhabdomyolysis.
○ Increased intracranial pressure can be seen.
○ Cerebral edema may occur, especially in children.

D. Etiology (Table 30.1)
- GCSE has different causes in patients with epilepsy compared to patients with no history of seizures.
- Most common cause of GCSE in patients with chronic epilepsy is discontinuation of or noncompliance with antiepileptic drugs (AEDs).
  ○ 15% of patients with epilepsy will develop SE during their lifetime.
- In patients without a history of epilepsy, the most common cause of GCSE is cerebrovascular (ischemic stroke, intracerebral hemorrhage).
- Other common causes are head trauma, anoxic injury, toxic/metabolic, and intracranial neoplasm.
- Causes also vary by age.
  ○ Half of GCSE cases in children are caused by infection and fever.

TABLE 30.1 Causes of GCSE

NEUROLOGIC CAUSES OF GCSE	NONNEUROLOGIC CAUSES OF GCSE

• Low AED levels
• History of epilepsy
• Cerebrovascular disease
  ○ Ischemic stroke, ICH, SAH, SDH
  ○ Venous sinus thrombosis
• Neoplasm
  ○ Primary or metastatic
  ○ Malignant or benign
  ○ Leptomeningeal carcinomatosis
  ○ Paraneoplastic
• Anoxic injury
• Head trauma
• CNS infections
  ○ Viral, fungal, parasitic, bacterial
  ○ Meningitis, encephalitis, abscess
  ○ Prion disease
• CNS inflammatory/ autoimmune disease
  ○ Neurosarcoidosis
  ○ Systemic lupus erythematosus
  ○ Primary CNS vasculitis
  ○ Multiple sclerosis
  ○ Hashimoto enephalopathy
	• Medication or substance related
	  ○ Alcohol withdrawal
	  ○ Illicits (amphetamines, cocaine, heroin, PCP, or ecstasy)
	  ○ Antibiotics (penicillins, fluoroquinolones, cephalosporins)
	  ○ Antidepressants (Buprorion and TCAs more likely to case SE than SSRIs and MAOIs)
	  ○ Theophylline
	  ○ Isoniazid (consider giving vitamin B6)
	  ○ Insulin
	  ○ Lidocaine
	• Metabolic
	  ○ Hypomagnesemia
	  ○ Hypocalcemia
	  ○ Marked shifts in plasma sodium levels
	• Eclampsia
	• Sepsis

○ In adults, the most common cause of GCSE is cerebrovascular disease (acute or remote ischemic stroke and intracerebral hemorrhage).

E. EEG During GCSE
- Largely based on animal models, GCSE has been described to occur in five stages (5).
- Stage 1: Discrete clinical and electrographic seizures.
- Stage 2: EEG evolves from discrete electrographic seizures into a waxing and waning pattern of rhythmic ictal discharges.
- Stage 3: Continuous epileptiform discharges are present.
- Stage 4: Continuous epileptiform activity is interrupted by periods of background suppression.
  ○ Epileptiform activity can be in the form of spikes, spike-and-wave, sharps, or rhythmic slow waves.
  ○ As this phase goes on, the periods of suppression become longer and the periods of epileptiform activity become shorter.
- Stage 5: Generalized Periodic discharges on a flat background.

II. BASICS

A. Need for Treatment
- GCSE is an emergency and must be aggressively treated.
- The longer an episode of GCSE persists, the more refractory the patient will become to treatment.
  ○ If treatment is not initiated until the patient is in subtle GCSE, then only 15% of those patients will respond to treatment.

B. Use of EEG
- Clinically evident seizures should be treated immediately without waiting for the EEG.
  ○ Neurocritical Care Society (NCS) guidelines for continuous EEG (cEEG) monitoring: indications in SE (Class I, level B evidence) (6).
    - SE without return to baseline greater than 10 minutes.
    - Coma, including post-cardiac arrest.
    - Epileptiform activity or periodic discharges on initial 30-minute EEG recording.
    - Patients with ICH, SAH, TBI.
    - Suspected nonconvulsive seizures in patients with altered mental status.
  ○ GCSE should also be managed with cEEG if a patient requires continuous paralytics after initial treatment with antiepileptic drugs (AEDs) (6).
- Approximately 30% of patients with GCSE will progress to nonconvulsive SE (NCSE) on EEG after clinical events cease (3).
  ○ In comatose patients, the duration of cEEG monitoring should be at least 48 hours to rule out the presence of nonconvulsive seizures (per NCS guidelines) (6).

- When a patient with refractory GCSE is being managed with phenobarbital, midazolam, or propofol, EEG should guide the degree of electrographic suppression desired.
  - Burst-suppression pattern is achieved when bursts of electrical activity are separated by 10 to 15 seconds of EEG suppression.
  - Electrographic seizures can still occur during burst suppression.
- When periodic discharges are observed, EEG monitoring should be continued, because these patterns have high epileptic potential.
  - It is controversial as to whether or not periodic discharges alone should be treated.
- EEG can also be helpful in identifying nonepileptic events that may mimic GCSE

C. General Medical Care
- Assessment and management of the patient's airway is important.
  - Apnea can occur with generalized seizures and intubation may be required.
  - If neuromuscular blockade is necessary for intubation, then use of a short-acting paralytic such as vecuronium (0.1 mg/kg) is preferable so that ongoing seizure activity will not be masked.
- Laboratory evaluation: finger stick glucose, complete blood count, basic metabolic profile, liver function test, magnesium level, phosphate level, urine toxicology screen, EtOH level, troponin, creatine kinase, urinalysis, and urine and blood bacterial cultures
- Check AED levels if the patient is known to take seizure medications.
- Administer IV thiamine before dextrose is given to avoid precipitation of Wernicke's encephalopathy.
- Severe acidosis can be treated with sodium bicarbonate.
- Hyperthermia is common (in up to 79% of patients) and can worsen neurologic injury from GCSE.
  - The treatment for hyperthermia in GCSE is intravascular cooling or passive, external cooling.
- Avoid hyperglycemia as it can worsen SE-induced brain injury.
- Initiate IV fluids as rhabdomyolysis is common.
- Lumbar puncture is indicated for SE of unknown etiology, if the patient is febrile, or if the patient is immunocompromised.
  - Empiric antibiotics and antivirals (vancomycin, ceftriaxone, acyclovir $\pm$ ampicillin) should be started while CSF studies are being obtained.
- Imaging:
  - A head CT should be obtained once the patient is stabilized and clinical seizures have stopped.
  - If the etiology of GCSE is unknown and the head CT is negative, then brain MRI should be obtained.
  - There can be changes in MRI from SE such as hippocampal edema, T2/FLAIR cortical hyperintensities (cortical ribbon pattern), and splenium lesions.

D. Medications (Table 30.2)
- Every hospital should have a GCSE treatment algorithm. A sample algorithm is presented in Figure 30.1.

TABLE 30.2   Summary of Various AEDs That Can Be Used to Treat GCSE

AED	DOSING	GOAL SERUM LEVEL	MECHANISM OF ACTION	ADVERSE REACTIONS
Diazepam	0.15–0.25 mg/kg IV with rate not to exceed 5 mg/min	n/a	GABA agonist	Respiratory depression, hypotension, and sedation
Lorazepam	0.1 mg/kg IV with rate not to exceed 2 mg/min	n/a	GABA agonist	Respiratory depression, hypotension, and sedation
Phenytoin	Load 20 mg/kg IV then 5–8 mg/kg/day divided TID	15–25 µg/mL	Sodium channel modulator	Drug rash, eosinophilia, purple-glove syndrome, irritative thrombophlebitis, and arrhythmias
Fosphenytoin	20 PE/kg then 5–8 PE/kg/day divided TID (PE = phenytoin equivalent)	15–25 µg/mL	Sodium channel modulator	Hypotension. Lower risk of infusion reaction than with phenytoin
Valproic acid	Load 20–40 mg/kg IV then 15–20 mg/kg/day divided BID or TID	>80 mg/L	Sodium channel inhibition, GABA potentiation, NMDA inhibition	Pancreatitis, hyperammonemia, thrombocytopenia and encephalopathy

Phenobarbital	Load 20 mg/kg IV then 1–4 mg/kg/day divided BID	30–50 μg/mL	Enhances GABA inhibition by modulating chloride currents	Long half-life (4 days), hypotension, respiratory depression, and sedation
Midazolam	Load 0.1–0.2 mg/kg IV then 0.75–10 μg/kg/min	n/a	GABA agonist	Respiratory depression, hypotension, sedation, and tachyphylaxis
Propofol	Load 1–2 mg/kg IV then 2–10 mg/kg/hr	n/a	GABA$_A$ agonist (may also inhibit NMDA receptors and modulate calcium channels)	Sedation, hypotension (3–10%), bradycardia, and propofol infusion syndrome
Pentobarbital	Load 5–20 mg/kg IV then 0.5–3 mg/kg/hr	10–20 μg/mL	Enhances GABA inhibition by modulating chloride currents	Sedation, hypotension, poikilothermia, and possibly immunosuppresion and higher infection rates
Levetiracetam	1000–2000 mg IV then daily dosing up to 4 g/day divided BID	n/a	Binds to synaptic vesicle-binding protein SV2A	Mild somnolence

Generalized Convulsive Status Epilepticus Treatment Algorithm

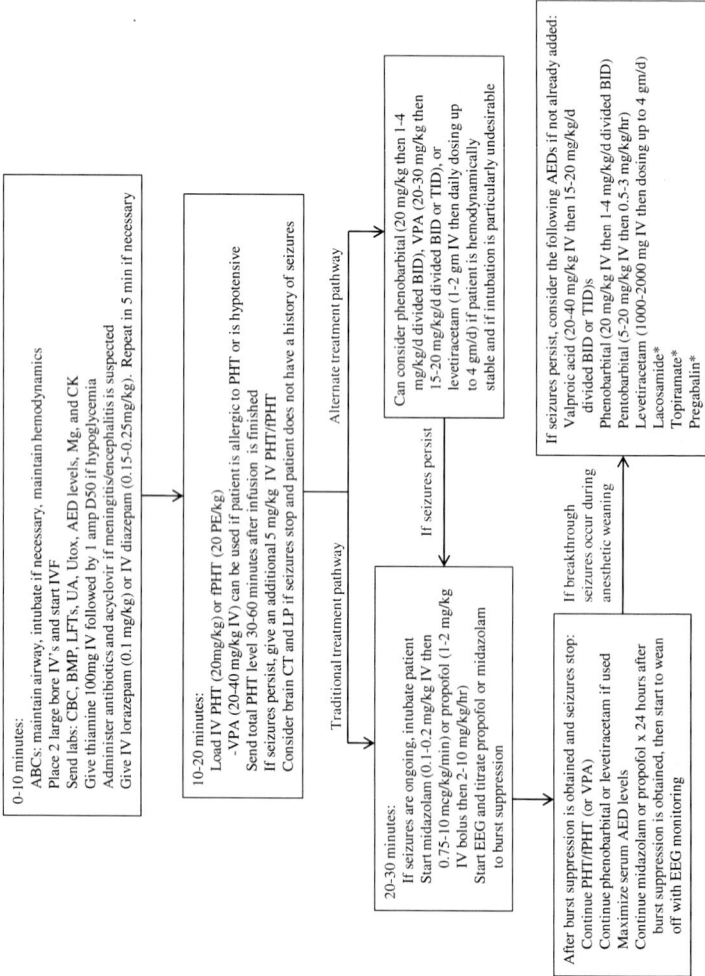

0–10 minutes:
ABCs: maintain airway, intubate if necessary, maintain hemodynamics
Place 2 large bore IV's and start IVF
Send labs: CBC, BMP, LFTs, UA, Utox, AED levels, Mg, and CK
Give thiamine 100mg IV followed by 1 amp D50 if hypoglycemia
Administer antibiotics and acyclovir if meningitis/encephalitis is suspected
Give IV Lorazepam (0.1 mg/kg) or IV diazepam (0.15–0.25mg/kg). Repeat in 5 min if necessary

10–20 minutes:
Load IV PHT (20mg/kg) or fPHT (20 PE/kg)
-VPA (20–40 mg/kg IV) can be used if patient is allergic to PHT or is hypotensive
Send total PHT level 30–60 minutes after infusion is finished
If seizures persist, give an additional 5 mg/kg IV PHT/fPHT
Consider brain CT and LP if seizures stop and patient does not have a history of seizures

Traditional treatment pathway

Alternate treatment pathway

If seizures persist

20–30 minutes:
If seizures are ongoing, intubate patient
Start midazolam (0.1–0.2 mg/kg IV then
0.75–10 mcg/kg/min) or propofol (1–2 mg/kg
IV bolus then 2–10 mg/kg/hr)
Start EEG and titrate propofol or midazolam
to burst suppression

If breakthrough
seizures occur during
anesthetic weaning

After burst suppression is obtained and seizures stop:
Continue PHT/fPHT (or VPA)
Continue phenobarbital or levetiracetam if used
Maximize serum AED levels
Continue midazolam or propofol x 24 hours after
burst suppression is obtained, then start to wean
off with EEG monitoring

Can consider phenobarbital (20 mg/kg then 1–4
mg/kg/d divided BID), VPA (20–30 mg/kg then
15–20 mg/kg/d divided BID or TID), or
levetiracetam (1–2 gm IV then daily dosing up
to 4 gm/d) if patient is hemodynamically
stable and if intubation is particularly undesirable

If seizures persist, consider the following AEDs if not already added:
Valproic acid (20–40 mg/kg IV then 15–20 mg/kg/d
divided BID or TID)s
Phenobarbital (20 mg/kg IV then 1–4 mg/kg/d divided BID)
Pentobarbital (5–20 mg/kg IV then 0.5–3 mg/kg/hr)
Levetiracetam (1000–2000 mg IV then dosing up to 4 gm/d)
Lacosamide*
Topiramate*
Pregabalin*

* Ideal dosing of newer AEDs in GCSE is unknown.

FIGURE 30.1 A sample algorithm for treating GCSE.

- Initial treatment of GCSE should occur rapidly and continue until clinical seizure cessation (per NCS guidelines: strong recommendation, high-quality evidence) (6).
- Emergent therapy with lorazepam, diazepam, and midazolam (NCS guidelines: strong recommendation, moderate quality evidence) (6).
  - Preferred initial therapy for GCSE
  - Potent and fast-acting
  - At higher concentrations, they limit repetitive neuronal firing.
  - Lorazepam is preferred given its longer duration of action (12–24 hours); duration of action of diazepam is 15 to 30 minutes.
  - Midazolam is the preferred drug for IM administration since IM absorption is most reliable with this benzodiazepine.
  - Rectal diazepam is given when there is no IV access and IM administration of midazolam is contraindicated.
- Phenytoin (PHT) and fosphenytoin (fPHT) (NCS guidelines: strong recommendation, moderate quality evidence) (6).
  - Used to maintain antiseizure effects after benzodiazepines terminate the seizures or for treatment of ongoing seizures after benzodiazepines have failed.
  - fPHT is a pro-drug and is preferable over PHT because it has less risk of severe thrombophlebitis and tissue necrosis and can be administered faster.
  - Infusion rate of PHT not to exceed 50 mg/min. fPHT can be administered up to 150 PE/min.
  - Re-load PHT or fPHT if total serum PHT level is les than 15 μg/mL or if free level is less than 1.5 μg/mL.
    - Re-loading dose when level is subtherapeutic = (desired level – current level) × weight (kg) × 0.64.
  - fPHT can also be loaded via I.M. route (10–20 PE/kg).
  - If a patient on PHT at baseline presents in GCSE, a PHT level should be obtained, but re-loading of PHT/fPHT should not be delayed while waiting for lab results.
  - Arrhythmias (bradycardia and ectopic beats) and hypotension are seen equally with both PHT and fPHT. Therefore, hemodynamic monitoring is necessary with both drugs.
  - Infusion-site reactions are less common with fPHT.
- Valproic acid (VPA) (NCS guidelines: strong recommendation, moderate quality evidence) (6).
  - Consider in patients when PHT is contraindicated, if patients are awake and avoidance of intubation is desirable, or in patients with primary generalized epilepsy.
  - Hypotension can occur but less so than with PHT.
  - Monitor liver function, complete blood count, amylase and lipase.
  - Contraindicated in patients with liver dysfunction.
- Anesthetic medications for refractory status epilepticus (RSE) (per NCS guidelines: strong recommendation, low-quality evidence) (6).
  - Midazolam
    - Used as a continuous infusion for RSE.
    - Infusion rate not to exceed 4 mg/min.

- Maintenance infusion is titrated to desired suppression of EEG.
- Rapid clearance makes midazolam preferable over barbiturates for iatrogenic coma.
- Preferred over propofol since midazolam has less hypotensive effects.
  - ○ Propofol
    - Used as a continuous infusion for RSE.
    - Has very short half-life (3 minutes), so must be used as a continuous infusion.
    - Maintenance dose is titrated to desired suppression of EEG.
    - Rapid clearance makes propofol preferable over barbiturates.
    - Propofol infusion syndrome can occur. It is a rare but fatal syndrome of cardiac failure, rhabdomyolysis, severe metabolic acidosis, and renal failure that occurs in patients receiving high propofol doses over long periods of time.
      - – Monitor plasma triglyceride levels and CK to prevent propofol infusion syndrome.
  - ○ Phenobarbital (PB)
    - Infusion rate not to exceed to 100 mg/min.
    - Typically used in RSE.
  - ○ Pentobarbital
    - In adequate doses, pentobarbital will almost always control seizures.
    - Used as a continuous infusion for RSE; can be titrated to desired suppression of EEG.
    - Infusion rate not to exceed 25 mg/min.
    - Can give additional 5 to 20 mg/kg boluses for breakthrough seizures.
    - Has a very long half-life of 144 hours and tends to cause prolonged hospital stays.
    - Usually used after propofol and midazolam fail.
    - Hypotension limits its use and requirement for pressors is common.
    - Known to cause poikilothermia and possibly immunosuppresion and higher infection rates.
- Newer-generation AEDs
  - ○ Levetiracetam
    - Ideal loading dose is unknown, but many studies have used 1,000 to 2,000 mg IV over 15 minutes with a maintenance dose of up to 4,000 mg daily divided BID.
    - Generally well-tolerated, but dose should be reduced for impaired renal function.
    - Favorable side-effect profile and lack of drug–drug interactions make it an attractive option for treatment of SE.
    - Case series and case reports have found mixed results for the treatment of RSE.
  - ○ Topiramate
    - Mechanism of action: blockade of sodium channels, enhancement of GABA-ergic transmission, and antagonizes AMPA/kainate receptors.
    - Case reports and small case series have shown termination of RSE with topiramate.
    - Use is limited because there is no IV formulation.

- Ideal starting dose is unknown.
- Studies have found efficacy with doses 300 to 1600 mg/d.
○ Pregabalin
  - Mechanism of action: binds to the alpha2delta subunit of the voltage-dependent calcium channel.
  - One small case series showed that pregabalin may be effective as an add-on agent for RSE at doses up to 600 mg/d.
  - Has a favorable side-effect profile, can be started at a high dose, and lacks drug–drug interactions but has no intravenous formulation.
  - Dosing in SE is unknown.
○ Lacosamide
  - Mechanism of action: enhancement of slow inactivation of voltage-gated sodium channels.
  - Found to be effective in animal models of SE.
  - Case reports and small case series show lacosamide might be effective as an add-on agent in RSE.
  - Ideal dosing in SE is unknown, but studies have used loading doses of 200 to 400 mg IV.
  - Studies report no serious adverse side effects.
  - IV formulation available.

E. Weaning of Anesthetic Medications After Resolution of GCSE
- Start weaning midazolam, propofol or pentobarbital after the patient has been in burst suppression for 12 to 48 hours (usually after 24 hours).
- Ensure adequate AED levels of other medications (PHT, VPA, PB) before weaning from burst suppression.
- Frequent EEG review during this phase is important to evaluate for breakthrough seizures.
- If breakthrough seizures occur, rebolus 30% to 70% of initial loading dose of the anesthetic agent, place patient back into burst suppression, and add additional AEDs before re-attempting to wean.

F. AED Interactions
- AEDs can interact with each other and with other medications used in critically ill patients.
- PHT is an inducer of the P450 system and decreases plasma levels of VPA.
- VPA is a P450 inhibitor and increases serum levels of PB.
- VPA levels are increased by salicylates, isoniazid, and erythromycin.
- PB initially increases, but later decreases, serum levels of PHT.
  ○ PB also reduces serum levels of benzodiazepines and VPA.
- PHT, VPA, and PB result in reduced warfarin levels.
- Numerous medications reduce serum PHT levels such as steroids, folic acid, rifampin, digitoxin, warfarin, VPA, and benzodiazepines.
- Numerous medications increase serum PHT levels such as omeprazole, cimetidine, trimethoprim, isoniazid, fluconazole, ketoconazole, and amiodarone.
- There are no drug–drug interactions with levetiracetam and lacosamide.

III. FURTHER CONSIDERATIONS/REMAINING QUESTIONS

A. How aggressive should treatment be when GCSE evolves into NCSE?
- There is no consensus on how NCSE should be treated, nor is it clear whether NCSE results in increased morbidity and mortality.
- Often, the patient's only physical manifestation of NCSE is altered mental status so it can be difficult to detect without EEG monitoring.

B. Which EEG patterns should be more aggressively treated?
- The EEG in NCSE may not reveal discrete, easily defined seizures.
- GPDs, LPDs or triphasic waves may represent different phases of SE.
- It is not clear if these EEG patterns are an epiphenomenon of the underlying disease or if they represent a pathologic disease entity that requires treatment.
- Continuous LPDs that do not change, but persist for long periods of time, are unlikely to represent epileptic discharges, but more likely to represent cortical injury.
- In contrast, LPDs that appear to evolve in amplitude and frequency are more likely to represent epileptiform activity.

REFERENCES

1. Treiman DM. Generalized convulsive status epilepticus. In: J Engel, Jr, TA Pedley. eds. *Epilepsy: A Comprehensive Textbook*. Philadelphia: Lippincott-Raven;1997:669–680.
2. Lowenstein DH, Alldredge BK. Status epilepticus. *N Engl J Med*. 1982;338:970–976.
3. Waterhouse, Elizabeth. Continuum. *Epilepsy* June 2010;16(3):199–227.
4. Treiman DM, Meyers PD, Walton NY, et al. A comparison of four treatments for generalized convulsive status epilepticus. *N Engl J Med*. 1998;339:792–798.
5. Trieman DM, Walton NY, Kendrick C. A progressive sequence of electroencephalographic changes during generalized convulsive status epilepticus. *Epilepsy Res*. Jan-Feb 1990;5(1):49–60.
6. Brophy GM, et al. Guidelines for the evaluation and management of status epilepticus. *Neurocrit Care*. 2012.

ADDITIONAL READING

Shorvon SD *Status Epilepticus: Its Clinical Features and Treatment in Children and Adults*. Cambridge: Cambridge University Press; 1994.

THIRTY-ONE

Nonconvulsive Status Epilepticus

Peter W. Kaplan

KEY POINTS

- Nonconvulsive status epilepticus is not one entity with a fixed prognosis and management paradigm but rather a heterogeneous group of disorders with variable outcomes and treatment strategies.
- Paramount to decision making is differentiation of rhythmic or evolving activity that should be *correctly* identified as seizures or status epilepticus from periodic, rhythmic, or interictal epileptiform activity which may not warrant treatment.
- Management decisions should include careful consideration of the ultimate prognosis of the individual patient with NCSE (eg, post-cardio-respiratory arrest; or multisystem failure in a frail ICU patient vs. subtherapeutic antiepileptic drug levels in a patient with epilepsy).
- Treatment should include utilization of the full range of AEDs with careful and expeditious titration of medication to clinical and EEG response while monitoring for adverse effects.
- Treatment is optimally conducted in an intensive care unit, with support of a critical care team when available.

I. BACKGROUND

A. Nonconvulsive Status Epilepticus (NCSE)
- Advances in neuro-intensive care EEG monitoring have uncovered many patients with nonconvulsive status epilepticus (NCSE) who were previously undiagnosed.
- NCSE is not a single entity with diagnosis and treatment options that can be generalized to all patients.
  - Rather, it is a group of heterogeneous disorders which are diagnosed and managed in a number of different clinical settings.
- The various types of NCSE have a wide range of prognoses.
- Diagnosis of NCSE is now being approached along three axes.
  - Ictal semiology

○ Etiology
○ EEG patterns (3rd London Colloquium on Status Epilepticus)
• Some types of NCSE are benign.
○ Seen with genetic absence epilepsy (typical absence status epilepticus) with no lasting morbidity.
• At the opposite extreme, electrographic status epilepticus with coma after cardio-respiratory arrest has an almost 100% mortality or nonreturn to consciousness (particularly if not managed with hypothermia).

II. BASICS

A. Animal Models of NCSE
• Animal models have not provided clear evidence of the potential for brain damage as a result of NCSE.
• No satisfactory model exists for typical absence status or for chronic epilepsy with NCSE triggered by low AED levels.
• Many animal models initially used for studying the effects of SE are created by inducing significant brain insults that themselves cause chronic neuronal damage.
○ Many models were initially used to investigate excitotoxicity, but were later also used "to replicate" complex partial status epilepticus in humans (1).
○ In these models, SE was induced in nonepileptic animals using powerful chemoconvulsants or prolonged high-frequency repetitive stimulation (1).
• Studies evaluating the effects of NCSE in humans are difficult to interpret
○ NCSE in humans is very different, usually involving lower frequency discharges.
○ AEDs and prior epilepsy may confer some neuroprotection.
○ It can be very difficult to distinguish damage resulting from the cause of SE from damage resulting from the seizures themselves (1,2).
○ Many case reports and small series in the literature include patients with NCSE from a wide variety of causes including preceding convulsive status epilepticus, encephalitis, stroke, or traumatic brain injury.

B. Studies of Cognition Before and After NCSE
• Few studies have directly measured possible cognitive consequences of NCSE.
○ Two studies of epilepsy patients who had cognitive evaluations after SE found no permanent decline in cognitive measures (3,4).
• In contrast to this reassuring "benign" outcome:
○ Two other studies investigated "pure" groups of patients with NCSE from a single etiology along with a control population.
○ Results suggest at least an additive adverse effect of seizures or SE on the initial insult in the case of subarachnoid hemorrhage or head trauma (5).
○ Patients in SE with these etiologies did worse than controls without these underlying etiologies.

C. Surrogates of Brain Damage
• Imaging of patients during and after NCSE:
○ Studies have demonstrated varying results.

- In patients with known idiopathic generalized epilepsy (childhood absence or juvenile myoclonic epilepsy) there is no evidence of CT or MRI changes following NCSE in patients who have not suffered additional insults from anoxia or trauma.
- Patients with a history of localization related epilepsy and NCSE:
  - Most cases show no lasting changes on imaging.
  - During the acute phase, MRI may show transient focal FLAIR changes.
  - There are clear reported cases of temporal lobe and hippocampal atrophy after temporal lobe NCSE, but it is not entirely clear whether these cases were triggered by a temporal lobe insult such as encephalitis.
- Other case series of NCSE in ICU settings:
  - Often there is evidence of cerebral damage associated with the onset and progression of NCSE, but without clear indication that the imaging changes are consequent to the NCSE proper (6).
- Significance of a serum neuron-specific enolase (NSE) level as a surrogate of brain damage
  - NSE is a serum marker of neuronal injury.
  - May rise during NCSE even without a concurrent, identifiable neurologic lesion.
  - NSE levels have been shown to rise following CPSE, partially related to the duration of SE (7).
  - Doubt has been raised regarding the specificity of these changes, as NSE may appear as a result of blood–brain barrier breakdown, and not necessarily reflect acute neuronal damage.
  - In published series some patients with good outcome had significantly increased NSE levels, whereas others with poor outcome had low levels.
  - Thus, the reliability of this test as a reflection of brain damage is debatable.

D. The Disadvantages of Treatment

- Clinical experience and the literature have informed us that treatment does *not* come without risk.
  - Treatment (particularly with benzodiazepines and anesthetics) can cause respiratory suppression, hypotension, prolonged ICU stays, concurrent infection, and death (8).
  - Such treatment cannot and should not be provided with a belief that there is "known safety and efficacy" in all cases.
  - A "one size fits all" treatment paradigm may tip the risk–benefit ratio away from the patient (2).

E. How to Approach the Diagnosis and Treatment of NCSE

- Several factors may underlie treatment decisions.
  - The degree of certainly regarding the diagnosis of NCSE.
  - The perceived prognosis for the particular case.
  - Whether treatment will improve prognosis or prevent deterioration.
- Clinical presentation of NCSE
  - The diagnosis of NCSE in large part depends on the clinician having a suspicion of seizures, triggering a request for an EEG.

- ○ Following convulsive SE, the patient may enter a state referred to as subtle SE in which it is hypothesized that there has been neuronal exhaustion producing an electro-clinical dissociation.
  - • This can result in few clinical indicators of status, but with seizures clearly seen on EEG.
  - • In this and other types of NCSE in coma that are frequently encountered in the ICU, the patient may show subtle facial, eye, head, neck, or limb myoclonus, changes in body or limb tone, or eye deviation and nystagmus.
  - • Even with these subtle clinical clues to possible NCSE, the clinician immediately encounters a further hurdle in the form of accurate interpretation of the EEG.
- • EEG diagnosis of NCSE
  - ○ Unfortunately, EEG misdiagnosis of NCSE is common.
  - ○ Inaccuracies range from an incorrect interpretation of EEG artifact (eg, due to bed vibration, physical therapy tapping, chewing of food), to the over-interpretation of interictal and periodic discharges.
  - ○ Triphasic waves of metabolic encephalopathic origin may resemble epileptic discharges.
  - ○ Much effort has been directed toward identifying EEG patterns believed to be diagnostic for NCSE (9).
    - • The optimal indicators for EEG evidence of NCSE include the appearance of epileptiform morphologies that evolve or change in frequency, amplitude or location, and typically faster than 1 to 2 Hz.
    - • However, the establishment of clear evidence of NCSE on EEG will miss a large intermediate segment of patients lying along the ictal–interictal spectrum.
    - • This unclear intermediate zone consists of EEGs that show little evolution, as well as activity that is less than or equal to 1 Hz without associated motor findings (eg, myoclonus, nystagmus).
  - ○ NCSE with EEG findings that show rhythmic changes and no spike component also pose diagnostic problems.
    - • Helpful clues, again, are an evolution in frequency or spatial distribution.
    - • Periodic waves that reflect cortical irritability include lateralized periodic discharges (LPDs); generalized periodic discharges (GPDs); bilateral independent periodic discharges (BIPDs); and stimulus-induced discharges (SIRPIDs).
    - • These patterns are often seen in temporal proximity to seizures—before or after—but are assumed by most to lie along the ictal–interictal spectrum and therefore, are not thought to represent "active" seizures.
    - • Others regard these patterns as the end stage of SE.
    - • Various strategies for the management of these controversial patterns have been proposed (10).
  - ○ Thus, much controversy surrounds whether periodic discharges should be suppressed with parenteral AEDs, given the morbidity associated with intensive anesthetic management (2).
- • Prognosis as a factor guiding management of NCSE.

○ Individual prognosis largely depends on semiology, level of consciousness, cause of NCSE, and in part on EEG patterns (eg, absence of background activity foreboding more marked underlying brain dysfunction) (Table 31.1).

  • For example, patients whose proximate cause of NCSE is low antiepileptic drug levels in chronic epilepsy have a low morbidity and mortality, in the range of 3% (12).

  • Conversely, a typical academic hospital will see a mortality rate of 30% to 50% in critically ill patients with NCSE as a result of an acute, severe brain insult.

F. Suggestions on How to Approach Treatment (Table 31.2)

• Treatment is optimally conducted in an intensive care unit with ventilator and intensivist support when possible.

• Clinician must titrate medication to the patient's clinical and EEG response while monitoring carefully for adverse effects.

• Drugs used include:
  ○ Oral AEDs
  ○ Benzodiazepines with potential respiratory and blood pressure suppressant effects
  ○ Parenteral use of phenytoin, valproate, or possibly newer agents such as levetiracetam or lacosamide
  ○ Anesthetic agents such as propofol, midazolam, or barbiturates

• Tailor treatment intensity to the perceived morbidity of the particular etiology and clinical setting of the case in question.
  ○ Use level of consciousness, age, and probable outcome as further guideposts.

• Avoid lowering the patient's level of consciousness to a level significantly below that present from the NCSE itself.

• Work expeditiously: benzodiazepines should work within 10 minutes; phenytoin, valproate, or levetiracetam within 20 to 30 minutes.

• If seizure activity persists, and if clinically indicated, consider proceeding to propofol, midazolam, or parenteral barbiturate but only with concurrent EEG monitoring (11).

• Careful ongoing assessment of EEG and clinical effect as well as treatment induced morbidity are paramount.

III. FURTHER CONSIDERATIONS/REMAINING QUESTIONS

A. Intensity and extent of treatment of NCSE is an open debate.

• Different types of NCSE have different prognoses in which case the risk/benefit of each treatment approach must be weighed.
  ○ Absence status epilepticus has no morbidity and oral agents can be considered.
  ○ On the other hand, there is evidence that NCSE in a patient with acute stroke confers additional morbidity such that more aggressive AED management would likely be justified.

• Experts do not agree on specific management strategies of NCSE.

• Continuous EEG monitoring is of high importance for the diagnosis of NCSE as well as monitoring therapeutic effect.

TABLE 31.1 Prognosis in Nonconvulsive Status Epilepticus

TYPES	PROGNOSIS	DIAGNOSIS	RESPONSE TO AEDs	RECURRENCE	OUTCOME
Typical absence status epilepticus (TAS)	Excellent	Frequently missed	Excellent	Frequent	No morbidity mortality
"De novo" absence status in the elderly	Excellent	Frequently missed	Good, but sometimes delayed	Occasionally (situation rated; triggers can be removed)	Excellent
Absence status with degenerative generalized epilepsies	Guarded to fair	Less frequently missed	Variable	Frequent	Variable, some with cognitive decline (difficulty in determining whether this is due to disease or to episodes of AASE)
Atypical absence status epilepsy (AASE)	Fair to poor	Less frequently missed	Relatively refractory (when seen in the setting of epileptic encephalopathy/mental retardation)	Frequent	Frequent cognitive morbidity, but it is difficult to differentiate this from the effects of disease progression and consequences

TYPES	PROGNOSIS	DIAGNOSIS	RESPONSE TO AEDs	RECURRENCE	OUTCOME
Simple partial non convulsive status epileptics (SPSE)	Usually good to excellent, occasionally poor	Frequently missed	Excellent	Frequent	Morbidity and mortality negligible to absent
Complex partial status epilepticus	When not associated with comorbid insults, good to excellent	Less frequently missed	Good to very good, but often delayed	Frequent	Only very rare cognitive sequelae (<1% of patients)
Electrographic seizures and coma	Very poor	Apparent if accompanied by myoclonus; covert (requiring EEG for diagnosis)	Often poor	Variable	Very poor — largely etiology-dependent

Adapted from Kaplan PW. Prognosis in non-convulsive status epilepticus. In: Jallon P, Berg A, Dulac O, et al eds. *Prognosis of epileptics*, Paris: John Libbey Euroest: 2003:311–325.

TABLE 31.2 Treatment Approaches for Nonconvulsive Status Epilepticus

Typical absence SE	Oral or IV benzodiazepines with supplementation of prior AED regimen
Atypical absence SE	Oral or IV benzodiazepines; valproate; levetiracetam; topiramate; supplement prior AED regimen
Complex partial SE	Oral or IV benzodiazepines; IV phenytoin, valproate or levetiracetam; supplement prior AED regimen
Nonconvulsive SE in coma	IV lorazepam; phenytoin; propofol, midazolam, pentobarbital; valproate; levetiracetam; topiramate; ketamine; lacosamide; ketogenic diet.

B. Which types of NCSE should be most aggressively treated?

- Obtunded patients with adequate respiratory and blood pressure support as well as patients with underlying stroke or head trauma should receive aggressive management of NCSE.
- Patients with minimal obtundation can often be managed my nonparenteral means and with less sedating agents.
- Frail and elderly patients require more careful management.
- Periodic discharges without motor manifestations or nystagmus when slower than 1/sec are usually not aggressively treated (ie, suppressed with sedating agents).
- There remains a large gray-zone of patterns that lie along the ictal–interictal continuum as well as clinical scenarios in which there is ongoing debate about the intensity of treatment and the perceived morbidity of nontreatment. These "syndromes" of NCSE should be subject to prospective, well-designed, therapeutic trials.

REFERENCES

1. Walker MC. Diagnosis and treatment of nonconvulsive status epilepticus. *CNS Drugs.* 2001;15:931–939.
2. Kaplan PW. Assessing the outcomes in patients with nonconvulsive status epilepticus. Nonconvulsive status epilepticus is underdiagnosed, potentially overtreated, and confounded by comorbidity. *J Clin Neurophysiol.* 1999;16:16:341–352.
3. Cockerell OC, Walker CM, Sander JWAS, et al. Complex partial status epilepticus: A recurrent problem. *J Neurol Neurosurg Psychiatry.* 1994;57:835–837.
4. Dodrill CB, Wilensky AJ. Intellectual impairment as an outcome of status epilepticus. *Neurology.* 1990;40:23–27.
5. Vespa PM, McArthur DL, Xu Y, et al. Nonconvulsive seizures after traumatic brain injury are associated with hippocampal atrophy. *Neurology.* 2010;75:792–798.
6. Young GB, Claassen J. Nonconvulsive status epilepticus and brain damage: Further evidence, more questions. *Neurology.* 2010;75:760–761.
7. DeGiorgio CM, Heck CN, Rabinowicz AL, et al. Serum neuronspecific enolase in the major subtypes of status epilepticus. *Neurology.* 1999;52:746–749.
8. Litt B, Wityk RJ, Hertz SH, et al. Nonconvulsive status epilepticus in the critically ill elderly. *Epilepsia.* 1998;39:1194–1202.

9. Kaplan PW. EEG criteria for nonconvulsive status epilepticus. *Epilepsia.* 2007;48 Suppl 8:39–41.
10. Claassen J. How I treat patients with EEG patterns on the ictal–interictal continuum in the neuro ICU. *Neurocrit Care.* 2009;11:437–444.
11. Claasen J, Hirsch LJ, Emerson RG, Mayer SA. Treatment of refractory status epilepticus with pentobarbital, propofol or midazolam: A systematic review. *Epilepsia.* 2002;43:146–153.
12. Shnecker BF, Fountain NB. Assessment of acute morbidity and mortality in nonconvulsive status epilepticus. *Neurology.* 2003;61:1066–1073.

THIRTY-TWO

Status Epilepticus in the Pediatric Population

James J. Riviello

KEY POINTS

- Status epilepticus (SE) and recurrent seizures in children are neurological emergencies that require an organized treatment approach.
- SE is considered refractory when seizures fail to terminate after administration of the first two antiepileptic drugs (AEDs), including the initial IV benzodiazepine.
- Special considerations exist for the treatment of seizures in children, especially children with febrile seizures or inborn errors of metabolism.
- The same approach used by adult epileptologists and neurocritical care specialists of initiating a continuous intravenous infusion after the failure of the first two AEDs should be extended to children.

I. BACKGROUND

A. SE and Recurrent Seizures Are Neurological Emergencies That Require an Organized Treatment Approach (1–3)

- In any critical situation, a standardized protocol ensures that treatment is delivered in a timely sequence. This is especially important in the intensive care unit where "time is brain."
- The most important goal in the treatment of SE is to immediately control all clinical and electrographic seizures, as prolonged seizures may result in neuronal injury.
- Of equal importance is to avoid iatrogenic injury (adverse effects) from the treatment itself.

B. Major Steps in SE Treatment

- Seizure identification
- Seizure treatment
  - Preserve vital signs by maintaining the airway, breathing, and circulation.
  - Administer AEDs without causing iatrogenic injury.

- If seizure recurrence is likely, administer a maintenance AED for prophylaxis.
- Identify and treat the underlying etiology and complications of seizures.

II. BASICS

A. Classification of Seizures as Focal or Generalized in Onset

- *Focal onset seizure*: initial clinical manifestations and EEG findings indicate activation of only a focal area, or one part of the cortex.
- *Generalized onset seizure*: more than minimal involvement of both cerebral hemispheres and initial activation of neurons occurs throughout both hemispheres.
- Consideration of whether seizures are focal or generalized in onset will aid in choosing the most effective AED, particularly in children who have a higher proportion of generalized onset seizures.

B. Etiology

- Failure to treat the precipitating cause of SE may make seizures more difficult to terminate.
- Some forms of SE such as those caused by underlying autoimmune or inflammatory conditions may require early consideration of alternative forms of treatment such as immunomodulation.
- A patient with known epilepsy may have seizure exacerbation precipitated by an acute illness or noncompliance.

C. Definitions, Stages of SE, and Compensatory Mechanisms

- Formerly, SE was considered refractory when the seizure lasted longer than 1 hour at which time treatment was switched from a standard AED to continuous infusion (cIV) of an IV anesthetic agent.
- SE is currently considered refractory when seizures fail to terminate after the first two AEDs administered, including the initial IV benzodiazepine (4).
  - This change in definition has led to a change in treatment sequence, with cIV agents given earlier.
- Determining the stage of SE helps with treatment decisions (1,5–6).
- Stages:
  - Incipient (0–5 minutes)
    - The beginning of any seizure could be the beginning of SE.
  - Early (5–30 minutes)
  - Transition
  - Late (established) (30–60 minutes)
  - Refractory (longer than 60 minutes)
  - Post-ictal
- It is no longer presumed that these stages have a fixed duration, as they vary depending upon specific characteristics of the individual patient.
- During all stages, including seizure onset, the brain's ability to compensate requires adequate airway, breathing, circulation, and cerebral blood flow.
- The systemic and brain metabolism abnormalities that occur with a prolonged seizure are well-described (7).
  - Decreased brain oxygen tension.
  - A mismatch between increase in oxygen and glucose utilization.

○ Fall in cerebral blood flow, followed by decrease in supply of brain glucose and oxygen.
- In a short seizure or the early stages of SE, brain compensatory mechanisms may protect against neuronal injury.
- However, compensatory mechanisms may become exhausted as the seizure progresses, increasing the risk of neuronal injury.
- Compensatory mechanisms may be further compromised when SE or new onset seizures occur in critically ill patients resulting in much higher mortality and morbidity (8).

D. Time Line for Treatment (Table 32.1)
- Most SE treatment protocols are based on a time line.
- At seizure onset, supportive measures include maintaining the airway, breathing, and circulation (the A, B, Cs).
  ○ Vital signs are taken, oxygen is administered, intravenous access is secured, and initial lab studies sent.
- Many seizures stop spontaneously while the above measures are implemented.
- If the seizure continues for greater than 5 minutes, the initial AED is given, referred to as first-line treatment.
- The first-line agent is usually IV lorazepam up to 0.1 mg/kg.
- If there is no IV access, midazolam, 0.2 mg/kg IM, fosphenytoin 20 mg/kg, or rectal diazepam (Diastat) can be used.
- In a large prospective, population-based study, seizures stopped after the first-line agent in 65% although of the patients that required a second-line agent, only 50% had seizure cessation (9).
- If the second-line agent does not work, the third-line agent is given, which also has a specific infusion time.
- Although there are no standardized guidelines, many use the following treatment sequence in children following failure of lorazepam:
  ○ Fosphenytoin
  ○ Followed by phenobarbital
  ○ Followed by midazolam
  ○ Pentobarbital if seizure activity continues (RSE)
- However, these predetermined infusion times can delay seizure termination so the approach used by adult epileptologists and neurocritical care specialists of initiating a continuous intravenous infusion after the failure of the first two AEDs should also be considered in children.

E. Diagnostic Studies
- Early laboratory evaluation is critical.
  ○ The American Academy of Neurology practice parameter on the diagnostic assessment of children with SE found the following abnormalities (5):
    - Abnormal electrolytes or glucose in 6%
    - Subtherapeutic AED levels in 32%
    - Positive blood cultures in 2.5%
    - CNS infection in 12.8%
    - Ingestion of toxic substances in 3.6%
    - Inborn errors of metabolism in 4.2%

TABLE 32.1   Treatment of SE in Children

DRUG	DOSE AND ROUTE	INFUSION RATE	ADVERSE EFFECTS
Lorazepam	0.1 mg/kg, IV	Do not exceed 2 mg/min, or .05 mg/kg over 2.5 min	Sedation, respiratory depression
If seizure(s) continues …			
Fosphenytoin	20 mg/kg, IV	No faster than 150 mg/min PE or 3 mg/kg/min	Hypotension, cardiac arrythmias, paresthesias, choreiform movements
If seizure(s) continues…			
Fosphenytoin	Additional 5–10 mg/kg IV[1]		
If seizure continues for 10 min after fosphenytoin …			
Phenobarbital	20 mg/kg, IV	No faster than 1 mg/kg/min, maximum 30 mg/min in infants and children	Sedation, hypotension, respiratory depression
If seizure(s) continues …			
Phenobarbital	Additional 5–10 mg/kg, IV		
Alternative second and third-line treatments			
Valproic acid	Loading dose: 20–40 mg/kg, IV; may give additional 20 mg/kg 10 min after loading dose	1.5–3 mg/kg/min	Hypotension, hepatitis, pancreatitis thrombocytopenia, usually with chronic administration
Levetiracetam	Loading dose: 20–50 mg/kg, IV Higher doses (240 mg/kg/day) used with good efficacy and limited adverse effects (19)	2–5 mg/kg/min Dosing in renal failure adjusted by glomerular filtration rate	
Lacosamide	Loading dose in adults: 200–400 mg; lower doses have also been used	40–80 mg/min for 15 min in one study	First-degree heart block

○ In the North London prospective study of new-onset SE (NLSTEPS), most cases of acute symptomatic SE had acute metabolic derangements (electrolyte imbalance, hypoglycemia, hypocalcemia, hypomagnesemia) or CNS infections (meningitis, encephalitis) (10).

- EEG monitoring
  - If seizures are clinically obvious, treatment should be initiated without EEG.
  - However, if convulsive movements stop but there is no clinical improvement, or if a patient has otherwise unexplained coma, EEG is needed to exclude nonconvulsive SE (NCSE).
    - In a study of children, NCSE occurred in 5/19 patients following control of convulsive SE (11).
    - In a study of all ages, NCSE was detected in 8% of all patients with unexplained coma (12).
  - In comatose patients, nonepileptic events can be confused with seizures unless EEG is used for confirmatory diagnosis.
    - In a study of 100 children in coma, nonepileptic events were misdiagnosed as seizures in 17 children, whereas epileptic seizures were documented in only 7 children (13).
  - An EEG should also be obtained as soon as possible if there is a strong suspicion for psychogenic nonepileptic seizures.
- Neuroimaging
  - Should be done on all new onset seizures in a critically ill patient and all new onset cases of SE.
  - The American Academy of Neurology practice parameter on the diagnostic assessment of children with SE found abnormal neuroimaging in 8% (5).
  - Not routinely recommended in a child with a known seizure disorder.
    - Exceptions include new focal deficit, persistent altered awareness, fever, recent head trauma, persistent headache, history of cancer, anticoagulation or HIV+ (14).
- Special diagnostic considerations
  - Children have an increased risk of a seizure from a fever, referred to as benign febrile seizures of childhood.
    - Typically lasts less than 15 minutes, but when one lasts longer than 15 minutes, it is called an atypical or complex febrile seizure.
    - In a recent prospective study of new onset seizures presenting with SE in children, 46 of 144 children (32%) were identified with febrile SE (15).
    - It is important to exclude meningitis in all cases of febrile SE.
      - In the NLSTEPS study, 4/24 with CSE and fever had bacterial meningitis (16).
  - Seizures may occur in a patient with a known metabolic disorder or may be the presenting manifestation of a metabolic disorder, especially in a younger child.
  - Special studies may be needed, such as serum lactic acid, serum amino acids, urine organic acids, pyruvic acid, ammonia, carnitene, and acylcarnitene.
  - Diagnosis of certain metabolic disorders may require a lumbar puncture to examine the CSF (17):
    - Glucose transporter defect
    - Disorders of lactic and pyruvic acid
    - Amino acid disorders such as hyperglycinemia
    - Serine deficiency syndrome
    - CNS folate disorders, folinic-acid responsive seizures, and neurotransmitter disorders

III. FURTHER CONSIDERATIONS/REMAINING QUESTIONS

A. How aggressively should seizures be managed?
- In deciding whether to change from a standard AED to a cIV infusion agent, consider the patient's condition and the type of SE.
  - For example, if absence SE occurs in the setting of childhood absence epilepsy, or if there are recurrent seizures in the setting of chronic epilepsy with stable vital signs, less aggressive treatment may be indicated compared to more aggressive treatment needed to immediately control the seizure activity with CSE.
  - The risk of neuronal injury is less likely in the setting of chronic epilepsy.

B. Treating Newborns
- A different treatment sequence is used for newborns.
- Phenobarbital is administered first line with a loading dose of 20 mg/kg with two additional 10 mg/kg doses if seizures continue (goal is a serum level of at least 40 μg/L).
- If seizures continue, either midazolam or fosphenytoin can be used next.
  - Midazolam: IV loading dose 0.15 mg/kg, with additional dose of 0.10 to 0.15 mg/kg given 15 to 30 minutes later if seizures continue.
  - Fosphenytoin: IV loading dose 20 mg/kg, given at a rate of 0.5 to 1 mg/kg/ minutes.
- Vitamin B6 and folinic acid should be used for refractory seizures in the newborn. Ideally, vitamin B6 should be administered during EEG monitoring to monitor for treatment response.

C. Refractory SE
- SE is considered refractory when the first two AEDs fail to terminate seizure activity.
- Treatment shifts from standard AEDs (fosphenytoin, phenobarbital, valproic acid, levetiracetam, and lacosamide) to the cIV agents (pentobarbital, midazolam, and propofol).
- In children, midazolam and pentobarbital are preferred agents as propofol has a higher incidence of adverse events such as propofol infusion syndrome.
- Infusion schedules
  - Midazolam: 0.2 mg/kg bolus (maximum 10 mg). If seizures continue for another 5 minutes, repeat dose at 0.2 mg/kg and start infusion of 0.1 mg/kg/ hr. If seizures continue, repeat midazolam bolus and then start pentobarbital (3 OK as is).
  - Pentobarbital: 5 mg/kg, followed by infusion of 1 mg/kg/hr, increase as needed to 3 mg/kg/hr.
  - Thiopental: 2 to 3 mg/kg IV bolus
  - Propofol: 1 to 2 mg/kg bolus, followed by 2 to 10 mg/kg/hr.
  - Consider vitamin B6 (pyridoxine) at a dose of 100 to 200 mg, IV.
    - Recommended for all cases of refractory SE in children from 18 months to less than 3 years old.
    - Consider folinic acid and Pyridoxal-5-phosphate for vitamin B6-resistant seizures.

D. New-Onset Refractory SE in a Previously Healthy Child
- Occurs in a previously healthy child with a nonspecific febrile illness, many times without a specific etiology identified.
- Because of its presentation, this syndrome is called FIRES (Febrile Illness-Related Epileptic Syndrome).
- Recent evidence suggests that the outcome may be improved if treated with the ketogenic diet rather than suppression with cIV agents (18).

E. Alternative Treatment of Refractory SE
- *High-dose phenobarbital*: Push to serum levels greater than 150 µg/mL.
- *Ketamine*: start 2 mg/kg with an infusion rate of 0.5 mg/kg/min. May cause increase in intracranial pressure (ICP) so avoid in patients with known elevated ICP.
- *Etomidate*: 0.3 mg/kg/IV. Avoid cIV infusion, which causes adrenal insufficiency.
- *Inhalational anesthetics*: Isoflourane
- *Verapamil*: effects calcium channels or is a known p-Glycoprotein inhibitor, which block AED transport dosing in children (from cardiac data: IV 0.1–0.3 mg/kg/ dose, maximum 5 mg/dose).
- *Topiramate (not available IV so administer through nasogastric tube)*: 10 mg/kg/ day for 2 days, followed by 5 mg/kg/day.
- Ketogenic diet, especially for FIRES
- Immune modulation
  - Corticosteroids, IV pulse of methylprednisolone, 30 mg/kg, maximum 1 g
  - Intravenous immunoglobulin (IVIG) 2 g/kg, usually administered over several days.
  - Plasmapheresis
- Hypothermia
- *Neurostimulation*: vagus nerve stimulation (VNS), transcranial magnetic stimulation (TMS), and electroconvulsive therapy (ECT)

REFERENCES

1. Riviello JJ Jr, Holmes GL. The treatment of status epilepticus. *Semin Pediatri Neurol.* 2004;11:129–138.
2. Riviello JJ Jr. Seizures in the context of acute illness. *Curr Opin Pediatr.* 2009;21:731–736.
3. Abend NS, Gutierrez-Colina AM, Dlugos DJ. Medical treatment of pediatric status epilepticus. *Semin Pediatri Neurol.* 2010;17:169–175.
4. Bleck TP. Refractory status epilepticus. *Curr Opin Crit Care.* 2005;11:117–120.
5. Riviello JJ, Ashwal Shirtz D, Glauser T, et al. Practice parameter: Diagnostic assessment of the child with status epilepticus (an evidence-based review): Report of the Quality Standards Subcommittee of the American Academy of Neurology and the practice committee of the Child Neurology Society. *Neurology.* 2006;67:1542–1550.
6. Goodkin HP, Riviello JJ Jr. Status Epilepticus. E Wyllie, eds. *The Treatment of Epilepsy: Principles and Practice*, 5th ed. Philadelphia: Lippincott Williams & Wilkins; 2011, pp. 469–485.
7. Lothman E. The biochemical basis and pathophysiology of status epilepticus. *Neurology.* 1990;40(Suppl 2):13–23.

8. Delanty N, French JA, Labar DR, et al. Status epilepticus arising de novo in hospitalized patients: An analysis of 41 patients. *Seizure.* 2001;10:116–119.

9. Chin RFM, Neville BGR, Peckham C, et al. Treatment of community-onset, childhood convulsive status epilepticus: A prospective, population-based study. *Lancet Neurol.* 2008;7:696–703.

10. Chin RFM, Neville BGR, Peckham C, et al. Incidence, cause, and short-term outcome of convulsive status epilepticus in children: Prospective, population-based study. *Lancet.* 2006;368:222–229.

11. Tay SKH, Hirsch LJ, Leary L, et al. Nonconvulsive status epilepticus in children: Clinical and EEG characteristics. *Epilepsia.* 2006;47:1504–1509.

12. Towne AR, Waterhouse EJ, Boggs JG, et al. Prevalence of nonconvulsive status epilepticus in comatose patients. *Neurology.* 2000;54:340–345.

13. Abend NS, Topjian AA, Gutierrez-Colina AM, et al. Impact of continuous EEG monitoring on clinical management in critically ill children. *Neurocrit Care.* 2010;15:70–75.

14. Practice parameter: Neuroimaging in the emergency patient presenting with seizure. *Ann Emerg Med.* 1996;27:114–118.

15. Singh RK, Stephens S, Berl MM, et al. Prospective study of new-onset seizures presenting as status epilepticus. *Neurology.* 2010;74:636–642.

16. Chin RFM, Neville BGR, Scott RC. Meningitis is a common cause of convulsive status epilepticus with fever. *Arch Dis Child.* 2005;90:66–69.

17. Hyland K, Arnold LA. Value of lumbar puncture in the diagnosis of genetic metabolic encephalopathies. *J Child Neuro.* 1999;14(Suppl 1):S9–S15.

18. Depositario-Cabacar DT, Peters J, Pong A, et al. High-dose intravenous levetiracetam for acute seizure exacerbation in children with intractable epilepsy. *Epilepsia.* 2010;51:1319–1322.

19. Nabbout R, Mazzuca M, Hubert P, et al. Efficacy of ketogenic diet in severe refractory status epilepticus initiating fever induced refractory epilepstic encephalopathy in school age children (FIRES). *Epilepsia.* 2010;51:2033–2037.

THIRTY-THREE

Alternative Therapies for Refractory Status Epilepticus

Nicolas Gaspard and Lawrence J. Hirsch

KEY POINTS

- The use of these alternative treatments is based on low levels of evidence from case series and reports only.
- Owing to the lack of randomized controlled trials (RCTs), the most effective titration rates, doses, and duration of treatment are unclear.
- Likewise, there is currently no established protocol to suggest when to select a particular agent over another, in what order these treatments should be attempted, and in which patient scenarios.
- Recent guidelines from the Neurocritical Care Society recommend the use of continuous EEG monitoring (cEEG) for the treatment of refractory status epilepticus (RSE) and to reserve alternative therapies for patients who do not respond to standard treatments. Consideration of transfer to a specialized center with cEEG and expertise in treatment of RSE is also recommended in these guidelines.

I. BACKGROUND

A. The Level of Evidence for the Choice and Use of Alternative Treatments Is Low

- There are No RCTs assessing the efficacy or safety of these treatments in RSE.
- The only available evidence comes from case series and case reports (Class IV).
- Efficacy is difficult to assess due to the use of multidrug regimens, the chance of spontaneous resolution of SE, and publication bias (positive experiences get published while negative series are typically not reported).
- Doses are based only on case series and therefore no methodical assessment of different dosing regimens has been performed (Table 33.1).
- Therapeutic levels and duration of treatment are largely unknown.

TABLE 33.1 Suggested Doses for Various Alternative Treatments in RSE

DRUG	INITIAL DOSE	MAINTENANCE	LEVEL	CLEARANCE	PROTEIN BINDING	REMOVED BY DIALYSIS	INTERACTIONS
Ketamine	1.5 mg/kg IV q 5 min until Sz control or maximal dose of 4.5 mg/kg	1.2 mg/kg/hr to be increased until SZ control or up to 7.5 mg/kg/hr cIV	?	Hepatic	45%	?	–
Vigabatrin	500 mg TID PO	Up to 1 g TID PO	?	Renal	No	Yes but dosage adjustment unknown	–
Felbamate	400 mg TID PO	Up to 1200 mg TID PO	40–100	Renal and hepatic	20–25%	?	PHB, PHT, VPA, and CBZ
Etomidate	0.3 mg/kg IV repeated until Sz control	1.2 mg/kg/hr to be increased until SZ control or up to 7.2 mg/kg/hr cIV	?	Hepatic	75%	?	–
Lidocaine	1–5 mg/kg (usually 100 mg) IV repeated until Sz control	Up to 6 mg/kg/hr	<5 mg/L	Hepatic	60–80%	No	Antiarrhythmic agent
Magnesium sulfate	2–4 g in 2 hr IV	2 g TID IV or 0.5–2 g/hr cIV	>2.0 mEq/L (up to 7.0 mEq/L?)	Renal	No	Varies with dialysis bath Mg^{2+} concentration	–
Steroids	Methylprednisolone 1 g qd IV for 3 days	1 mg/kg per day then taper?	–	Renal	>90%	No	Ketogenic diet
IVIg	0.4 g/kg qd for 5 days	No	–	–	–	No	–
Plasmapheresis	1 session qod for 5–7 days	?	–	–	–	–	Possible clearing of antiepileptic drugs

B. General Guidelines

- Prognosis and mortality following RSE depend primarily on the underlying etiology and type of status epilepticus (SE).
- Outcome can be good even after protracted RSE, especially when there is no evidence of definite, widespread, and irreversible injury on neuroimaging.
- Aggressiveness and duration of treatment should be tailored to the type and etiology of SE.
- To choose an appropriate treatment and dose, alterations in pharmacokinetics must be noted in the following patient situations:
  - Organ failure (renal failure, liver failure, paralytic ileus, etc)
  - Organ replacement therapy (hemofiltration, hemodialysis, etc)
  - Other therapies (plasma exchange)
- Possible treatment interactions exist, not only pharmacokinetic interactions but additive side effects as well.
- Awareness of side effects can avoid unnecessary toxicity.

II. BASICS

A. Ketamine (KET)

- Acts as N-methyl-D-aspartate (NMDA) receptor antagonist.
  - Theoretical neuroprotective effects
  - However, one case of possible long-term cerebellar neurotoxicity has been published.
- Animal models
  - KET appears more effective in the maintenance phase than in earlier SE, suggesting a unique role in the treatment of RSE.
- Case series and reports
  - Two series, published as abstracts only, report use of intravenous KET in 21 adults with RSE.
    - SE was permanently controlled in 12/14 patients in one series but only transiently controlled in 4/7 patients in another series.
  - In a third series (five children), NCSE resolved in all cases with oral administration of KET.
- KET is not associated with cardiorespiratory depression or hypotension.
  - However, there is a risk of hypertension, which can be beneficial in some patients, particularly those that cannot tolerate high doses of other SE treatments due to low blood pressure.
- KET may also elevate intracranial pressure (ICP) and should be used cautiously in patients with high ICP.
- Animal data suggest a possible synergistic action with benzodiazepines.

B. Etomidate (ETO)

- A nonbarbiturate GABA receptor agonist
- One case series reports successful use in eight adults with RSE, with permanent control of SE.
- Associated with only mild cardiorespiratory depression but blocks adrenal cortisol production.

○ This reduces stress response and requires dexamethasone supplementation until at least 48 hours after its withdrawal.
- Other side effects include nonepileptic myoclonus, which can be confused with seizures.
- May also induce epileptiform discharges.
- No significant drug interactions but tachyphylaxis may occur.

C. Lidocaine
- A fast voltage-gated sodium channel blocker
- Used mainly as an antiarrhythmic drug (class Ib).
- Extensive use in the pediatric and neonate population, often in nonrefractory SE.
  ○ Three large series in children (306 patients) report a success rate of 36% to 69%.
  ○ Sixty adult cases published in six series, with a success rate of 29% to 100%.
    - Lidocaine was used for RSE or when sedative anesthetics were contraindicated (patients with chronic respiratory diseases, etc).
    - Few adverse events were noted.
    - Use was found to be safe in patients with chronic respiratory disease for whom the use of sedative drugs was judged to be too risky.
- Despite a similar mode of action to that of phenytoin (PHT), lidocaine showed evidence of efficacy in PHT-resistant SE.
- Few major adverse events have been reported, however, lidocaine might cause seizures or cardiac arrhythmias at serum levels higher than 5 mg/L.
- May interact with other antiarrhythmic drugs.

D. Magnesium
- NMDA receptor and voltage-gated calcium channel (VGCC) antagonist properties.
- Treatment of choice for seizures in eclampsia and hypomagnesemia (which appears to be more frequent after TBI).
  ○ Efficacy in preventing seizures in eclampsia is likely related to direct treatment of the underlying condition via effects on the endothelium.
- The only evidence in non-eclampsia-related SE is one small case series of two patients with Alpers' syndrome.
- Should be used with caution in renal failure, neuromuscular disease, or heart block.
- Main advantage is the safety profile with only rare instances of hypotension, cardiac arrhythmia, and neuromuscular weakness reported.
- No significant drug interactions.

E. Immunotherapy: Steroids, IV Immunoglobulin (IVIG), and Plasma Exchange (PE)
- Treatment of choice in cases where SE was proven to be secondary to underlying immune dysfunction (autoimmune brain or systemic disease).
  ○ Since some cases of RSE may be due to an occult immune-mediated process, may also be used in refractory SE of undetermined cause.
  ○ May act on epileptogenic inflammatory pathways, even if the underlying cause is not inflammatory.
  ○ Use has been reported in 10 small case series of patients with idiopathic (presumed autoimmune) RSE and four case reports.

- In total, 37 patients received steroids, 24 IVIG, and six PE therapy. Response to treatment was difficult to assess due to the multidrug regimen used and severity of the cases. With rare exceptions, outcome was disappointing.
- There are anecdotal reports with other immunosuppressive drugs such as cyclophosphamide or mycophenolate mofetil.
  - There have been no clinical trials evaluating immunotherapy in SE, and in particular, no direct comparison of the three available immunomodulatory treatments in SE.
  - Available reports suggest that immune treatments may be tried sequentially in case of failure of one modality.
- Steroids
  - Glucocorticoids have inhibitory effects on a broad range of immune pathways.
  - Various formulations of steroids have been used: dexamethasone, prednisolone, methylprednisolone, and ACTH (primarily in infants).
  - Methylprednisolone is most frequently used.
  - Risks include infection, hyperglycemia, fluid retention, and electrolyte disturbances.
  - The gluconeogenic effect of steroids may prevent ketosis when used concomitantly with the ketogenic diet.
- IV Immunoglobulin (IVIG)
  - Multiple mechanisms of action, most of which are incompletely understood.
  - Known to suppress inflammatory and autoimmune processes.
  - Multiple products are available, with comparable efficacy.
  - Usually well-tolerated but risks include:
    - Acute renal failure
    - Fluid overload
    - Cardiac failure
    - Hematological disturbances
    - Aseptic meningitis syndrome
    - Fever and chills
  - No significant drug interactions
- Plasma exchange therapy (PE)
  - Clears circulating antibodies and immune complexes from blood.
  - Requires fluid replacement by albumin solution or fresh frozen plasma, as well as anticoagulation with heparin/citrate.
  - A significant volume of fluid is exchanged (typically $1-1.5$ times the plasma volume).
    - Should be used with caution in cases of hypotension or hemodynamic instability.
  - Must be performed by an experienced team, as it carries significant risks:
    - Hypo or hypertension
    - Citrate-induced hypocalcemia or alkalosis
    - Bleeding due to heparin or heparin-induced thrombocytopenia (first 12 hours) or thrombosis due to hypercoagulable state (24–72 hours after)
    - Hypokalemia
    - Bacterial infections
  - Note: PE can clear antiepileptic and other drugs from circulating blood.

- Although there is not enough data available, significant clearance is expected when protein binding is greater than 80% and $V_d < 0.2$ L/kg.
- Most likely to affect PHT, valproate, and benzodiazepines.
- Levels should be checked before and after PE and doses adjusted.

F. Ketogenic Diet (KD)
- A high fat-to-protein (4:1), glucose-free diet (thus glucose should be avoided in IV fluids).
- Available in soluble preparation for enteral administration.
- Requires an experienced dietician.
- Shown effective and safe in the control of RSE in three small case series (two adult patients and 15 children) and three single case reports.
- Contra-indicated in rare cases of inborn errors of metabolism (β-oxidation defects, primary and secondary carnitine deficiency, carnitine cycle defects, electron transport chain defects, ketogenic defects, ketolytic defects, pyruvate carboxylate deficiency, and pyruvate dehydrogenase phosphatase deficiency).
- Risk of hypoglycemia, electrolyte and acid–base imbalance, and fluid loss.
  - Blood sugar and urinary ketosis should be regularly checked.
- KD interactions
  - A negative interaction with steroids is possible as steroids may prevent ketosis.
  - One case of fatal propofol (PRO) infusion syndrome has been documented so that the concomitant use of KD and PRO should be avoided or used with extra caution.
  - Acidosis is expected to be more pronounced when KD is used in conjunction with carbonic–anhydrase inhibitors (topiramate, zonisamide, and acetazolamide).
    - Therefore, it is reasonable to regularly monitor acid–base balance or to taper off the carbonic anhydrase inhibitor.

G. General Hypothermia
- General hypothermia with endovascular cooling aims to achieve body temperature between 32°C and 35°C, which decreases brain metabolism, reduces seizure activity, and is theoretically neuroprotective.
- Three case series (nine adults, three children), and two case reports showed some efficacy although often transient.
- Associated with a major risk of:
  - Acid–base and electrolyte disturbances
  - Coagulation disorders and thrombosis
  - Infection
  - Cardiac arrhythmia
  - Bowel ischemia and paralytic ileus
- Acid–base balance and serum lactate should be routinely monitored.
- Possible potentiation of side effects with barbiturates, especially ileus.

H. Focal Brain Cooling
- Objective is to achieve seizure control by cooling focal or global brain regions through surgical (cortical or intraventricular) or intravascular application of cold saline or ethyl chloride.
- Avoids the adverse events associated with general hypothermia.

- Efficacy has been demonstrated in animal models with no evidence of neuronal damage as well as several case reports and series in humans with chronic epilepsy (not SE).
- Three cases have been reported in SE in humans.
  - Two of the three patients had a good outcome.

I. Inhalational Halogenated Anesthetics (desflurane, isoflurane)
- Act as fast-acting nonbarbiturate GABA agonists.
- Evidence from five case series (24 adult patients) and six case reports suggests some efficacy, albeit transient.
  - However, use of these agents presents major logistic issues in the ICU.
- Associated with hypotension, cardiorespiratory depression, paralytic ileus, and deep venous thrombosis.
- May induce epileptiform discharges.

J. Vagus Nerve Stimulation (VNS)
- An approved treatment for refractory epilepsy.
- Mechanism of action remains debated.
- Usually requires several months of therapy to reach full efficacy.
- Four cases have been reported in which RSE was controlled by VNS.
- Implantation of the device requires surgery (chest and neck, not brain).
- Side effects include:
  - Bradyarrhythmia
  - Infection at implantation site
  - Voice change
  - Inability to obtain body MRIs after implantation

K. Electroconvulsive Therapy (ECT)
- Induces presynaptic GABA release and a refractory period to seizures.
- One case series of three adult patients, and two single case reports support its use in RSE.
- Weaning off antiepileptic drugs (or very high stimulation settings) might be required to achieve the desired effect, which usually entails an induced generalized tonic–clonic seizure.

L. Transcranial Magnetic Stimulation (TMS)
- Low-frequency (1 Hz) repetitive TMS reportedly increases the neuronal refractory period.
  - Effect outlasts the treatment period.
  - On the basis of preliminary data from patients with chronic epilepsy, multiple treatments per week may have a lasting effect of decreasing excitability.
- The only available evidence of its use in SE stems from two case series (nine children) and two case reports (one adult patient and one child) with epilepsia partialis continua. Most patients experienced transient improvement and a minority had a sustained (more than 1 day) benefit.
- Most likely to be effective with a superficial and well-defined ictal focus.

M. Vigabatrin (VGB)
- Irreversibly inhibits GABA transaminase, increasing GABA levels in the brain.

- No published series or reports have described its use for RSE, although the authors are aware of at least two anecdotal cases of apparent efficacy in this setting.
- Available only as an enteral formulation.
- Opposed to its risk in chronic epilepsy patients, no retinal toxicity is expected during short-term treatment (less than 3 months).
- No major side effects are expected with short-term use.

N. Felbamate (FBM)

- Mechanism of action is largely unknown.
- FBM has some affinity for the glycine binding site of the NMDA receptor, which may be a potential mechanism of action in the treatment of RSE.
- Some evidence of efficacy from animal studies of SE.
- Successful use was reported in one case of anti-NMDA receptor antibody encephalitis in humans.
- Available only as an enteral formulation.
- Associated with significant increased risk of aplastic anemia and with rare cases of hepatic failure.
- Metabolized by and is a weak inducer of CYP3A4 and inhibitor of 2C19; thus, there are possible pharmacokinetic interactions with valproate, PHT, phenobarbital, and carbamazepine.

O. Neurosurgery

- Resective surgery as well as subpial transections, hemispherotomy, and corpus callosotomy have been tried and described in five case series (25 patients) and six case reports, most of which were in children with focal epileptogenic lesions.
- Presurgical evaluation requires multiple investigations (MRI, PET) for localization of the seizure focus and intra-operative electrocorticography.
- Should be considered an alternative in RSE when a focal lesion is seen on neuroimaging and/or focal epileptogenic region is clearly identified.

III. FURTHER CONSIDERATIONS/REMAINING QUESTIONS

A. Randomized Controlled Trials

- Required to establish the efficacy of alternative treatments, as well as to define the doses to be used, the levels to be reached, and the timing of the treatment.

SUGGESTED READING

1. Bleck TP, Quigg MS, Nathan BR, et al. Electroencephalographic effects of ketamine treatment for refractory status epilepticus. *Epilepsia.* 2002;43(Suppl 7):282.
2. Pascual J, Ciudad J, Berciano J. Role of lidocaine (lignocaine) in managing status epilepticus. *J Neurol Neurosurg Psychiatry.* 1992;55(1):49–51.
3. Visser NA, Braun KP, Leijten FS, et al. Magnesium treatment for patients with refractory status epilepticus due to POLG1-mutations. *J Neurol.* 2011;258(2):218–222.
4. Van Baalen A, Häusler M, Boor R, et al. Febrile infection-related epilepsy syndrome (FIRES): A nonencephalitic encephalopathy in childhood. *Epilepsia.* 2010;51(7):1323–1328.

5. Van Lierde I, Van Paesschen W, Dupont P, et al. De novo cryptogenic refractory multifocal febrile status epilepticus in the young adult: A review of six cases. *Acta Neurol Belg.* 2003;103(2):88–94.

6. Wusthoff CJ, Kranick SM, Morley JF, et al. The ketogenic diet in treatment of two adults with prolonged nonconvulsive status epilepticus. *Epilepsia.* 2010;51(6):1083–1085.

7. Nabbout R, Mazzuca M, Hubert P, et al. Efficacy of ketogenic diet in severe refractory status epilepticus initiating fever induced refractory epileptic encephalopathy in school age children (FIRES). *Epilepsia.* 2010;51(10):2033–2037.

8. Corry JJ, Dhar R, Murphy T, et al. Hypothermia for refractory status epilepticus. *Neurocrit Care.* 2008;9(2):189–197.

9. Karlov VA. Focal cooling suppresses continued activity of epileptic focus in patients with partial status epilepticus. *Epilepsia.* 2003;44(12):1605.

10. Kofke WA, Young RS, Davis P, et al. Isoflurane for refractory status epilepticus: A clinical series. *Anesthesiology.* 1989;71(5):653–659.

11. Mirsattari SM, Sharpe MD, Young GB. Treatment of refractory status epilepticus with inhalational anesthetic agents isoflurane and desflurane. *Arch Neurol.* 2004;61(8):1254–1259.

12. Kamel H, Cornes SB, Hegde M, et al. Electroconvulsive therapy for refractory status epilepticus: A case series. *Neurocrit Care.* 2010;12(2):204–210.

13. Alexopoulos A, Lachhwani DK, Gupta A, et al. Resective surgery to treat refractory status epilepticus in children with focal epileptogenesis. *Neurology.* 2005;64(3):567–570.

ADDITIONAL READING

Shorvon S, Ferlisi M. The treatment of super-refractory status epilepticus: A critical review of available therapies and a clinical treatment protocol. *Brain.* Oct 2011;134(10):2802–2818.

Foreman B, Hirsch LJ. Epilepsy emergencies: Diagnosis and management. *Neurol Clin.* Feb 2012;30(1):11–41.

Robakis TK, Hirsch LJ. Literature review case report, and expert discussion of prolonged refractory status epilepticus. *Neurocrit Care.* 2006;4(1):35–46.

Brophy GM, Bell R, Claassen J, et al. Neurocritical care society status epilepticus guideline writing committee. Guidelines for the evaluation and management of status epilepticus. *Neurocrit Care.* 2012 Aug;17(1):3–23.

THIRTY-FOUR

Prophylaxis of Seizures in the ICU Population

Gretchen M. Brophy and Eljim P. Tesoro

KEY POINTS

- Seizure prophylaxis should be considered in high-risk critically ill patients, such as those with acute neurological injury (eg, head trauma, subarachnoid hemorrhage (SAH), intracranial hemorrhage), or those undergoing surgery for brain tumors.
- The duration of prophylaxis should be limited to 3 to 7 days after the initial injury or surgery unless seizures occur during the prophylaxis period.
- Antiepileptic agents used for seizure prophylaxis should be chosen based on individual patient characteristics (including concomitant medications) in order to avoid drug interactions and severe adverse effects.
- Many of the newer antiepileptic drugs (AEDs) are better tolerated than the traditional agents.

I. BACKGROUND

A. Seizure Prophylaxis in High-Risk Critically Ill Patients
- Seizures are considerable complications in the critically ill that may affect patient outcomes and increase length of hospital stay.
- Patients with neurological injury, undergoing intracranial surgery, or diagnosed with brain tumors are at highest risk and should be considered for prophylactic antiepileptic drug therapy.
- However, the adverse effects of AEDs in these intensive care unit (ICU) patients can also be significant and include:
  - Severe rash (eg, Stevens-Johnson syndrome)
  - Fever
  - Hematological and neurobehavioral abnormalities (eg, slow cognition and inattention)

B. Limiting seizure prophylaxis therapy to those at risk, and choosing the appropriate AED and duration of therapy, are extremely important.

II. BASICS

A. Seizure Prophylaxis Overview
- Seizure prophylaxis should be reserved for critically ill patients who are at high risk of seizures that could further complicate their clinical course (Table 34.1).
- Many AEDs are associated with significant adverse effects (Table 34.2) and therapy should be individualized based to help avoid further complications.
- To rapidly achieve therapeutic AED concentrations, some AEDs can be loaded intravenously, whereas others can only be orally administered.

B. Seizure Prophylaxis in Traumatic Brain Injury
- Prophylaxis appears most effective for early-onset seizures (ie, within the first 7 days post-injury), but not for late-onset seizures (1).
- Duration of therapy should be limited for most patients unless early seizures are observed.
- Risk factors that may increase the risk of posttraumatic seizures:
  ○ Glasgow Coma Scale (GCS) < 10
  ○ Presence of a cortical contusion
  ○ Depressed skull fracture
  ○ Epidural, subdural, or intraparenchymal hemorrhage
  ○ Penetrating head injury
  ○ Seizure within 24 hours of injury (2)

C. Subarachnoid Hemorrhage
- Seizures most commonly occur within 24 hours of SAH.
- Seizure prophylaxis may be considered in the immediate post-SAH period, with duration of therapy of approximately 3 to 7 days (3–5).
- For patients at higher risk of seizures (eg, prior seizures, history of hypertension, intraparenchymal hematoma, infarction, or middle cerebral artery aneurysm) extended prophylaxis may be considered (4).
- The type of intervention for securing an aneurysm in SAH patients appears to play a role in the incidence of seizures.
  ○ Endovascular coiling is associated with a lower risk of seizures compared to open craniotomy for surgical clipping (6).
- In SAH patients, first-generation AED (ie, phenytoin and phenobarbital) use has been associated with poor patient outcomes as well as complications such as fever (7).
- Prolonged exposure to phenytoin has been associated with poor neurological and cognitive outcomes and should be limited to patients at high risk or those who have failed other AEDs (8).

D. Intracerebral Hemorrhage
- These patients commonly present with clinical seizures.
- Patients at highest risk are those with higher National Institute of Health Stroke Scale (NIHSS) score, midline shift, or lobar hemorrhage (9).
- The use of traditional AEDs (especially phenytoin) for seizure prophylaxis has been associated with poor outcomes and appears to provide no benefit in this patient population (10). However, the effect on outcome of modern AEDs used for prophylaxis has not been evaluated.

TABLE 34.1 Seizure Prophylaxis for High-Risk Patients

NEUROLOGICAL INJURY	DURATION OF PROPHYLAXIS	CONSIDERATIONS
Traumatic brain injury	1) *SEVERE* TBI (GCS 3–8): 7 days 2) *MODERATE* TBI (GCS 9–13): 7 days for the following: depressed skull fracture, penetrating TBI, EDH/SDH/IPH, traumatic SAH 3) *MILD* TBI (GCS 14–15): No prophylaxis needed (2)	Antiepileptic agents suggested based on available data (1,2,13): Phenytoin and levetiracetam
Aneurysmal SAH	3–7 days	Phenytoin associated with poor cognitive outcomes (7,8)
Intracerebral hemorrhage	No prophylaxis for basal ganglia or cerebellar hemorrhages Consider 7 days of prophylaxis for *lobar* hemorrhages reaching the cortical surface	Seizures generally occur within 24 hours of ICH
Brain tumor	No prophylaxis *unless* the patient presents with seizures Patients undergoing supratentorial tumor resection and without seizures: Start therapy preoperatively and discontinue after 7 days if the patient remains seizure-free	Avoid phenytoin in patients receiving radiation therapy (12); consider drug interactions with chemotherapeutic agents
General craniotomy Burr-hole washouts Acute ischemic stroke Meningitis	No prophylaxis indicated	

EDH, epidural hematoma; GCS, Glasgow Coma Scale; ICH, intracerebral hemorrhage; IPH, intraparenchymal hemorrhage; SAH, subarachnoid hemorrhage; SDH, subdural hematoma.

TABLE 34.2   Adverse Effects of AEDs Most Commonly Used for Seizure Prophylaxis

ANTIEPILEPTIC DRUG	POTENTIAL ADVERSE EFFECTS	CONSIDERATIONS

Phenytoin (Dilantin®)	Arrhythmias hypotension
	Phlebitis
	Purple glove syndrome
	Drowsiness
	Ataxia
	Rash
	Fever
		• Multiple drug interactions
		• Target concentrations:
		  Total phenytoin: 10–20 µg/mL
		  Free phenytoin: 1–2 µg/mL

Fosphenytoin (Cerebyx®)	Paresthesias Hypotension	• IV prodrug of phenytoin • IV preparation is better tolerated than phenytoin
Levetiracetam (Keppra®)	Aggression somnolence Dizziness	• Low incidence of cognitive side effects • No significant drug interactions • Not hepatically metabolized • Renal dosing adjustments required
Valproic acid (Depacon®, Depakote®)	Thrombocytopenia Hyperammonemia Pancreatitis	• Not recommended for posttraumatic seizure prophylaxis • Multiple drug interactions • Carbapenem antibiotics may decrease concentrations • Target concentrations: 50–100 µg/mL

IV, intravenous; SIADH, syndrome of inappropriate antidiuretic hormone.

- Current guidelines do not recommend seizure prophylaxis.
- Treatment should be reserved for patients with clinical seizures or electrographic seizures on EEG with changes in mental status (9).

E. Brain Tumor
- Owing to the potential for serious adverse effects with AEDs, seizure prophylaxis in newly diagnosed brain tumor patients should be reserved for those who present with seizures.
- Post-operative seizure prophylaxis (for up to 7 days) may be considered in patients undergoing tumor resection (11).
- Second-generation AEDs are generally better tolerated and lack the drug interactions and severe adverse effects seen with the first-generation agents.
- Phenytoin has been associated with severe rash in patients undergoing radiation therapy and drug–drug interactions between first-generation AEDs and chemotherapeutic agents may cause significant complications (12).

III. FURTHER CONSIDERATIONS/REMAINING QUESTIONS

A. Cognitive Deficits and Prophylaxis
- In critically ill patients, cognitive deficits may be exacerbated by AEDs.
- Therefore, the benefits and risks of seizure prophylaxis need to be carefully weighed.
- It may be reasonable to delay AED therapy until seizures occur.

B. Undiagnosed Nonconvulsive Seizures
- Critically ill patients with neurocognitive impairment are at risk for nonconvulsive seizures.
- To prevent prolonged seizure activity and further complications, EEG monitoring should be considered in all critically ill ICU patients if there is any suspicion of nonconvulsive seizures.

C. Paralyzed Patients at High Risk of Seizures
- EEG monitoring should be implemented to monitor depth of sedation and exclude the possibility of nonconvulsive seizures.
- Consider AED prophylaxis until paralytic agents are fully reversed and there is no evidence of seizure activity.

D. When to Discontinue Seizure Prophylaxis
- Discontinue AEDs if no seizures occur during the prophylaxis period.
- Failure to discontinue this therapy could lead to future drug interactions, serious adverse effects, and further complications.

REFERENCES

1. Temkin NR, Dikmen SS, Wilensky AJ, et al. A randomized, double-blind study of phenytoin for the prevention of post-traumatic seizures. *NEJM*. 1990;323:497–502.

2. Bratton SL, Chestnut RM, Ghajar J, et al. Antiseizure prophylaxis. *J Neurotrauma.* 2007;24:S83–S86.

3. Chumnanvej S, Dunn IF, Kim DH, et al. Three-day phenytoin prophylaxis is adequate after subarachnoid hemorrhage. *Neurosurgery.* 2007;60:99–102.

4. Bederson JB, Connolly ES, Batjer HH, et al. Guidelines for the management of aneurysmal subarachnoid hemorrhage: A statement for healthcare professionals from a special writing group of the Stroke Council, American Heart Association. *Stroke* 2009;40:994–1025.

5. Diringer MN, Bleck TP, Hemphill JC, III, et al. Critical care management of patients following aneurysmal subarachnoid hemorrhage: Recommendations from the Neurocritical Care Society's Multidisciplinary Consensus Conference. *Neurocrit Care.* 2011;15:211–240.

6. Molyneux AJ, Kerr RS, Yu LM, et al. International Subarachnoid Aneurysm Trial (ISAT) Collaborative Group. International subarachnoid aneurysm trial (ISAT) of neurosurgical clipping versus endovascular coiling in 2143 patients with ruptured intracranial aneurysms: A randomized comparison of effects on survival, dependency, seizures, rebleeding, subgroups, and aneurysm occlusion. *Lancet.* 2005 Sep 3-9;366(9488):809–817.

7. Rosengart AJ, Huo D, Tolentino J, et al. Outcome in patients with subarachnoid hemorrhage treated with antiepileptic drugs. *J Neurosurgery.* 2007;107:253–260.

8. Naidech AM, Kreiter KT, Janjua N, et al. Phenytoin exposure is associated with functional and cognitive disability after subarachnoid hemorrhage. *Stroke.* 2005;36:583–587.

9. Morgenstern LB, Hemphill JC, 3RD, Anderson C, et al. Guidelines for the management of spontaneous intracerebral hemorrhage: A guideline for healthcare professionals from the American Heart Association/American Stroke Association. *Stroke* 2010;41:2108–2129.

10. Messe SR, Sansing LH, Cuccchiara BL, et al. Prophylactic antiepileptic drug use is associated with poor outcome following ICH. *Neurocrit Care* 2009;11:38–44.

11. Milligan TA, Hurwitz S, Bromfield EB. Efficacy and tolerability of levetiracetam versus phenytoin after supratentorial neurosurgery. *Neurology.* 2008;71:665–669.

12. Ahmed I, Reichenberg J, Lucas A, et al. Erythema multiforme associated with phenytoin and cranial radiation therapy: A report of three patients and review of the literature. *Int J Dermatol.* 2004;43:67–73.

13. Szaflarski JP, Sangha KS, Lindsell CJ, et al. Prospective, randomized, single-blinded comparative trial of intravenous levetiracetam versus phenytoin for seizure prophylaxis. *Neurocrit Care.* 2010;12:165–172.

ADDITIONAL READING

Liu KC, Bhardwaj A. Use of prophylactic anticonvulsants in neurologic critical care: A critical appraisal. *Neurocrit Care.* 2007;7:175–184.

THIRTY-FIVE

Billing and Coding for ICU EEG Monitoring

Marc R. Nuwer

KEY POINTS

- CPT Code 95956 for continuous ICU EEG monitoring can be used if all of the following conditions are met:
  - A nurse or technologist is observing for changes;
  - A physician can interpret the record during the ongoing recording and change patient care as needed;
  - At least 16 channels are recorded;
  - The goal is the identification of a seizure focus if present;
  - The recording lasts at least 12 hours.
- CPT Code 95951 can be used if all of the above criteria are met AND continuous video is also monitored and recorded.

I. BACKGROUND

A. Regulation of Reimbursement
- Performed through U.S. health care public policy systems.
- Coding systems are used for medical, surgical, and diagnostic procedures.

B. Coding Systems Include:
- Current Procedural Terminology (CPT)
  - A codified listing of medical, surgical and diagnostic procedures and quality measures.
- National Correct Coding Initiative (NCCI or CCI) edits
  - A list of which pairs of CPT codes cannot be used with each other
- International Classification of Diseases (ICD)
  - A codified listing of diagnoses, symptoms and other conditions that may affect a patient.
- Linkage tables
  - An insurance company's listing of which ICD codes are considered medically necessary reasons for conducting a CPT procedure.

II. BASICS

A. Current Procedural Terminology (CPT®) Codes and Modifiers
- CPT is a numerical coding system for each medical, surgical, and diagnostic procedure.
  - It allows for more accurate communication between providers and carriers.
  - CPT is a trademarked product of the American Medical Association (AMA).
- Codes for continuous ICU EEG
  - The most common codes used for EEG in the ICU.
    - 95813: EEG extended monitoring greater than 1 hour.
    - 95951: Monitoring for localization of cerebral seizure focus by cable or radio, 16- or more-channel telemetry, combined EEG and video recording and interpretation, each 24 hours.
    - 95956: Monitoring for localization of cerebral seizure focus by cable or radio, 16 or more channel telemetry, electroencephalographic (EEG) recording and interpretation, each 24 hours, attended by a technologist or nurse.
- Modifiers for continuous ICU EEG
  - The 2-digit modifiers describe special circumstances.
    - 26: *Professional Component*: use this modifier with inpatient EEG services to denote that you are billing only for the professional fee.
    - 52: *Reduced Services*: use this modifier with a 24-hour code when recording less than 12 hours.
    - 59: *Distinct Procedure*: use this modifier when two similar services were needed on the same day, for example, a routine EEG was performed in the morning and continuous EEG monitoring was started in the evening.
- Coding instructions for continuous ICU EEG
  - Time-based codes
    - These CPT codes use recording time as a basis for code use.
    - Recording time is when the recording is underway and data are being collected.
    - Recording time excludes set-up and take-down time.
    - If recording for less than 12 hours, use modifier 52 with codes 95951 or 95956.
  - Continuous codes
    - Codes 95951 and 95956: for recordings in which interpretations can be made throughout the recording time, with interventions to alter or end the recording or to alter the patient care during the recordings as needed.
  - 16 channels
    - Codes 95951 and 95956 require recording from at least 16 channels.
  - To localize a seizure focus
    - Codes 95951 and 95956 require the goal of localizing a seizure focus, if one is present.
  - Automated spike and seizure detection
    - Included in Codes 95951 and 95956.
    - Do not code separately for these features.
- Distinguishing among codes
  - Code 95951 has video; code 95956 does not have video.

○ Do not use code 95951 when simply adding video to a routine EEG recording.
○ Use code 95813 if some required parts of codes 95951 or 95956 are missing (eg, too few channels) but at least 1 hour in duration.
- Disallowed code pairs
  ○ Do not bill the baseline 20 to 30 minutes EEG recording separate from the continuous ICU EEG monitoring.
  ○ NCCI disallows billing the routine EEG on the same day as the continuous EEG monitoring.
  ○ If both were medically necessary, for example, a routine EEG in the morning and start of continuous ICU EEG in the evening, use modifier 59 with the continuous monitoring code.

B. International Classification of Diseases (ICD)
- Lists codes for diagnoses, symptoms, and other conditions
  ○ U.S. currently uses a Code Modification (CM) of the ninth international system, known as ICD 9-CM.
  ○ U.S. will switch to ICD-10 in the next few years.
- ICD-9-CM codes for seizures and epilepsy
  ○ Generalized epilepsies
    - 345.00: nonconvulsive epilepsy, not intractable
    - 345.01: nonconvulsive epilepsy, intractable
    - 345.10: convulsive epilepsy, not intractable
    - 345.11: convulsive epilepsy, intractable
  ○ Status epilepticus
    - 345.2: petit mal status
    - 345.3: grand mal status
  ○ Localization-related (focal) epilepsy and epileptic syndromes
    - 345.40: with complex partial seizures, not intractable
    - 345.41: with complex partial seizures, intractable
    - 345.50: with simple partial seizures, not intractable
    - 345.51: with simple partial seizures, intractable
  ○ Other syndromes
    - 345.6: infantile spasms
    - 345.7: epilepsia partialis continua
    - 345.80: other forms of epilepsy, not intractable
    - 345.81: other forms of epilepsy, intractable
    - 333.2: myoclonus
  ○ Epilepsy, unspecified
    - 345.90: not intractable
    - 345.91: intractable
  ○ Convulsions (as a symptom)
    - 780.31: febrile convulsions
    - 780.39: other convulsions
  ○ Alteration of consciousness
    - 780.01: coma
    - 780.02: transient alteration of awareness

- 780.09: drowsiness, somnolence, unconscious, semicoma, or stupor
- 780.2: syncope and collapse
- There are two definitions of intractable:
  ○ Patient who has had seizures during the past year.
  ○ Patient whose seizures interfere with life's activities.
  ○ In general, a patient having seizures in the ICU would be considered intractable.

C. Linkage Tables

- Carriers create policies about the ICD diagnoses for which particular CPT codes are considered medically necessary.
  ○ This automates decisions about whether a procedure is "medically necessary" for a given diagnosis.
  ○ These ICD-CPT lists are called "linkage tables."
- The epilepsy ICD codes are generally accepted to justify providing EEG CPT codes.
  ○ Other diagnoses are variably accepted.
  ○ As a result, it is important to consider the ICD code used when providing EEG services.
- Medicare carriers linkage table are online.
  ○ Some states require all carriers to make available the linkage tables and other rules used for coverage determinations.
- The statement "not medically necessary" by a carrier often means, "That ICD is not on our linkage table for that CPT procedure."

III. RESOURCES

- CPT is a trademarked product of the American Medical Association.
  ○ The book *Current Procedural Terminology* (CPT) is available from AMA CPT Product Catalogs at www.ama-assn.org/ama/pub/category/3116.html
- Medicare coverage information is available at www.cms.hhs.gov/mcd
  ○ A particular physician resource area is at www.cms.hhs.gov/physicians
  ○ The specific linkage tables are found in Local Carrier Decisions at: www.cms.gov/DeterminationProcess/04_LCDs.asp#TopOfPage
- The American Academy of Neurology (AAN) at www.aan.com publishes a useful ICD coding book specially designed for neurologists.

THIRTY-SIX

Report Generation and Effective Communication With the ICU Team

Stephen Hantus

KEY POINTS

- Efficient and timely communication is essential to a successful ICU EEG monitoring program.
- EEG monitoring reports are traditionally written once daily, but in the ICU, where EEG findings may change several times per day, seizures and other clinical changes may be inadequately treated if EEG findings are not communicated to treating physicians more frequently.
- Continuous EEG (cEEG) reports should be organized, concise, and relay a clear clinical impression to the ICU team.
- Communication with the ICU team takes multiple forms, including the written copy of the EEG report, urgent updates on select patients, and detailed explanation of the clinical significance of complicated EEG findings.
- A joint conference between the EEG and ICU teams is valuable to establish the foundation of shared patient care, promote better understanding of complicated EEG patterns, foster research, and obtain consensus on management of specific EEG findings.

I. BACKGROUND

A. The Method of EEG Reporting Has Evolved From Routine EEGs Performed in the Outpatient Clinic.

- Outpatient EEG reports routinely written and finalized within 1 to 5 days of recording.

B. EEG Monitoring of Epilepsy Patients for Diagnostic or Presurgical Evaluation Led to the Need for More Immediate Video-EEG Monitoring Reports.

- EEG monitoring reports often condense findings from multiple days of monitoring into a single report.

- Reports are often not immediately available due to lag time for dictation and uploading to the patient's chart.

C. EEG Monitoring in the ICU Setting Requires a Different Level of Reporting.
- Seizures or other clinically significant EEG changes can occur at any time of the day or night.
- A delay in diagnosis and treatment of seizures can lead to increased morbidity and mortality.
- After seizures are diagnosed, the ICU team needs frequent feedback on the effectiveness of the treatment.
- These needs are met only if EEG results are reported multiple times per day.
- However, no standards for ICU EEG reporting exist outside of individual institutional protocols.
- EEG findings are often reported in paragraph format that is full of EEG jargon and difficult for the ICU team to interpret.

II. BASICS

A. A study by Young and colleagues evaluating outcomes following nonconvulsive status epilepticus (NCSE) suggests that there is an urgency for diagnosis and treatment that exceed many current standard practices (1).
- NCSE lasting less than 10 hours was associated with discharge home with minimal disability.
- By comparison, NCSE of 10 to 20 hours in duration was associated with significant disability.
- NCSE lasting longer than 20 hours was associated with death in most cases.
- Thus, a single report generated once every 24 hours would not allow for timely diagnosis and treatment of clinically significant events in order to prevent morbidity and mortality.

B. Digital Technology Allows the Generation of Multiple Daily Reports as Well as Enhanced Communication With the ICU Team.
- The ability to view EEG files remotely (from home, at a distant office, etc) has decreased the response time for EEG interpretation.
- Electronic medical records make reports instantly available regardless of location.

C. EEG Reports Should Be Organized in a Standard Way for Ease of Interpretation (Figure 36.1).
- The **introduction** contains the clinical history as well as technical recording information.
  - Indication for EEG monitoring
  - Primary neurological or medical diagnosis
  - Comorbid medical conditions
  - Current medications and sedatives
  - Number of electrodes and montage
  - Type of electrodes
  - Duration of the recording

I. Patient Information
    Name, Date of Birth, Patient Location
    Referring Physician, Interpreting Physician, EEG Technologist

II. Technical Details
    Number and type of electrodes
    Montage
    Skull defect present?
    Duration of the recording
    Video recording (yes or no)

III. Clinical Background
    Indication for EEG monitoring
    Primary neurological or medical diagnosis
    Comorbid medical conditions
    Medications and sedatives
    Intubation status, ICP monitoring

IV. EEG Description
    Background
        Frequency, voltage, symmetry
        Variability and reactivity
        Continuous versus periods of suppression (Burst-suppression pattern)
    Seizures
        EEG findings
            Location, duration, frequency
        Clinical Correlate
    Rhythmic or Periodic Patterns
        Generalized or lateralized pattern
        Periodic discharges or rhythmic delta activity
        Frequency, duration, and persistence of rhythmic or periodic patterns
        Are patterns stimulus induced? (yes or no)

V. EEG Impression and Clinical Correlation

FIGURE 36.1 Example of an ICU EEG monitoring report.

- The "body" of the EEG report contains the **description** of the electrographic findings.
  - Presented in an objective, organized format such as a table or with bulleted sections.
  - Should be written in technical and detailed language that is understandable to electroencephalographers.
  - Includes description of background including frequency, voltage, reactivity, and presence or absence of rhythmic or periodic patterns, and seizures.
- The EEG **interpretation** and impression summarizes the important EEG abnormalities.
  - Contains important findings from the body of the report that are worth pointing out to the intended audience of the report (the ICU physician who ordered the study).
  - Details such as voltage and background frequencies are contained in the description only and do not need to be repeated in the EEG impression.

○ Example
  - "Sharp waves: right temporal region"
  - "Seizure: right temporal region at 0630, no clinical signs"
- Finally, a **clinical correlation** is required to convey your interpretation of the findings outlined in the EEG impression.
  ○ This should be straight forward and supply information to help guide the ICU team in clinical management.
  ○ Example of how a clinical correlation based on the above EEG impression of right temporal sharp waves and right temporal seizures with no clinical signs might read:
    - "Continuous EEG was reviewed between the hours of 5 a.m. until 11 a.m. on 5/17/2012 and contains interictal epileptiform activity arising from the right temporal region. One electrographic seizure was recorded at 6:30 a.m. arising from the right temporal region with no apparent clinical signs."

D. A Protocol for Urgent Communication With the ICU Team Is Necessary.
- In addition to written reports, there needs to be a method in place for urgent communication of clinically significant EEG changes regardless of when they occur.
- This additional communication can be verbal (face to face) or via a text message or page.
- The method of reporting urgent findings will likely differ from weekdays to weekends and weeknights depending on the staffing of the EEG monitoring unit and the ICU team.
- It is important that a protocol is in place so that both the EEG and ICU teams are aware of who the "contact" person is for communication of urgent findings for a given day or shift.

E. Regularly Scheduled Joint Conferences Between the Epilepsy Service and the ICU Service Improve the Communication Process.
- The EEG service is typically staffed by neurologists, fellows, and EEG technologists with expertise in EEG monitoring while the ICU service may include neuro intensivists, critical care pulmonologists, and mid-level providers without specific training in EEG.
- The meeting can address the care of shared patients.
  ○ Helps with sharing knowledge and perspectives on the case that may not be appreciated by each individual service.
  ○ Can also address concerns if needs of one service are not being met.
  ○ Clinical discussion also helps solidify an approach to difficult cases such as refractory SE when there are no clear treatment guidelines and a consensus on management is needed.
- Promoting education about the field ICU EEG monitoring is vital to the survival of the cEEG program.
  ○ For most efficient EEG monitoring, residents as well as staff physicians need education on the appropriate indications for cEEG monitoring, appropriate duration of cEEG monitoring, and significance of the EEG patterns detected.
  ○ Joint discussions among different services often result in better appreciation of the gaps in clinical knowledge that can lead to research collaborations.

- Each service has different resources and talents and a regular meeting to discuss research possibilities can advance their commitment as well as further knowledge in the field.

III. FURTHER CONSIDERATIONS/REMAINING QUESTIONS

A. What Are the Advantages of Improved Communication of ICU EEG Findings?

- A standardized database of cEEG findings utilizing standardized EEG terminology as well as standard reporting format would help build a common language among medical centers.
- This would make multicenter studies more feasible and promote cross-institution communication.

B. How Feasible Is Continuous, Live Monitoring of cEEG by Trained EEG Personnel?

- This would be the most responsive and thorough method of reviewing EEG data.
- Developing the tools and determining the personnel needed and financial feasibility for such real-time monitoring and reporting of EEG findings will require additional investigation.

REFERENCE

1. Young GB, Jordan KG, Doig GS. An assessment of nonconvulsive seizures in the intensive care unit using continuous EEG monitoring: An investigation of variables associated with mortality. *Neurology.* 1996;47:83–89.

THIRTY-SEVEN

Multimodality Monitoring

Emily Gilmore and Jan Claassen

KEY POINTS

- In critically ill comatose patients, the clinical exam is often extremely limited and traditional physiological assessments such as heart and respiratory rate, oxygen saturation, and blood pressure lack sufficient sensitivity and specificity for detecting changes in neuronal function.
- In contrast, invasive multimodality brain monitoring (MMM), allows assessment of intracranial pressure (ICP), partial brain tissue oxygen tension ($PbtO_2$), jugular bulb venous saturation ($SjVO_2$), interstitial brain chemistry, intracortical electroencephalography (ICE), regional cerebral blood flow (rCBF), and brain temperature.
- MMM can detect secondary brain injury in "real time"; however, more widespread implementation is limited in practice by the complexities of data visualization and analysis.
- There are no guidelines addressing the placement of invasive monitoring devices. As for other neurosurgical procedures, general recommendations by the National Institutes of Health and the College of American Pathologists should be followed.

I. BACKGROUND

A. Traditional Assessment in Critically Ill Comatose Patients

- Clinical examination is often extremely limited and may miss secondary brain injury.
- Such events of secondary injury impact outcome and are potentially amenable to treatment if diagnosed in a timely fashion.
- Routine physiologic monitoring such as heart and respiratory rate, oxygen saturation, blood pressure, cardiac output, and central venous pressure lack sensitivity and specificity for detection of neuronal injury.
- Imaging studies are limited due to poor temporal resolution.

- EEG allows continuous monitoring, but has limited spatial resolution and is subject to artifact.

B. Uses of Invasive MMM
- MMM allows assessment of multiple physiological parameters (Table 37.1)
  - Intracranial pressure (ICP)
  - Regional cerebral blood flow (rCBF)
  - Partial brain tissue oxygen tension (PbtO$_2$)
  - Brain temperature
  - Intracortical electroencephalography (ICE)
  - Interstitial brain chemistry using microdialysis (MD)
- ICP monitoring is the most established component of MMM followed by the assessment of PbtO$_2$.
- Although combining devices that assess different physiologic measures allows more comprehensive assessment and improved detection of secondary brain injury, such benefits must be carefully weighed against the risks of invasive monitoring which includes bleeding and infection.
- MMM technology is most applicable to critically ill neurology and neurosurgical patients with:
  - Poor-grade subarachnoid hemorrhage (SAH)
  - Intracerebral hemorrhages (ICH)
  - Severe traumatic brain injury (TBI)
  - MMM may also help management of patients with large vessel acute ischemic strokes (AIS), refractory status epilepticus (SE), and cardiac arrest (CA).

C. Ongoing Concerns Regarding MMM
- There is controversy regarding preferred placement of monitoring devices.
  - Many practitioners place probes in at-risk or penumbral tissue such as the area surrounding a mass lesion after TBI, a vascular territory most likely to be affected by vasospasm after SAH, or a vascular territory most at risk of herniation in the setting of large AIS.
  - Monitoring contralateral to the injury may be of limited value and monitoring in the center of the pathology (ie, inside a blood clot) is of no value.
- MMM appears to be able to detect secondary brain injury in "real time."
  - However, more widespread implementation of MMM is limited by lack of integrated software that allows for easy analysis and interpretation in real time at the bedside.

D. Guidelines for MMM
- Currently, no guidelines address the placement of invasive monitoring devices.
- For every probe placement, the risk–benefit ratio must be considered, particularly in the setting of coagulopathies.
- As for other neurosurgical procedures, general recommendations by the National Institutes of Health and the College of American Pathologists should be followed.
- In one institution's experience in 61 patients, complications of MMM placement were rare and included hemorrhage (immediate 2%, delayed 1%), and ventriculitis (5% in patients with concurrent external ventricular drain, EVD, and 4% in patients without an EVD) (1).

TABLE 37.1 Summary of MMM Techniques

PARAMETER[A]	DEVICE	NORMAL RANGE	PATHOLOGICAL RANGE	MRI SAFE
ICP	Ventriclear™ EVD (Medtronic™, Goleta CA)	<20 mmHg	≥20 mmHg	Yes
	Ventrix NL960-V™ (Integra Neurosciences™, Plainsborough, NJ)			Yes
	Camino 110 4B™ (Integra™)			Yes
	ICP Express (Codman™)			Yes
	Micro Ventricular Bolt Pressure Monitoring Kit™ (Integra™)			No
CPP	A-line, ICP monitor	≥60 mmHg	≤60 mmHg	Yes
CBF	Bowman Perfusion Monitor™ (Hemedex™, Cambidge, MA)	50 mL/100 g/min	≤20 mL/100 g/min; loss of neuronal function and threshold for ischemia	No
Brain temp	LICOX C8.Bv with IT2 Tunneling Kit™ (Integra™)	Correlates with core body temperature (normal 37°C)	37.2	No
	LICOX PMO™ Kit (Integra™)			No
SjVO$_2$	Baxter–Edwards Vigilance Continuous Oximetry Monitor	50–75%	<50%, indicative of ischemia > 75%, indicative of hyperemia	No
PbtO$_2$	LICOX CCI.SB IT2TM with IT2 Tunneling Kit™ (Integra™)	20 mmHg in white matter	≤15 mmHg or 5 mmHg drop in 1 hour, sustained for 15 minutes	No
	LICOX CCI.SB™ with IM3 Bolt Kit™ (Integra™)	35–40 mmHg in gray matter		No
	LICOX PMO™ Kit (Integra™)			

(continued)

TABLE 37.1 Summary of MMM Techniques *(continued)*

PARAMETER[a]	DEVICE	NORMAL RANGE	PATHOLOGICAL RANGE	MRI SAFE
MD[3,4]	CMA 70™MD catheter (CMA/Microdialysis™, North Chelmsford, MA)			No
Glucose		1.7 ± 0.9 –2.1 ± 0.2 mmol/L	≤1.1 mmol/L(20 mg/dL) or 50% below baseline in 2 hours	
Lactate		2.9 ± 0.9–3.1 ± 0.2 mmol/L	6.7 ± 1.1	
Pyruvate		166 ± 47–151 ± 12 µmol/L	84.3 ± 35.8	
LPR		19 ± 2–23 ± 4	Controversial: > 40 or more than 50% above baseline	
Glutamate		16 ± 16–14 ± 3.3 µmol/L	Unknown	
Glycerol		82 ± 44–88 ± 14 µmol/L	Unknown	
EEG				
Scalp	Ives EEG Solutions Inc.™ Conductive plastic cup or subdermal wire electrodes	Variable	Variable	Yes
Depth	Spencer™ 8-contact depth electrode (Ad-Tech™, Racine, WI)		Unknown	No

[a]Note that normal and pathologic ranges are often controversial, depend on site-specific considerations, and may differ from patient to patient. Possibly relative changes may be much more important than crossing a predefined threshold of abnormality.

Adapted from Stuart MR, et al. Intracranial multimodality monitoring for acute brain injury: A single institution review of current practices. *Neurocrit Care.* 2010;12:188–198.

II. BASICS

A. Intracranial Pressure (ICP)
- Physiology and pathology
  - Measures pressure in millimeters of mercury (mmHg) via a parenchymal or ventricular device.
  - ICP thought to reflect the global pressure of the entire cranial vault as the intracranial volume is determined by the sum of brain tissue (80%), blood (10%), and CSF (10%) volumes.
  - Monroe–Kellie doctrine: although these percentages may change through intrinsic regulatory mechanisms, the total volume is constant since the bony skull does not allow for expansion.
    - As in other parts of the body, compartment syndromes can develop.
    - Thus, it is possible to develop pressure gradients between the intracranial hemispheres or fossas which can lead to herniation even in the setting of "normal" ICP.
  - Through waveform analysis, ICP monitoring provides information about autoregulation of cerebral blood flow (CBF) and volume as well as compliance of the CSF system.

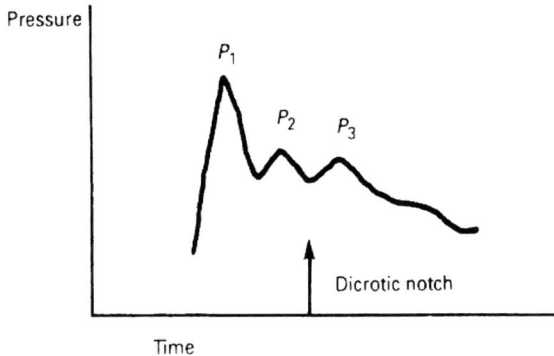

Normal ICP waveform: P1 = percussion wave; represents arterial input; P2 = tidal wave; represents retrograde venous pulsation/intracranial volume; P3 = dicrotic wave; represents venous drainage

  - Pathologic waves (Lundberg waves)
    - A waves (Plateau waves)
      - Rapid rise in ICP from normal to peak levels at 50mmHg for 5 to 20 minutes followed by a spontaneous reduction.
      - Reflect intact autoregulation in a poorly compliant brain.
      - Characteristically associated with reductions in cerebral perfusion pressure (CPP).
      - When severe, also can be associated with reduced CBF leading to global hypoxic–ischemic damage.

- B waves
  - Sharply peaked waves to levels 30mmHg with rapid reduction within seconds that recur every 1 to 2 minutes.
  - Classically associated with changes in respiratory pattern.
  - Useful marker of abnormal intracranial compliance.
- C waves
  - Rhythmic elevations occurring every 10 to 12 minutes but to a lesser extent than the A and B waves.
  - Often associated with fluctuations in blood pressure.
  ○ With intact autoregulation, there is a wide range of CPP over which large changes in the systemic blood pressure will produce small changes in the ICP.
  ○ ICP is a surrogate for cerebral blood volume and reflects the reserve of arterioles to constrict and dilate in response to changes in arterial blood pressure.
- Measurement of ICP
  ○ ICP is probably the most commonly measured parameter in neurocritical care units and can be obtained via a variety of methods.
    - Invasive probe inserted into the brain parenchyma through a burr hole.
    - External ventricular drain (EVD) attached to an external pressure transducer, which may serve as both a diagnostic and therapeutic monitoring device. However, EVDs have an associated 5% infection risk, which is not always reduced by antibiotic coating.
    - Microtransducers can be placed in the ventricular, subdural, or epidural space or in the parenchyma. The most reliable and most widely used method is placement into the brain parenchyma, which may have lower infection rates than EVD catheters.
  ○ Estimations of ICP changes can be analyzed through ICP waveform analysis, transcranial dopplers (TCDs), and duplex recordings.
    - Although these measures reflect changes in ICP rather accurately, they unfortunately do not allow accurate estimation of the absolute ICP level and therefore are still at the investigational stage.
- Management
  ○ The Brain Trauma Foundation recommends that ICP be measured in all salvageable patients with severe TBI defined as a Glasgow Coma Scale (GCS) score of 3 to 8 after resuscitation and an abnormal CT scan (Level II).
  ○ Additionally, ICP monitoring may be indicated in patients with severe TBI with a normal CT and at least two of the following (Level III):
    - Age > 40
    - Unilateral or bilateral motor-posturing
    - Systolic blood pressure (SBP) <90 mmHg on admission
  ○ When should treatment be initiated for elevated ICP?
    - Controversial, but experts often recommend treating if ICP is elevated (greater than or equal to 20−25 mmHg).
    - However, herniation may occur even at an ICP < 20 mmHg depending on the locations of the intracranial mass and the pressure monitor.
  ○ ICP management protocols may include the following:

- Surgical decompression: Consider repeat CT scanning and definitive surgical intervention or ventricular drainage.
- Sedation: Intravenous sedation to attain a motionless, quiet state.
- CPP optimization: Vasopressor infusion if CPP < 70 mmHg, or reduction of blood pressure if CPP > 110 mmHg.
- Osmotherapy: Mannitol 0.25 to 1.0 g/kg IV (repeat every 1–6 hours as needed).
- Hyperventilation: Target $PaCO_2$ levels 28 to 32 mmHg acutely as a temporizing measure, otherwise target 35 mmHg.
- Hypothermia: Cool core body temperature to 33°C to 35°C.
- Pentobarbital: Load with 5 to 20 mg/kg with maintenance infusion at 1 to 4 mg/kg/hr.
- Further discussion
  - Despite its widespread use, there is no randomized controlled trial that demonstrates the benefits of ICP monitoring.

B. Partial Brain Tissue Oxygen Tension ($PbtO_2$)

- Physiology and pathology
  - Maintaining adequate oxygenation of end organs including the brain is a fundamental principle in the management of critically ill patients.
  - $PbtO_2$ probes can provide regional information about "at risk" brain tissue.
  - $PbtO_2$ can be thought of a direct measure of brain tissue oxygenation and a marker of the balance between regional supply and demand.
  - However, the underlying physiology that $PbtO_2$ measurements reflect is complex and includes:
    - O_2 saturation in the arterial blood
    - CO_2 level
    - Partial arterial pressure of oxygen (PaO_2)
    - MAP (manifold absolute pressure)
    - CPP
    - Regional CBF
    - Hemoglobin concentration
    - Diffusion distance between the capillaries and cells
    - Proportion of arterioles and venules surrounding the probe
      - Thus, changes in the $PbtO_2$ are difficult to interpret in isolation.
- Measurement of $PbtO_2$
  - Invasive monitor is placed through a burr hole or at the time of craniotomy.
  - $PbtO_2$ is a regional measure reflecting a cube of 14 to 17 mm^3 of brain tissue.
- Management:
  - In patients with TBI and a normal CPP and ICP, $PbtO_2$ values usually lie between 20 and 30 mmHg.
  - $PbtO_2$ values less than 15 mmHg for more than 10 to 15 minutes, or a drop of 5 mmHg over an hour, warrant exploration since this is associated with ischemia and poor outcome in TBI patients (Level III).
- Further discussion
  - Low $PbtO_2$ is associated with worse outcomes but does treatment result in clinical improvement?

- A multicenter randomized trial to evaluate whether targeted therapy will improve outcomes is currently underway (Brain Tissue Oxygen Monitoring in Traumatic Brain Injury (BOOST 2)).
  - A recent study in poor-grade SAH patients showed an increased risk of vasospasm when the $PbtO_2$ is dependent on CPP in the setting of autoregulation failure (2).
    - Unlike the threshold effect as seen in glucose metabolism, this recent data revealed a graded response of $PbtO_2$ to mild reductions in CBF and substrate delivery.
    - This suggests that $PbtO_2$ monitoring may be "best-suited" for assessing autoregulation status and thus target patients who will be particularly vulnerable to hypoperfusion (2).

C. Jugular Bulb Venous Saturation (SjVO₂)

- Physiology and pathology
  - Measures oxygen content of venous blood in the jugular veins with a sensor in the jugular bulb, the dilated portion of the vein at the skull base.
  - Measurements are global as opposed to regional or focal.
    - Hence, smaller desaturations are prone to washout from better perfused areas as well as from mixed venous contamination.
  - Jugular venous oxygen saturation is influenced by CBF, arterial blood saturation, and the relative oxygen extraction of the brain (OEF).
  - Normal $SjVO_2$ is greater than or equal to 60%.
    - Values less than 50% reflect ischemia.
    - Increased saturations greater than 75% may reflect hyperemia or infarcted tissue.
  - Large differences in the arterial jugular venous oxygen content likely reflect global cerebral ischemia, whereas small differences reflect cerebral hyperemia ("luxury perfusion").
  - Poor outcome is associated with recurrent or persistent desaturations, as well as with elevations above the threshold of 75%.
- Measurement of $SjVO_2$
  - Relatively noninvasive
  - Complications similar to those of any central line placement in the jugular vein:
    - Puncture of carotid artery
    - Hematoma formation
    - Thrombosis
    - Rarely, elevated ICP
  - Measured continuously or intermittently via a fiberoptic catheter.
  - Catheter is placed retrograde near the origin of the internal jugular vein.
  - Placement is confirmed with a lateral and/or an antero-posterior neck x-ray demonstrating the catheter tip above the disc of C1/C2.
  - Poor placement can lead to inaccurate values, especially if distal to the jugular bulb where superficial facial veins may cause false elevations.
- Management
  - After anemia, hypoxia, and hypotension, increased ICP or decreased CPP have been excluded, abnormally low or high values should prompt initial recalibration with a jugular and arterial blood gas assessment.

- ○ High SjVO$_2$ is seen with cell death or infarction.
- ○ Importantly, sedation also decreases oxygen utilization by suppressing cerebral metabolism and may result in a high SjVO$_2$.

D. Microdialysis
- Physiology and pathology
  - ○ PET and magnetic resonance spectroscopy (MRS) allow visualization of brain metabolism at isolated points in time.
    - However, physiologic states in acutely brain-injured patients change rapidly and continuous measures are therefore desirable.
    - Obtaining imaging studies may be logistically difficult and can pose a risk to critically ill or unstable patients.
  - ○ MD measures the concentration of metabolites and cell breakdown products in brain tissue extracellular fluid.
    - It thus provides information about local energy metabolism and cellular integrity as well as regional substrate delivery.
    - Lactate–pyruvate ratio (LPR) is the best known measure.
  - ○ Chemical markers routinely monitored:
    - Glucose
    - Lactate
    - Pyruvate
    - Glycerol
    - Glutamate
  - ○ Brain metabolism basics
    - During the anaerobic part of glycolysis, pyruvate is formed from glucose, forming two ATP molecules.
    - In the presence of adequate oxygen supply, pyruvate enters the citric acid cycle to yield 32 molecules of ATP.
    - However, if the supply of oxygen is diminished as in ischemia, ATP production from this cycle decreases.
    - In an effort to compensate, cells shift toward the anaerobic portion of glycolysis where pyruvate gets converted into lactate.
    - As a result, both lactate and LPR increase.
  - ○ As supply of oxygen and energy substrates decreases (eg, during ischemia):
    - Both pyruvate and glucose reach very low levels leading to a further rise of the LPR.
    - Recent studies have postulated that brain may not only utilize glucose but also be able to metabolize lactate as an energy substrate.
  - ○ Glycerol, an important cell membrane phospholipid
    - In the setting of energy failure, calcium moves intracellularly.
    - This leads to phospholipase activation and ultimately cell membrane breakdown, with the release of glycerol into the interstitium.
  - ○ Glutamate, an excitatory neurotransmitter, may be dysregulated in acute brain injury
    - Glutamate's excitotoxicity is mediated by excessive calcium influx into brain cells through glutamate-mediated ion channels.
    - May ultimately lead to secondary brain injury.

- Measurement of MD
  - ○ Invasive, via a small probe placed through a burr hold or at the time of craniotomy.
  - ○ CSF-like fluid is circulated via a small pump and allowed to equilibrate via passive diffusion with the extracellular fluid through a 20–100 kDa dialysis membrane.
  - ○ Dialysate is collected and then analyzed at regular intervals depending on the pump speed, typically not more often than every 20 to 60 minutes.
  - ○ Regional measure: reflects 2 to 3 mm of brain tissue surrounding the probe.
  - ○ Relative measure: recovery rate of extracellular fluid is dependent on the fluid perfusion rate and membrane pore size.
  - ○ Placement is important as injured or at-risk tissue is metabolically distinct from remote or normal tissue.
- Management
  - ○ Exact cutoffs for MD measurements and particularly the interpretation of abnormal values are somewhat controversial.
  - ○ As a guide for normal values, using a 10 mm membrane, pore size of 20 kDa, and flow rate of 0.3 μL/min, the following normal values have been proposed (3–5):
    - Glucose—1.7 ($\pm$0.9)– 2.1 ($\pm$0.2) mmol/L
    - Lactate—2.9 ($\pm$0.9)–3.1 ($\pm$0.2) mmol/L
    - Pyruvate—166 ($\pm$47)–151 ($\pm$12) μmol/L
    - L/P ratio—19 ($\pm$2)–23 ($\pm$4)
    - Glutamate—16 ($\pm$16)–14 ($\pm$3.3) μmol/L
    - Glycerol—82 ($\pm$44)–88 ($\pm$12) μmol/L
  - ○ LPR reflects the redox state of the cell's energy metabolism
    - Tracks with states of secondary metabolic stress, including but not limited to ischemia, hypoxia, vasospasm, intracranial hypertension, seizure activity, and hyperthermia.
  - ○ In cerebral ischemia, MD typically reveals increased lactate, decreased glucose and pyruvate, and increased LPR and lactate–glucose ratios (5).
  - ○ Elevated LPR is a sensitive but not specific marker of ischemia
    - In ischemia, glutamate usually increases first, followed by LPR and, ultimately, the glycerol level.
    - These increases in metabolic markers have been shown to precede other measures capable of detecting ischemia (ie, TCD) (6).
  - ○ Glutamate
    - Increases with decreased CBF and during seizures.
    - Interpretation of glutamate changes is made easier when additional MMM parameters such as $PbtO_2$ are available.
    - Studies show correlation between increased glutamate levels and poor outcome in TBI and SAH patients.
    - However, there is wide variability of glutamate levels within and among patients, making it difficult to draw definitive conclusions about the use of glutamate as an outcome marker in these patient populations.

- To date, the relationship between glutamate dysregulation and acute brain injury remains unclear.
  ○ Glycerol
    - Since it reflects cell membrane degradation, may be a useful marker of tissue hypoxia and cell damage in the setting of acute brain injury.
    - Increased levels can also occur with increased systemic levels or via the formation of glycerol from glucose.
    - Glycerol levels are typically elevated in the first 24 hours after TBI and are considered representative of the primary injury.
    - Glycerol levels decline exponentially after the initial 24 hours following TBI, so any glycerol spikes during this time are thought to be associated with secondary injury or seizures (7).

E. Cerebral Blood Flow (CBF)
- Physiology and pathology
  ○ The critical variable for brain function and survival
  ○ Brain requires a certain CBF to meet its metabolic demands
    - This can be estimated by cerebral metabolic rate of oxygen ($CMRO_2$).
    - Imaging studies such as CT or MR perfusion studies using contrast agents or arterial spin labeling sequences can estimate CBF but cannot be repeated frequently.
      – Thus, such studies have very poor temporal resolution.
  ○ Obtaining continuous CBF measures is challenging.
  ○ However, indirect estimates of perfusion can be made as part of the invasive MMM approach such as those based on thermal dilution measurements.
  ○ CBF and CPP (discussed above) are related and CPP is at times used as a surrogate for CBF measures.
- Measurement of CBF
  ○ Placement:
    - Invasive probe inserted into brain parenchyma through a burr hole.
    - Preferred probe placement is controversial but mirrors the discussion above on ICP measurement probes.
  ○ Devices:
    - Laser-Doppler flowmetry (LDF)
      – Invasive subcortical fiberoptic probe that measures the shift of reflected laser light.
      – Relative regional measure.
    - Thermal dilution flowmetry: invasive probe placed in gray or white matter that measures heat conduction between two electrodes.
      – Regional measure
      – May reflect true CBF.
- Further discussion
  ○ CBF monitoring is used less frequently than other neuromonitoring tools.
  ○ One measure called FRx (flow-related autoregulation index) has been proposed recently as an assessment of autoregulatory status (8).
    - Relates regional CBF to MAP.
    - Similar to the more established autoregulatory measures derived from ICP measurements.

- ○ CBF measuring devices have not been validated clinically and thus remain as research tools.

F. Brain Temperature
- Physiology and pathology
  - ○ Brain temperature is usually 1°C to 1.5°C warmer than core temperature.
  - ○ The brain-to-core temperature ratio is quite predictable and constant, even in acute brain injury.
  - ○ Marked changes in the association between core and brain temperature may be an indicator of cerebral injury, but this is still under investigation.
- Technical aspects
  - ○ Invasive probe inserted into brain parenchyma through a burr hole.
  - ○ Temperature measured with a thermocouple probe.
  - ○ Often used in conjunction with other invasive monitoring measures including ICP and $PbtO_2$.
- Management
  - ○ Can be used to guide fever control and induced hypothermia.
  - ○ Fever is associated with worse outcomes for many acute brain injuries, including stroke, TBI, and SAH.
- At this time, brain temperature measurements are a research tool.

G. Intracortical Electroencephalography (ICE, or "depth" electrode):
- Used in conjunction with scalp cEEG monitoring.
- Allows for an improved signal-to-noise ratio and detection of seizures that may not be visualized on scalp EEG.
- May be useful in detecting ischemia.
- Technical aspects
  - ○ Ideal placement
    - Determined on a case-by-case basis after factoring in the patient's anatomy and pathology.
    - Goal: placement into brain tissue at maximal risk of secondary injury.
  - ○ Regional: reflects the electrical activity in the region of the probe.
- Clinical findings
  - ○ A recent study showed that most patients (10/16; 62.5%) had highly epileptogenic patterns or seizures in the ICE recording that were not detectable on the scalp.
    - – Additionally, two patients who suffered significant nonseizure-related secondary neurological complications had prominent ICE-specific changes that were detected hours before other monitoring modalities (9).
  - ○ A more recent small case series of five patients showed improved signal-to-noise ratio compared to conventional scalp EEG in the detection of ischemia from vasospasm.
    - – In all three patients with vasospasm confirmed by angiography, a sustained drop in the alpha–delta ratio (ADR) was observed during 1 to 3 days prior to angiography (10).
- However, the clinical significance of EEG findings seen on depth electrodes that are not visualized on scalp EEG remains uncertain.

III. FUTURE CONSIDERATIONS/REMAINING QUESTIONS/ CHALLENGES

A. MMM Utilization
- Although MMM is in use at several medical centers in the United States and Europe, it is not part of routine clinical care of neurologically critically ill patients at most centers.
- Some techniques are used by just a few centers, whereas others (eg, partial brain tissue oxygenation) have been recommended for more widespread use in patients with TBI by the Brain Trauma Foundation.

B. Impact of MMM on Outcome
- Knowledge of relationship of MMM parameters and outcome is in its infancy.
- Answers depend both on performance of devices as well as the therapeutic intervention and the timing of its implementation.

C. Large Multicenter Prospective Trials Are Needed
- Results could drive algorithmic approaches to physiologic, metabolic, and electrical consequences of acute brain injury.
- Lacking such trials, each patient for who MMM is employed should be treated on a case-by-case basis.

D. Promise of MMM
- Invasive brain monitoring holds great promise for the future.
- May not only add additional insight into the clinical state of the patient but may completely change treatment approaches for critically brain-injured patients.
- The high-time resolution and the (theoretical) ability to get instantaneous feedback about brain physiology in response to interventions may allow the development of patient-specific treatment paradigms based on observed physiologic effects.
- May also provide insight into the critical mechanisms of brain injury that would otherwise remain poorly understood.

E. Major Goals for the Future
- Development of automated alarm systems that are sensitive and specific enough to identify secondary injury when permanent damage can still be prevented.
- Combining MMM with other techniques, including proteomics or imaging, may offer further insights into mechanisms underlying acute brain injury.
- The future of MMM lies in the ability to visualize and computationally analyze patient-specific "physiologic profiles" that can be trended over time and used in "real time" to anticipate, treat, and ideally prevent further insults in the unresponsive, acutely brain-injured patients.

CASE VIGNETTES

Detecting Ischemia With ICE

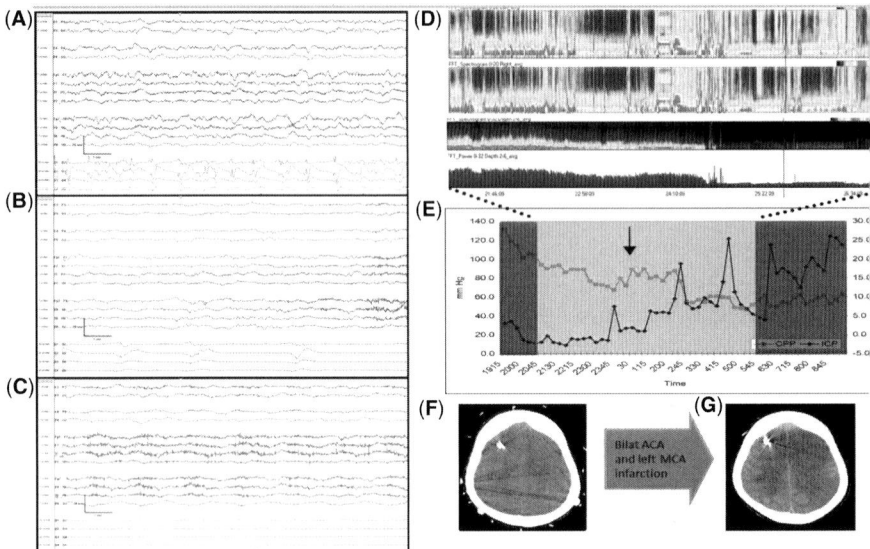

A 70-year-old woman with subarachnoid hemorrhage, and systemic hypotension leading to diffuse intracerebral infarction: (A–C) Sequential raw EEG tracings compare concurrently recorded scalp and intracortical findings (bottom 4 channels) . An evolution can be seen from the highly epileptiform baseline EEG on ICE (A) to a burst-suppression pattern (B) and ultimately nearly complete attenuation (C), whereas the scalp recording did not demonstrate an obvious change. (D) Quantitative EEG analysis of a 6-hour period. The top three rows are derived from scalp EEG, and the bottom two rows from the intracortical electrode. A significant and permanent decline in EEG total power is seen in the intracortical electrode (arrow) with a similar change in the ICE spectrogram. This event was associated with progressive decline in cerebral perfusion pressure (CPP; gray line), as well as a significant increase in intracranial pressure (ICP; black line) (E). Computed tomographic imaging before (F) and after (G) the ICE-specific changes demonstrating infarction. With permission from Waziri A, et al. Intercortical Electroencephalography in Acute Brain Injury. Ann Neurol 2009;66:366–77.

Detecting Ischemia With Multimodality Monitoring

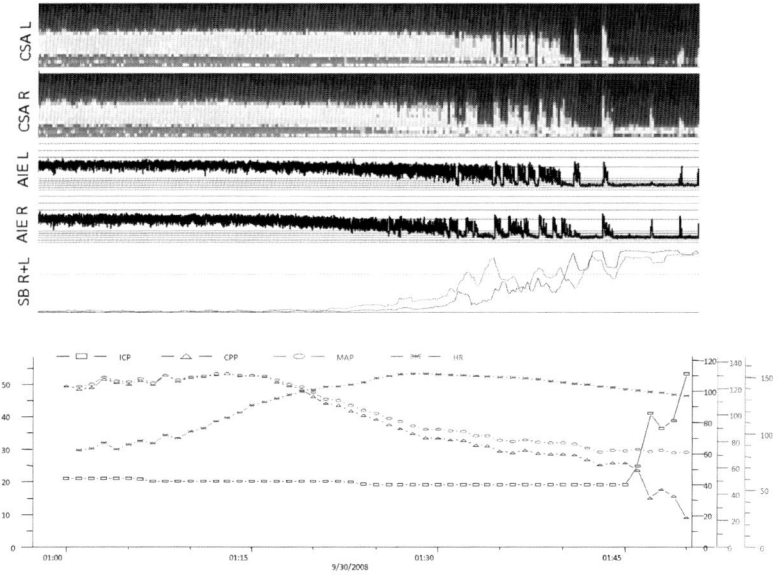

A 55-year-old man admitted with intraventricular hemorrhage in setting of phencycli-dine abuse who developed refractory hypotension resulting first in a drop in mean arterial pressure (MAP) and a delayed increase in the intracranial pressure (ICP; bottom graph). Quantitative electroencephalography (EEG) analysis demonstrates attenuation of all frequencies in the compressed spectral array (CSA; top graph), par-ticularly on the right. The amplitude-integrated EEG (AIE) reveals a drop in the maximum amplitude per epoch and the suppression-burst ratio (SB) depicts increas-ingly suppressed EEG background. L = left hemisphere, R = right hemisphere. With permission from Kurtz P, Hanafy KA, Claassen. J Cur Opinion Crit Care 2009;15:99–109, Figure 13–2, pages 101–102.

Detecting Seizures With Multimodality Monitoring

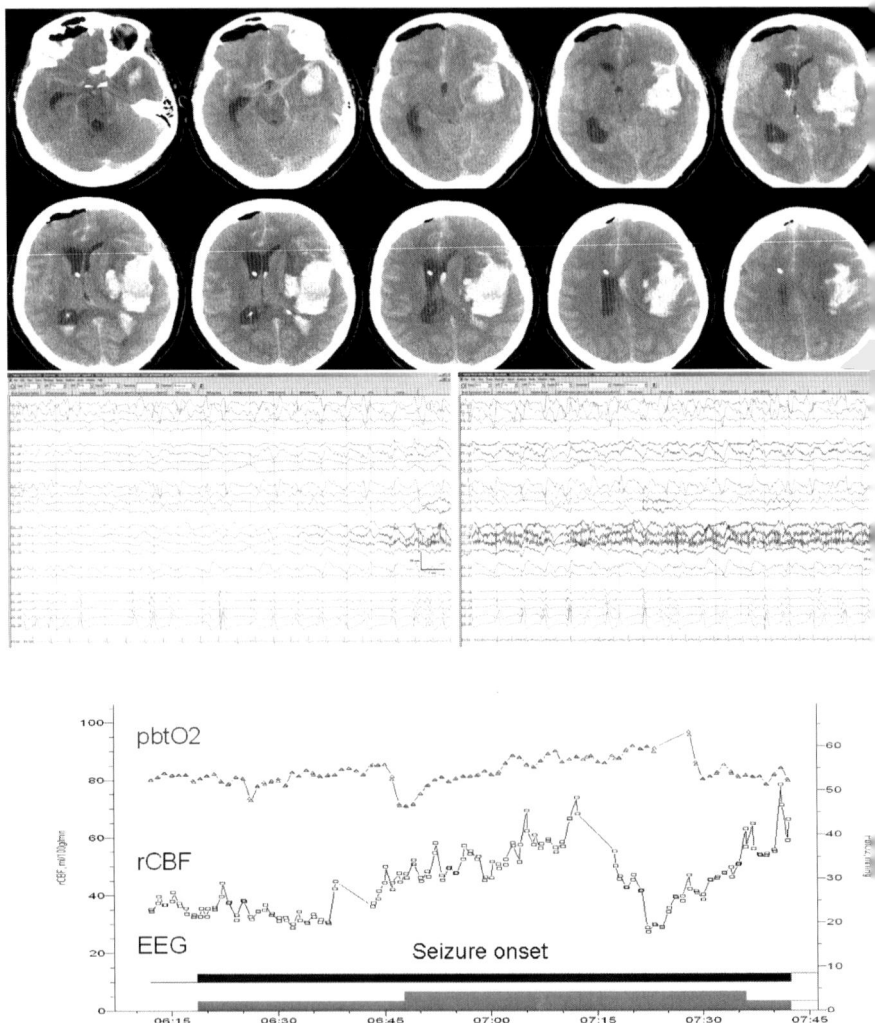

A 62-year-old woman with a Hunt Hess 5, left middle cerebral artery (MCA) aneurismal SAH underwent a left hemicraniectromy for hematomal evacuation and clip placement. She developed a pattern on scalp EEG suggestive of seizure activity, but is much more clearly seen on the depth electrode (Bottom channels, D1–D6). Additionally, there are changes in the PbtO$_2$ and regional CBF that correlate to the onset of seizures.

REFERENCES

1. Stuart RM, Schmidt M, Kurtz P, et al. Intracranial multimodal monitoring for acute brain injury: A single institution review of current practices. *Neurocrit Care.* Apr 2010;12(2): 188–198.
2. Schmidt JM, Ko SB, Helbok R, et al. Cerebral perfusion pressure thresholds for brain tissue hypoxia and metabolic crisis after poor-grade subarachnoid hemorrhage. *Stroke.* May 2011;42(5):1351–1356.
3. Schulz MK, Wang LP, Tange M, Bjerre P. Cerebral microdialysis monitoring: Determination of normal and ischemic cerebral metabolisms in patients with aneurysmal subarachnoid hemorrhage. *J Neurosurg.* Nov 2000;93(5):808–814.
4. Reinstrup P, Stahl N, Mellergard P, et al. Intracerebral microdialysis in clinical practice: Baseline values for chemical markers during wakefulness, anesthesia, and neurosurgery. *Neurosurgery.* Sep 2000;47(3):701–709; discussion 709–710.
5. Hillered L, Vespa PM, Hovda DA. Translational neurochemical research in acute human brain injury: The current status and potential future for cerebral microdialysis. *J Neurotrauma.* Jan 2005;22(1):3–41.
6. Nilsson OG, Brandt L, Ungerstedt U, et al. Bedside detection of brain ischemia using intracerebral microdialysis: Subarachnoid hemorrhage and delayed ischemic deterioration. *Neurosurgery.* Nov 1999;45(5):1176–1184; discussion 1184–1175.
7. Tisdall MM, Smith M. Cerebral microdialysis: Research technique or clinical tool. *Br J Anaesth.* Jul 2006;97(1):18–25.
8. Barth M, Woitzik J, Weiss C, et al. Correlation of clinical outcome with pressure-, oxygen-, and flow-related indices of cerebrovascular reactivity in patients following aneurysmal SAH. *Neurocrit Care.* Apr 2010;12(2):234–243.
9. Waziri A, Claassen J, Stuart RM, et al. Intracortical electroencephalography in acute brain injury. *Ann Neurol.* Sep 2009;66(3):366–377.
10. Stuart RM, Waziri A, Weintraub D, et al. Intracortical EEG for the detection of vasospasm in patients with poor-grade subarachnoid hemorrhage. *Neurocrit Care.* Dec 2010;13(3): 355–358.

THIRTY-EIGHT

EEG Monitoring in the ICU: Future Directions

Nicolas Gaspard and Lawrence J. Hirsch

KEY POINTS

- Better understanding of EEG patterns in critically ill patients will lead to improvement in patient care.
- Data regarding the utility of EEG monitoring (cEEG) for indications other than seizure detection is currently limited. However, cEEG monitoring represents a significant opportunity for identifying causes of secondary injury other than seizures, particularly ischemia.
- Advances in quantitative EEG (QEEG) analysis will not only improve detection of clinically significant EEG changes but also allow for more rapid and efficient screening and interpretation of cEEG.
- Considerable potential exists for both real-time EEG monitoring (neurotelemetry) and invasive multimodality monitoring to guide treatment decisions.

I. BACKGROUND

A. The interpretation of EEG in critically ill patients is challenging. Many EEG patterns exist that are of unclear significance and whose interpretation is controversial.

- These include periodic discharges (PDs), stimulus-induced rhythmic, periodic and ictal discharges (SIRPIDs); rhythmic delta activity (RDA); and triphasic waves (TW).

B. The availability of cEEG monitoring is currently limited to large hospitals and academic institutions with adequate technical resources.

- cEEG hookups are very time consuming and require EEG technologists with expertise.
- Significant collaboration with information technology is needed for proper networking and remote access, which is essential for physician review of important events in a timely manner.
- Considerable technical support is also required for maintaining and storing the large amount of data that cEEG produces.

- In most institutions, EEG interpretation is limited to intermittent retrospective review of CEEG, rather than real-time review.
  - It has been demonstrated that EEG has the potential to identify background changes secondary to evolving ischemia and prior to irreversible neuronal injury. However, real-time monitoring is crucial for this purpose.
- As a result, cEEG is not yet widely used for purposes other than recording seizures in patients known to be at high risk for seizures.

C. The best treatment options and optimal level of aggressiveness have not been determined for:
- Seizure prophylaxis
- Treatment of nonconvulsive seizures (NCS)
- Treatment of status epilepticus (SE), especially nonconvulsive SE (NCSE) and refractory SE (RSE)

II. BASICS

A. A better understanding of EEG patterns seen in critically ill patients and their relationship to brain injury is needed. Examples:
- Cortical spreading depression/peri-injury depolarization
- Periodic and rhythmic patterns without clear evolution
- Stimulus-induced patterns

B. NCS have been associated with worse outcome in intracranial hemorrhage (ICH), subarachnoid hemorrhage (SAH), and traumatic brain injury (TBI), but randomized clinical trials are needed to determine whether aggressive treatment actually improves outcome.
- Such studies would benefit greatly from the adoption of standardized EEG terminology and correlations with other physiological parameters.
- Biological markers of brain injury are needed, whether from serum (neuron-specific enolase), brain microdialysate (lactate, glucose, glutamate), structural neuroimaging (MRI with diffusion-weighted imaging), or functional imaging (PET or SPECT).
- Ultimately, the goal is to develop multimodality brain monitoring to allow the parallel recording and analysis of electrical and biological markers that can signal significant pathophysiological changes and guide patient-specific treatment.

C. The utility of cEEG for detection of nonictal events requires further study.
- Small, retrospective studies have shown that QEEG parameters are able to detect delayed cerebral ischemia in SAH prior to changes seen on clinical exam or transcranial Doppler.
  - Prospective, randomized controlled trials are needed to determine whether these changes can also be detected with real-time cEEG monitoring with improved sensitivity, more cost-effectiveness and less risk than standard detection methods of transcranial Doppler or angiography.
- QEEG is able to identify other clinically significant events, including increased intracranial pressure, expanding ischemia in acute stroke, and systemic

abnormalities (hypoxia, hypercapnia, and hypotension), but sensitivity and specificity for these purposes is unknown.

D. The current practice of using cEEG with intermittent retrospective review should be replaced with real-time EEG monitoring (neurotelemetry).

- Advances in EEG technology are required to display raw EEG, QEEG, and video data for multiple patients in a format that allows for easy visual assessment.
- Additional staffing, presumably from advanced EEG technologists, will be needed for around-the-clock screening.
- MRI- and CT-compatible electrodes will allow for fewer interruptions in cEEG since this patient population frequently undergoes neuroimaging procedures. Although these electrodes currently exist, they are more expensive than conventional electrodes and have not been widely adopted.
- Advances in QEEG analysis methods will aid in optimizing the detection rate and defining sensitive and specific combinations of QEEG parameters for the identification of acute brain events (seizures, ischemia, increased ICP, etc).
- The design of online QEEG analysis with user-friendly interface and alarm systems will make 24/7 real-time neurotelemetry useful for EEG technologists, ICU nurses, and neurointensivists.

E. Multicenter randomized controlled trials utilizing cEEG will need to address several questions regarding the treatment of SE.

- Most Class I data regarding the treatment of SE focuses on convulsive SE. Studies addressing the treatment of NCSE are required, especially to define how aggressive to treat various NCSE patterns.
- Several newer antiepileptic drugs (AEDs) have been used for treatment of SE but none has been the object of a prospective, randomized controlled trial.
- There are essentially no data better than class IV evidence to guide the treatment of RSE.
- A direct comparison of the available anesthetic agents for the treatment of RSE is needed.

F. Predicting and preventing epileptogenesis remains the ultimate goal.

- Early markers (EEG patterns or other biomarkers) of epileptogenesis need to be identified.
- Animal models of epileptogenesis need further characterization to identify such biomarkers, pathophysiological changes, and therapeutic goals.

III. FURTHER CONSIDERATIONS/REMAINING QUESTIONS

A. The efforts required to make significance advances in cEEG will require multicenter collaborations.

B. Advances in the understanding of EEG patterns and their significance, both at a global level and for the individual patient, will require combining cEEG with other physiological parameters, including data derived from multimodality monitoring.

C. Widespread use of standardized terminology is essential for the conduct of such multicenter studies.

D. Guidelines outlining technical and professional standards for continuous EEG monitoring are needed for medical centers wishing to develop cEEG programs.

E. Continuous EEG with real-time monitoring (neurotelemetry) is time and resource intensive and therefore studies of cost-effectiveness will be required to better define the scope of their indications. However, the full clinical benefit of these technologies can only be fully realized after real-time neurotelemetry has been implemented.

F. The ultimate aim is to develop an efficient method for individualized, real-time decision-making based on both clinical and neurophysiologic monitoring data.

ADDITIONAL READING

1. Friedman D, Claassen J, Hirsch LJ. Continuous electroencephalogram monitoring in the intensive care unit. *Anesth Analg.* 2009;109(2):506–523.
2. Claassen J. How I treat patients with EEG patterns on the ictal–interictal continuum in the neuro ICU. *Neurocrit Care.* 2009;11(3):437–444.
3. Stewart CP, Otsubo H, Ochi A, et al. Seizure identification in the ICU using quantitative EEG displays. *Neurology.* 2010;75(17):1501–1508.

Index

Note: Page number followed by 'n' denotes Footnote

Handbook of ICU EEG Monitoring